Big Medicine from Six Nations

The Iroquois and Their Neighbors

Christopher Vecsey, Series Editor

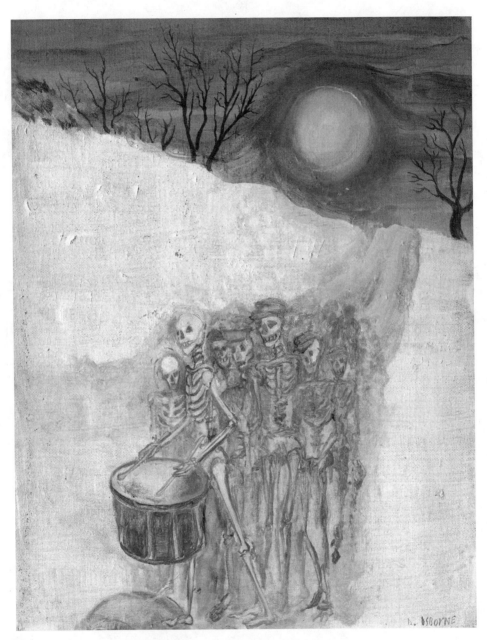

Ghost Drummers.
Painting by Diana Osborne Williams.
Used by permission of the artist.

Big Medicine
from Six Nations

• • •

Ted Williams

Edited and with an Afterword by Debra Roberts

Foreword by Christopher Vecsey

SYRACUSE UNIVERSITY PRESS

First Edition 2007

07   08   09   10   11   12   6   5   4   3   2   1

The paper used in this publication meets the minimum requirements of
American National Standard for Information Sciences—Permanence of
Paper for Printed Library Materials, ANSI Z39.48–1984∞™

For a listing of books published and distributed by Syracuse University Press,
visit our Web site at SyracuseUniversityPress.syr.edu.

ISBN-13: 978-0-8156-0863-9

ISBN-10: 0-8156-0863-2

Library of Congress Cataloging-in-Publication Data

Williams, Ted C., 1930–

Big medicine from six nations / Ted Williams ; edited and with an afterword
by Debra Roberts ; foreword by Christopher Vecsey.—1st ed.

p. cm.—(Iroquois and their neighbors)

ISBN 978–0–8156–0863–9 (hardcover : alk. paper)

1. Tuscarora Indians—Medicine. 2. Tuscarora Indians—Religion.
3. Tuscarora Indians—Rites and ceremonies. 4. Traditional medicine—East (U.S.)
5. Shamanism—East (U.S.) 6. Healing—East (U.S.) 7. Six Nations—History. I. Title.

E99.T9W55 2007

299.7'855092—dc22

2007001112

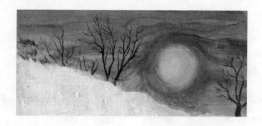

This book is dedicated

to the Little People,

and to all the False Faces,

and to all Benevolent Entities of this

and all other galaxies,

and to the Periodic Table

Ted Williams was born April 6, 1930, on the Tuscarora Indian Reservation near Niagara Falls, New York. His father, Eleazer Williams, was an Indian doctor and Sachem Chief of the Turtle Clan at Tuscarora. His mother, Amelia Chew Williams, served time as the Clan Mother of the Wolf Clan.

Upon graduation from La Salle High School (1948, Niagara Falls), Ted joined the military and spent four years as a paratrooper in the Eighty-second Airborne during the Korean conflict. He then used G.I. Bill funding to attend the Knapp School of Music in Chicago, playing trumpet and doing small band jazz arrangements.

After marriage in 1954, Ted returned to Niagara Falls and tried his hand as a crane operator at the new large construction project New York State Electric Power Project. The job paid so well that Ted pursued this occupation, transferring his trade to the Eastman Kodak Company in 1966 and retiring there in 1990.

In the 1970s, Ted began doing healings, using herbal remedies, healing-with-hands, and ceremony. The famous seer Daisy Thomas told him that he must join the False Face Society for protection, which led to Ted's participation in the traditional "Longhouse Way of Life." In 1976, Ted wrote the book *The Reservation* (Syracuse University Press).

Always active in sports, Ted won many championships in archery, both as an amateur and as a professional. By age seventy-five, he had also won five consecutive pro disc golf world championships in his age group division (seventy and older), called the Legends.

He and his wife, Diana, lived for years in the Pisgah National Forest area of Madison County, North Carolina, in a White Pine home they built with storm-fallen trees. In September 2005, Ted gently passed away into the arms of his beloved Divine and Harmonious Universe.

Contents

How We Have Lived, Small Incidences

Propriety and Derangement

Six Nations, One Humanity

New Age and Ancient Wisdom

Closing

Illustrations

Foreword

When Arpena Mesrobian handed me *The Reservation* in 1981, she told me that it was her proudest achievement as director of Syracuse University Press (and hers was a distinguished career). I brought the book home, opened it up, started reading, and the laughter began, then the tears.

Ted Williams touched you like that. This Tuscarora man—member of his mother's Wolf Clan, son of a Turtle Clan Sachem Chief, and an accomplished artist and musician—had composed an album of love songs to his people and place. They may have had the appearance of an improvised set of droll, sometimes macabre tales, but they were possessed of an aesthetic unity, telling as they did of Ted's coming to consciousness of his imperiled Tuscarora culture.

On the pages of this book, the reader got to meet Ted's family, his neighbors, and the nonhuman persons who populated the Tuscarora environment. People visited one another and shared stories. They argued, and sometimes they damaged each other and themselves. Death was ever present. Rituals offered opportunities for all manner of interaction, and the outside world provided challenges that shook the foundations of the reservation community.

The Reservation closed with a passage, set in Ted's young adulthood, that explained that book's genesis (and, it might be said, this one's, too) in the deaths of the culture bearers of his parents' generation:

> "The Tellers" were all dead or dying. I didn't feel very good. I wasn't even walking anymore. Right next to me was a young pine tree. It was one of the 4H trees that I had planted. It was almost as tall as I was now. I put my hand on its sappy little trunk.
>
> "OoKHREHHéweh," I said to the little pine, "who's going to be 'The Tellers' now, now that 'The Tellers' are dead?"
>
> At first the little tree didn't answer, but I waited. After a while it

said, "You and I will be 'The Tellers.' Someday children will say, 'What did the Old Folks say?' and they will be asking about US—about what YOU and I are talking about right now."

Ted Williams had become a Tuscarora Teller, and *The Reservation* was his home-grown tale.

I told my students to read this book in order to learn about American Indian life in the twentieth century. Over the years I have assigned it many times, and they have often told me that they had expected to find a set of Indian stories, but instead were taken by Ted's transcending humanity.

They should meet him, then.

And they did, when he came to my class. He told them how he had been breast-fed after his birth for many years, until he started asking his mother for cookies with his milk. That got the students laughing, and they questioned him about his life, his writing, his people, and his beliefs. When they inquired about today's Tuscaroras, Ted replied (and I wrote it down), "Beliefs are where it's at, and if you believe, you can do anything. Believe in yourself, and only good things can happen." He seemed to be addressing his audience as well as his tribe. Then he added, "If the Tuscaroras need something and want it back, it will come back." Here he seemed to be describing his own lifelong project to keep alive the traditional wisdom of his people. He told the class about his enduring "quest for spiritual knowledge," his search for "Higher Consciousness," his desire to learn all he could about Medicine in all its forms.

It did not surprise me, when the class was over, that several students sought Ted out privately for advice and guidance.

Another time, in another school setting, students wanted to know why there were so many disfigured characters in *The Reservation*. Ted told about his childhood fascination with deformity: "When I wanted to see cripples, I would ask to go with my parents to Niagara Falls, and I'd sit in the parked car and 'watch the parade.' " But more, for Ted, disablement gave rise to thoughts about Medicine.

At the White Corn Ceremony, he explained, each person got one ear to open. If it was normal, that was all you got. If one was "deformed"—and there were names for all the different types of abnormalities, such as having one missing row of kernels—you received more corn, which was considered a Medicine as well as food.

Several years ago my students sent Ted some love letters, laced with queries. They wanted to know what he was doing these days. He wrote back, "Much of the time [the interim] since the publication of *The Reservation* 'til now has been spent learning and doing ceremony and participating in the Longhouse ceremonies at Onondaga. I belong to the semisecret False Face Society for the protection of myself and my Medicines. I was instructed to become a member by the late and great Daisy Thomas. (Great, great 'reader' from the Six Nation Rez at Osweken, Ontario.)"

He continued that he was writing another book, postponed by the building of his house in North Carolina, about the "ESP-type experiences of Indians of the Six Nation Confederacy." He planned to call the book something like "Indian Medicine." Ted enclosed several of his "Love, Ted" poems, inspired by Lakota rituals, which he intended to include in the Medicine book he had in mind.

As series editor of "Iroquois and Their Neighbors," I immediately had to write back and invite him to consider Syracuse University Press as his once and future publisher. Thus, Ted's Dear Readers, you have before you *Big Medicine from Six Nations*, a Telling of Ted's experiences in gathering Medicines and Medicine lore both near and far.

When the 4H pine tree told Ted to collect the necessary information to become a Teller, he began his especial search for Medicine among the Six Nations of Iroquois and beyond—from Utes, Lakotas, Australian Aborigines, Natives, and non-Natives—wherever "Higher Consciousness" could be fathomed.

Readers will not be disappointed if they hope to gain insight regarding Six Nation Medicine, broadly conceived: not just herbal cures, but charms, spells, prayers, omens, feasts, games of chance and skill, vision quests, Sweat Lodges, loci of power, ghosts, skeletons, spirits, shape-shifting, witchery, humor, masks, the Great Law of the Six Nation Confederacy—all the hidden and apparent powers that manifest themselves to the Iroquois. But readers will also find that there is more to this book, more about the "spiritual mechanics" of humankind writ large: Sundances, crystal balls, ouija boards, channelings, teacup readings, past-life regression sessions, auras, odds, premonitions, serendipity, sexuality, femininity, generosity, telekinesis, electricity, homeopathy, exorcisms, fears, assurances, UFOs, and ESP.

Ted refers regularly to the Enneagram, developed by Don Richard Riso and

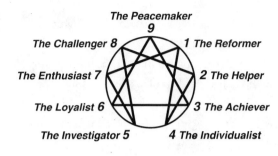

The Enneagram with Riso-Hudson names. Courtesy of the Enneagram Institute.

Russ Hudson and explicated in their book *Discovering Your Personality Type*, published (among other books) by the Enneagram Institute.

When I penned this preface in July 2005 and sent it off to Ted for inclusion in the manuscript, I closed with a roadside exchange from the old-time song "The Arkansas Traveler":

"Howdy, stranger."

"Howdy, stranger."

"Have you lived here your whole life?"

"Not yet." —

I mentioned earlier that this book was a Telling, but not a culmination, and certainly not the last word from Ted Williams.

And it wasn't. Not quite.

In August, Ted wrote back with a heartfelt note, which I am quoting here at length:

> There is something I must tell you about. — For the last year and a half or so I have suffered bouts of 'total loss of memory.' The first big notice-able one came when, one evening, I drove (50 min.) into Asheville and when I got there I could NOT remember why I was there. I spent $1\frac{1}{2}$ hours in grocery stores, hardware and building supply places but never did remember WHY I was there. It all struck me as very funny even though I knew that it could have happened at a crucial occasion. I drove home and later (maybe even the next day) I found out that I was supposed to be at a disc-golf meeting. (Now THAT IS SERIOUS!)

Well, I say that because this year's World Championship at Allentown, Pennsylvania—as the time of it approached—became a more and more exciting prospect. Last year, at Des Moines, Iowa, Dr. Stancil Johnson, a psychiatrist from California, and I were TIED with only 4 holes to do (18 holes a day, Mon-Fri, and now on the final 9 on Saturday) and he would be at Allentown seeking revenge.

Then—my son discovered, on the internet, that a 'new guy' (only 70 years old to my 75 and therefore now eligible to compete in 'my' division called 'The Legends') was entered and had a rating higher than mine (877 to my 855). His name is Ragnar Overby from Virginia and stands 6'5" to my 5'7".

On day one, July 25, Stancil and Rag were assigned a different foursome than I was so I had to wait that whole day to find out what scores we each ended up with. Ragnar a 75, me a 75 and Stan only strokes off at 77 (same scoring as 'ball' golf).

On Tuesday my 'afterburners came on' and I got a 64 to Rag's 71. Stan had a near heat stroke from the record high temperatures and ended up with 81 and had to withdraw from the tournament.

(The reason I'm telling you all this is because the activity of disc golf keeps me alive and excited to be alive.)

On Wednesday I got a 66 to Rag's 75. So now I had a 16 stroke lead. I was 'running away' with it.

But then came Thursday. It was MY turn to succumb to the heat. I had no 'sick' symptoms. No dizziness. No nausea. No fever—just a complete inability to think. I remember hearing members of my foursome saying 'HEY TED! IT'S YOUR TURN.' I ended up with an 82. My lead went from 16 to 7. Dehydration.

On Friday 2 of my sons arrived. One from near the Tuscarora Reservation, Tom age 49 and Bob (Richmond, Virginia) age 46. They carried a chair, umbrella, and ice water. 'SIT DOWN!'—'GET UNDER THE UMBRELLA!'—'DRINK SOME MORE WATER!'

Ragnar still got me by 2 more strokes to cut my lead to 5.

On Saturday, the FINAL 9 HOLES, with the help of my boys, I tied Ragnar (who, by the way, can throw $1\frac{1}{2}$ times farther than I can) and won $800 for 1st place. Rag got $500 for 2nd. So, if I only won by 4 strokes last year and 5 this time, I'm getting better with age.

"OK," he ended, "back to the book. . . . I'll stay closer in touch with you from now on."

Ted Williams died in September 2005, having just finished his book about Big Medicine.

Christopher Vecsey
Colgate University

Acknowledgments

Credit is owed for any contributions, in any form, that came to this book from any of the Elements of our universal family, as well as from the Little People and the Medicine spirits of any of the Medicine societies of the Longhouse.

I want to mention my wife, Diana, part Onondaga, who has the name Je gon sa se(t) ("She Takes Care of the Garden," meaning including the garden of people because she is a homeopathic doctor). She is also a painter, a poet, and a mover and a shaker as the "Echo" in the Standing Quiver Stomp Dance. I better acknowledge her, too, for doing the painting for the cover of the book, or I could see the inside of a doghouse.

Daughter Rhiannon (cum laude grad in art at Buffalo State University), thanks for the woodcuts that appear throughout the book.

Then there's Fairy Godmother, Debra Roberts, who fed my yellow tablet scribbles into the computer.

Professor Chris Vecsey did the intro, bless his hide.

And what about Syracuse University Press? Real people. Real pros. Real class acts to follow by any other press.

If I forgot anybody or anything, put yourself in here.

Love,
Ted

Opening

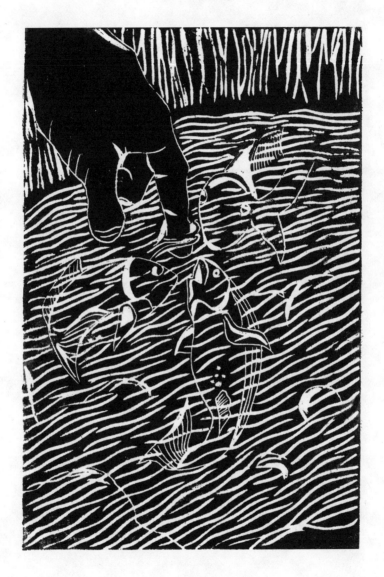

Overleaf: Uncle Charley's finger attracting the fish; see "Uncle Charley," pp. 35–39.
Woodcut by Rhiannon Miles Osborne.

Dear Readers

Dear Readers,

I hear that the older I get, the farther I will have walked to school as a boy. I was born on April 6, 1930. My mother, Amelia, was a Tuscarora, as was my father, Eleazer. The Tuscarora Nation is part of the Six Nation Iroquois Confederacy. The other five nations are "charter" members of the original Five Nation Iroquois Confederacy, which formed under the persuasion of an enlightened person called the Peacemaker. The laws of the confederacy say that whatever the mother's nationality is, her children are that nationality. So if my father, Eleazer, had been Mohawk or Oneida or Seneca or Cayuga or Onondaga (original members), I would still be a Tuscarora.

We consider the designation "Iroquois" as being improper because it did not come from any of our six languages. At the same time, people of the English-speaking "world" who have gone through quite a bit of schooling and who would like people to use the "proper" naming of things don't want us to call ourselves "Indians." But we do anyway because Columbus, not wanting to admit to a boo-boo in navigation, said we were.

In the early days of my life, we didn't have electricity, so we didn't have any radios or telephones. Today, if someone were to visit without first telephoning, we might think they were barging in on us. Back then, it was exciting to hear the dog bark and see someone coming to our house, for any reason. Maybe they had news.

This was a magical time. Time? There is no Tuscarora word for time (and likely in no other Indian language either). If we asked anyone the time, we said, "Det de waa ni(t) deh?" What we were saying was, "How many times does the iron strike?" So that phrase must have come about after the hearing of grandfather clocks tolling out chimes. But there were very few man-made noises.

There was a church bell in the Baptist church. If someone died, the bell ringer would be told. We would first hear a rapid "ding-dong-ding-dong-ding-dong . . ." and then silence. Then single tolls would come. We counted them because each toll represented a year of the dead person's life. We often easily guessed who it was that died. Again, "How many times did the iron strike?"

Two or three generations before my time, the federal government began wondering what to do with all these Indians (of the whole United States of America). Federal Indian schools were set up, and Indian children were forced to attend them. The idea was that there would be a subtle assimilation of these Indians into the mainstream society. Part of the message to the Indians was, "We will educate you. Hey, you might even become the president some day." The other part of the message was, "You are pagans, heathens, but we will rescue you. You won't have to go to hell if you renounce your traditional beliefs and ceremonies." No speaking of a native tongue allowed. No traditional songs or dances allowed. This system was close to legal genocide. Many kidnapped children died of heartbreak and homesickness.

My father attended Carlisle Indian School, but my mother went to public school. She became so adept at reproducing the sound of the English language that she would be asked to "read" to the class though she had no idea what she was saying.

Someone told me that at one school a teacher was determined to get an Indian boy to read. "Look at the words in this book. I'll say three or four words, reading from left to right, then you repeat aloud right after me those same words."

All went well for a few sentences when suddenly there was a disturbance by two other children in the room.

"You be QUIET back there!" the teacher said.

"You be QUIET back there," the boy read.

My father was fifty years old when I was born. His friends, of his age and older, could therefore be two generations ahead of mine.

At night, when I was supposed to be in bed asleep, I'd be on the floor with my ear over the grille of the air register, listening to the talk between my father and his friends. My father was an "Indian doctor," so many of his friends, even from other reservations, would be talking "Medicine talk." Today, we might describe that kind of talk as "extrasensory perception (ESP) oriented."

Most of the experiences in which Indians drifted out of physical consciousness (went into ESP mode) took place before television, music-playing devices, video games, and the computer began occupying everyone's daily time schedule.

Nevertheless, it is very interesting how the ancient concept that the Universe is one big family touches base with "discoveries" made by science.

With the thought that if I studied hard enough I might become president of the United States, I dug into my grade school studies. My father's brother, Theodore, like many other Indians, could not assimilate the forced textbook path to enlightenment and came back from Carlisle Indian School neurotic, a polite way of saying "crazy." A sister, Minnie, made the grade and became a registered nurse. Another sister, Lizzie, though she became a schoolteacher, had a nervous breakdown and became more like Theodore than Minnie.

Minnie told me about Confucius and Taoism, and that people studying this philosophy had reached enlightenment. But she said that there were other ways to enlightenment. One was "the textbook way." Einstein had taken it. A physicist was considered "the brains" of our society.

Although the Longhouse became my way, I tried to keep track of Einstein's way, too. When I heard that subatomic particles exhibited a behavior that didn't jive with mathematical formulas, and when physicists came up with "the Uncertainty Principle," I said, "Goody! They're back to square one." "Square one" to me was Medicine people saying a thousand years ago, "All things are alive and have a consciousness of their own. We are all part of the Great Cycles of All Things."

So, because I like the verification of the Six Nation Great Law by science, my references to some scientific orientation in my version of the Thanksgiving Address will likely be considered "too modern" by some traditionalists. But I have recited an approximate version of this Thanksgiving Address every morning and every night for the past four years and am in good "touch" with these Elements, and they have given me only encouraging feedback.

I also feel that humor is good Medicine, and I spend a lot of my time in my "child." One time, at the great Native American Writers Conference at Oklahoma State University in Norman, a little Eskimo woman recited her poetry to us. So beautiful was it that we excitedly leaped to our feet and gave her a standing ovation. Three hundred Indians clapping and whistling and doing the Indian "Lalalalala . . ." accolade salute.

It was too much for her. She stood there transfixed for a moment, and then she acknowledged our kudos by going into her "child." She began racing around the stage with her arms out, "playing airplane."

I think we all cried. But we also screamed our approval. We all became "children." And pandemonium ensued.

So maybe "a child shall lead them" . . . and we will place within the sod each sacred kernel of white corn . . . when the Red Oak's leaves resemble a squirrel's hand.

Love,
Ted

Prelude to the Prelude

In each of the Six Nation (Iroquois) areas of the United States and Canada, each nation or reservation that observes the traditional activities of the Great Law of the Great Peace has a sacred meeting place called the Longhouse. Before any traditional event takes place within these buildings, a powerful statement is recited, at both the preceding and closing of each day's event. This statement is called the Thanksgiving Address. Its importance is pronounced by a sort of "drum roll," a prelude of words that has (by someone) been interpreted in English as "The Words Before All Else."

The opening and closing can be embellished by the speaker, or it can be shortened (sticking to its essence)—for example, when the twenty-one-day Midwinter Ceremony is ending near the witching hour with a social dance, and everyone is sleepy, and babies are whining.

The version given here is just a skeleton of what can be said in the various Indian languages with their more deeply spiritual meanings.

Pretend, when you open this book, that you are entering one of the Longhouses, that you understand all six languages. If you are a man, when you get through the door, turn to the left, sit down and behave yourself. If you're a woman, sit on the right side.

Maybe the ghost of Emerson Waterman will holler, "SI 'DITE!" Then, in the quiet that prevails, someone will stand up and in a sedate manner recite the Prelude (opening words) and then the Thanksgiving Address.

Prelude to the Thanksgiving Address

As you know . . . as we all inherently know . . . we are all just part of the Great Cycles of All Things.

And because we are all from the same Cosmology, we are all part of one great family, not only within the Element called People, but as intimate kin to all the Elements of this Divine and Harmonious Universe.

So tremendous, so magical is this Divine and Harmonious Universe, that the greatest of scholars . . . physicists . . . philosophers . . . astronomers . . . have not been able to calculate the immensity and complexity of this Great Mystery; but our Faithkeepers tell us that "GRATITUDE IS THE BEGINNING OF KNOWLEDGE AND UNDERSTANDING."

And so . . . before any significant occasion, we always open and close each day's ceremony with the Thanksgiving Address; and so powerful is it that the Faithkeepers say it is the life force of their teaching . . . because:

When we do the Thanksgiving Address, as it progresses into Divineness, it automatically brings forth the Creator or the Essence of the Creator or that Highest of Consciousness into our midst.

And when this happens, some of our secular thoughts, engulfed in unworthiness, and in awe of such a Presence, automatically drift off, leaving room for some of what we call the Good Mind to come in.

And when this happens, if we have decisions to make, they won't be made by our own know-it-all selves, but with some of that Divine intervention.

As Creation became completed, we, the Element called People, being the last Element to be created, have been given the task of caretaker of all the other Elements of our Divine and Harmonious Family.

And we have been given four tools to do this with:

We have our Good Thoughts
We have our Good Feelings
We have our Good Words
We have our Good Deeds

Because our ancestors used these tools admirably to make this a better Universe for the unborn, they have left us with a great good feeling.

And so it is, then, with happy hearts, we thank Soong gwi oo dee sut eh (Creator) that this is so.

The Thanksgiving Address

In the interest of not giving away the sacred secrets of our philosophy, this version of the Thanksgiving Address is meant for the reader to get a basic grasp of why it is so important to us. The speaker may expound to any length or just hit the "high points" in a late-at-night closing. The Thanksgiving Address "starts" and "ends" each day's ceremonial event. Also, the order of first-to-last-spoken-about has no hierarchy, but rather, for easier memory and so as to not skip some Element, we start with the surface of the Earth and go upwards. Some of our ancestors are "planted" underground, so that's where we start. Also, in each Longhouse, after the "Thank you" to each Element, the audience responds with a word meaning "agreed," which in this version is omitted.

Let us awaken to our duty to always be thankful . . . and so we greet and introduce into the consciousness and gratitude of our mind and spirit, the Element People . . . for, first of all, if it weren't for our ancestors, we wouldn't be here . . . they have strived to make this a better world for us and all living things . . . and for their having prayed seven generations ahead for our welfare, we must especially be grateful to those who prayed for us, seven generations ago.

And they have passed on to us the Medicine knowledge that cured and healed and kept them alive and healthy so that we were able to be born.

Part of this Medicine came in the form of the great ceremonies in which we were taught the explicit songs and dances . . . including instructions for induction into the various healing societies and other important societies for those of us who received the calling.

We must also be grateful for the instructions regarding the power and the use of all the great variety of food plants . . . and the explicit ones to be used in each of the ceremonies called the Feast . . . also the reverence and use of the great Sacred Tobacco.

And for the many other things we were taught . . . how to communicate with the other family-member Elements . . . to regulate the weather . . . to shape-shift . . . and we must be most grateful to have had expounded to us the Great Law of the Great Peace.

And so we open our hearts to you and tell you, "We love you and wish to thank you for all that you have done for us and for all you have given us."

UH SEH DE UH SEH DE UH SEH DE WA G'YEAH HANNEE'GIH N'YOWWEH HOI(T) . . .

OO'NIH TWEANT IT'NWO(T) DE YOO'REAH DUH'GIHH G'WIN-NEE(T) G'WIHH EHH'JEEH.

(*Translation:* Three times three times three large, enthusiastic "Thank yous" . . .

Now all of us universal family members, in our Urehdeh—life, energy, Divine Consciousness in all things—are as one.)

(*Note:* The word *Urehdeh* is sometimes seen spelled *U-renta*. Mike Bastine [Algonquin] says that some Indian nations forbid the speaking out loud of that word as being too holy for human usage.)

And so we greet and introduce into the consciousness and gratitude of our mind and spirit the next Element, our Mother Earth . . . and we can see our Mother as we may have seen her in a vision quest . . . the same as the picture taken by Apollo 17 . . . a blue-and-white opalescent orb . . . gliding gracefully and effortlessly through space . . . as though on a spiritual mission . . . so, so beautiful . . . the blue of the oceans . . . the misty white cloud cover . . . and the white polar caps. So beautiful.

That is our Mother . . . never telling a lie . . . no ulterior motives . . . and she has given us everything we would ever need . . . air, water, food, clothing, shelter, Medicine, love, a Divine Consciousness . . . a wonderful place to live.

So we open our hearts, and we say to her, "Mom . . . we love you very much, and we wish to thank you for all you have given us and for continuing to do so."

UH SEH DE UH SEH DE UH SEH DE WA G'YEAH HANNEE'GIH N'YOWWEH HOI(T) . . .

OO'NIH TWEANT IT'NWO(T) DE YOO'REAH DUH'GIHH G'WIN-NEE(T) G'WIHH EHH'JEEH.

◆ ◆ ◆

And so we greet and introduce into the consciousness and gratitude of our mind and spirit the next Element, Plant Life.

From the bottom of the deepest ocean to the top of the highest mountain, we have all of these green growing things . . . billions and billions of leaves . . . each producing pure oxygen in photosynthesis with the Day Sun that we may breathe more healthfully . . . billions and billions of leaves . . . each waiting for us to exhale carbon dioxide . . . that they, too, may breathe . . . that this exchange can be perpetual . . . and we know, then, that we are indeed an intricate part of this Divine and Harmonious Universe.

So we honor, first, the Medicine plants . . . knowing that the amount of cure that we can get from them is directly related to the amount of reverence we have for them . . . and knowing that they have always gladly given their lives for ours, and for our ancestral health and ceremonial usage we owe them a great amount of gratitude. Among them the great see-into-the-future Medicine, the great Ga noo du(t) oit . . . the baby-never-die Medicine, the great D'yeh g'yeh guh tu(t) uh . . . the great Sacred Tobacco, the Joss hoo(t) eh weh . . . and many more magical Medicine plants.

And so we open up our hearts and say, "We love you, and we wish to thank you for saving the lives of us people and for all the other magical things that you have done for us."

UH SEH DE UH SEH DE UH SEH DE WA G'YEAH HANNEE'GIH N'YOWWEH HOI(T) . . .

OO'NIH TWEANT IT'NWO(T) DE YOO'REAH DUH'GIHH G'WIN-NEE(T) G'WIHH EHH'JEEH.

And so we greet and introduce into the consciousness and gratitude of our mind and spirit the next Element, the Food plants . . . and they are powerfully represented by the many varieties of the three Sacred Sisters . . . the Corn . . . the Beans . . . and the Squash.

Not only have they been our sustenance and preventative Medicine . . . but they provide the exact ingredients needed to produce the supernatural results of the various Medicine feasts.

And so we say to both the domestic and the wild Food plants, "We love you very much, and we wish to thank you for keeping us alive and well."

UH SEH DE UH SEH DE UH SEH DE WA G'YEAH HANNEE'GIH N'YOWWEH HOI(T) . . .

OO'NIH TWEANT IT'NWO(T) DE YOO'REAH DUH'GIHH G'WIN-NEE(T) G'WIHH EHH'JEEH.

And so we greet and introduce into the consciousness and gratitude of our mind and our spirit the next Element, Water . . . and we can see that water in so many different forms . . . icicles and snowflakes . . . moondogs and sundogs . . . rainbows and clouds . . . glaciers and icebergs . . . oceans and rivers and streams . . . water fountains and waterfalls . . . fog and little droplets of dew on a spiderweb . . . sweat on our brow and steam in a Sweat Lodge . . . and when we become out of balance . . . too materialistic . . . here comes a flood . . . to put us on our knees . . . and balance is restored . . . and when we realize that we ourselves are 85 percent water or more . . . we realize how vital water is to us and to all living things.

So we open our hearts, and we say, "Oh beautiful and precious water, we love you very much, and we wish to thank you for all you mean to us."

UH SEH DE UH SEH DE UH SEH DE WA G'YEAH HANNEE'GIH N'YOWWEH HOI(T) . . .

OO'NIH TWEANT IT'NWO(T) DE YOO'REAH DUH'GIHH G'WIN-NEE(T) G'WIHH EHH'JEEH.

And so we greet and introduce into the consciousness and gratitude of our mind and our spirit the next Element, all Creaturehood, both on land and in the sea . . . from the amoeba to the zebra . . . from the seahorse to the Clydesdale . . . from the lightning bug to the electric eel to the elephant . . . and this enormous family membership is symbolized by the principal member, the deer, whose antlers represent the awareness and alertness of the aggregate of that great family . . . and they have faithfully given themselves that we may have food . . . clothing . . . shelter . . . Medicine . . . companionship . . . oracles . . . a Divine Consciousness, and more.

For all this, we open our hearts to all Creaturehood, and we say, "Oh dear loving family members . . . we love you very much, and we wish to thank you for all you have given us."

UH SEH DE UH SEH DE UH SEH DE WA G'YEAH HANNEE'GIH N'YOWWEH HOI(T) . . .

OO'NIH TWEANT IT'NWO(T) DE YOO'REAH DUH'GIHH G'WIN-NEE(T) G'WIHH EHH'JEEH.

And so we greet and introduce into the consciousness and gratitude of our mind and our spirit the next Element, the Trees . . . and they have given us so much . . . the aesthetic pleasure of the taste of various fruits and nuts . . . the syrup and confections from the sap, or lifeblood of the principal tree, the Sugar Maple . . . the symbolism and Medicine of the Tree of Peace, the great White Pine, which the mere touch of cures depression . . . the Medicine tree, the Basswood, from which the False Faces are made . . . the many other Medicine trees .. and their providing of shade, building material, firewood, love, peaceful companionship, the prevention of landslides, and great beauty, especially in the coloring of autumn.

For this and much more, we open our hearts, and we tell them how much we love them and that we wish to thank them.

UH SEH DE UH SEH DE UH SEH DE WA G'YEAH HANNEE'GIH N'YOWWEH HOI(T) . . .

OO'NIH TWEANT IT'NWO(T) DE YOO'REAH DUH'GIHH G'WIN-NEE(T) G'WIHH EHH'JEEH.

And so we greet and introduce into the consciousness and gratitude of our mind and our spirit the next Element, the Birds . . . and what a drabness would beset our world if it were not for the aesthetic pleasures of the music of their voices . . . the beauty of the colors of their feathers . . . the great grace that they exhibit in flight . . . and they have provided us with food . . . an astounding oracular talent . . . an example of peace and alertness as exemplified in the symbol of the eagle atop the Tree of Peace, guarding the Six Nation Confederacy . . . their contributing portion of the great, great Medicine, the Na go(t) na gaww, the never-die Medicine . . . their example of a Divine Consciousness.

For this and more we open our hearts to all birds and tell them that we love them very much and wish to thank them for all they mean to us.

UH SEH DE UH SEH DE UH SEH DE WA G'YEAH HANNEE'GIH N'YOWWEH HOI(T) . . .

OO'NIH TWEANT IT'NWO(T) DE YOO'REAH DUH'GIHH G'WIN-NEE(T) G'WIHH EHH'JEEH.

And so we greet and introduce into the consciousness and gratitude of our mind and our spirit the next Element, our great family member, the Great Grandfathers, the Thunderers . . . and they have faithfully guarded and protected us against any intruding out-of-balance forces that emerge from time to time to beset us . . . and we have heard them vehemently scolding such existences away so that we would not be influenced . . . and we have even seen the fire with which they do that . . . but we can only imagine the joy and anticipation of the green growing things for the ionized rain that follows to make sure that everything is clean again.

So we open our hearts and say to our Grandfathers, "Oh dear Grandfathers, we love you very much for your protecting us, and we wish to thank you."

UH SEH DE UH SEH DE UH SEH DE WA G'YEAH HANNEE'GIH N'YOWWEH HOI(T) . . .

OO'NIH TWEANT IT'NWO(T) DE YOO'REAH DUH'GIHH G'WIN-NEE(T) G'WIHH EHH'JEEH.

And so we greet and introduce into the consciousness and gratitude of our mind and our spirit the next Element, the Four Winds . . . and we know that they travel about, keeping track of things and aiding the Grandfathers and the rain to reach their destinations . . . and when we again get out of balance for any of many reasons, here comes a hurricane or tornado to frighten us back into balance and to remind us that we are not infallible . . . and though we might see parts of our abode flying up into the sky, we can also wonder how long we would live without air.

So we open our hearts to the Four Winds, and we tell them how precious they are to us and that we wish to thank them:

UH SEH DE UH SEH DE UH SEH DE WA G'YEAH HANNEE'GIH N'YOWWEH HOI(T) . . .

OO'NIH TWEANT IT'NWO(T) DE YOO'REAH DUH'GIHH G'WIN-NEE(T) G'WIHH EHH'JEEH.

•   •   •

And so we greet and introduce into the consciousness and gratitude of our mind and our spirit the next Element, the Four Directions . . . a subtle doorway between the physical consciousness and the ethereal world . . . members of our universal family that transcend molecular structure . . . the means by which nesting birds can fly south in winter and return unerringly to their nesting places . . . the means by which lost ships can be found at sea . . . a miraculous means by which we travel . . . always constantly at our disposal . . . the cornerstone of our equilibrium.

So we must not unconsciously take for granted this great family membership . . . but instead open our hearts and say, "Oh great Four Directions, we love you for your everlasting faithfulness, and we wish to thank you."

UH SEH DE UH SEH DE UH SEH DE WA G'YEAH HANNEE'GIH N'YOWWEH HOI(T) . . .

OO'NIH TWEANT IT'NWO(T) DE YOO'REAH DUH'GIHH G'WIN-NEE(T) G'WIHH EHH'JEEH.

And so we greet and introduce into the consciousness and gratitude of our mind and our spirit the next Element, the Night Sun, our Grandmother Moon . . . and she loves us and, if she could, would like to bounce us on her knee . . . and when we get too take-it-for-granted of her, she would like to remind us that she is not just up there whistling Dixie . . . that she is there to remind us that she will not allow us to be forgotten as a species . . . for she has given females a time-cycle period called a moon . . . and at a special time in that cycle they can become fertile and reproduce . . . and for those of us who may not believe that there is a powerful attraction between our Grandmother and us and the earth, we can be reassured by watching the rising and the falling of the tides . . . and we are reminded by the natal ties we have with our beautiful Grandmother Moon that we are indeed an intricate part of this Divine and Harmonious Universe.

So we open our hearts and say, "Oh dear Grandmother, we love you very much and wish to thank you for all you mean to us."

UH SEH DE UH SEH DE UH SEH DE WA G'YEAH HANNEE'GIH N'YOWWEH HOI(T) . . .

OO'NIH TWEANT IT'NWO(T) DE YOO'REAH DUH'GIHH G'WIN-NEE(T) G'WIHH EHH'JEEH.

♦   ♦   ♦

And so we greet and introduce into the consciousness and gratitude of our mind and our spirit the next Element, our elder brother, the Day Sun . . . and if it were not for the steadfast love and warmth embracing us each day, we would not exist . . . we would be cast in the darkness and frozen . . . and we don't know the vast amount of beneficial vitamins, minerals, and trace Elements that have been radiated to us throughout our existence . . . and so this magical life-giving source is responsible not only for our existence but for the existence and growth of all of our family and therefore all of the other necessary benefits that we derive from our other family members.

So we open our hearts, and we say, "Oh dear elder brother, we love you very much, and we wish to thank you for all you have given to us and for all you mean to us."

UH SEH DE UH SEH DE UH SEH DE WA G'YEAH HANNEE'GIH N'YOWWEH HOI(T) . . .

OO'NIH TWEANT IT'NWO(T) DE YOO'REAH DUH'GIHH G'WIN-NEE(T) G'WIHH EHH'JEEH.

And so we greet and introduce into the consciousness and gratitude of our mind and our spirit the next Element, the Stars . . . and their awesome nightly beauty evokes the astrological influences they have upon us . . . and we can be en-tranced by them when we lay in the soft summer grass and peer into the sky . . . a myriad of diamonds, twinkling and winking at us, as though they had some se-cret to tell us . . . then after a while it comes to us that there just have to be thou-sands of other solar systems like our own . . . with Day Suns and celestial bodies orbiting about them . . . then after a while it becomes clear . . . that what we are looking at . . . is nothing but a replica . . . of the molecular structure of all other things . . . even the internal workings of an atom . . . of neutrons . . . protons . . . ions . . . electrons . . . photons . . . each orbiting . . . each smaller particle less physical than the other . . . until we are speaking of pure energy and Divine Consciousness . . . the recipe of all that there is, including ourselves . . . and we can feel a Divine responsibility for the caretaking of this Divine and Harmonious Universe.

So we open our hearts and say, "Oh beautiful, beautiful stars, we love you very much, and we wish to thank you for all you mean to us."

UH SEH DE UH SEH DE UH SEH DE WA G'YEAH HANNEE'GIH N'YOWWEH HOI(T) . . .

OO'NIH TWEANT IT'NWO(T) DE YOO'REAH DUH'GIHH G'WIN-NEE(T) G'WIHH EHH'JEEH.

And so we greet and introduce into the consciousness and gratitude of our mind and our spirit the next Element, the Four Protectors, sometimes called the Four Messengers . . . and now it behooves us to be aware of this great connection with the ethereal world . . . our own intuitive link with the vast dynamic intelligence of the Universe . . . a mystical family membership with no molecular structure . . . and we don't know how many times our lives have been saved by these alert messengers . . . for instance, at times when we were leaving the safety of our homes to do an errand, something stopped us at the door, ostensibly to see if we remember to take everything we might need . . . when we reach the intersection where another vehicle would have struck us . . . THAT vehicle would have already passed through . . . and these great Elements stand ever ready to help transport the supplications of our ceremonies.

So we open our hearts and say, "Oh dear Four Protectors, we love you very much, and we wish to thank you for all you have done for us."

UH SEH DE UH SEH DE UH SEH DE WA G'YEAH HANNEE'GIH N'YOWWEH HOI(T) . . .

OO'NIH TWEANT IT'NWO(T) DE YOO'REAH DUH'GIHH G'WIN-NEE(T) G'WIHH EHH'JEEH.

And so we greet and introduce into the consciousness and gratitude of our mind and our spirit the ultimate Element, Soong gwi oo dee sut eh . . . Creator of this Divine and Harmonious Universe . . . the manifestation of supreme power, goodness, intelligence, and forgiveness . . . and so we owe a great gratitude for there being all that there is . . . and for the constant watching over us . . . and for reminding all things of their duties.

So we open our hearts to this Highest Consciousness, and we say, "We love you very much, and we wish to thank you for all that there is and for all of your benevolence."

UH SEH DE UH SEH DE UH SEH DE WA G'YEAH HANNEE'GIH N'YOWWEH HOI(T) . . .

OO'NIH TWEANT IT'NWO(T) DE YOO'REAH DUH'GIHH G'WIN-NEE(T) G'WIHH EHH'JEEH.

If we have forgotten any Elements and left them out, let them speak for themselves, for all the Elements are more Divine than we are, being as they are unable to tell a lie or have ulterior motives.

Medicines and Poisons

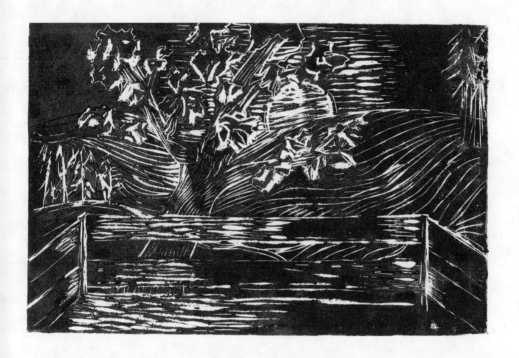

Overleaf: Tree that blocked the view and, when cut without ceremony, broke Ted's back; see "One Time This Happened," pp. 140–51. Woodcut by Rhiannon Miles Osborne.

The Second Death of Bill Uh

Life, for me, not counting the gestation period, started on the Tuscarora Indian Reservation near Niagara Falls, New York, on April 6, 1930.

Three years later my father, Eleazer, who did what we call Indian Medicine, took me to the eighty-eighth annual Tuscarora National Picnic. It took place in the heat of summer. That spring, on March 18, my sister, Freida, had been born. Our mother, Amelia Chew Williams, was of the Wolf Clan, so, following the matriarchal traditions of the Six Nation Iroquois, Freida and I automatically became little wolves, too. Father was of the Turtle Clan and would soon become Sachem (roughly, "senior") Chief of that clan. He was fifty-three years of age when Freida was born. Amelia was thirty-four.

At the picnic, Father held on to my three-year-old hand to keep me from cruising about, which I was wont to do. I felt trapped as father would stop and talk at length to his friends, some of whom were Six Nations Elders from Canada, where he had spent time learning Medicine. (I capitalize the word *Medicine*, meaning the kind of Medicine that is within the influences of a universally Divine Consciousness.)

There was plenty of noise, and that's what I would have wandered toward if I could. I could hear a white man hollering, "PEANUTS, POPCORN, WATER-MELON, FIVE CENTS!"

Just about the time I was reaching the height of boredom, however, something came to my rescue. I saw a man crying and talking, and I thought he was about to fall over from grief. Father was busy talking and paid no attention.

What I was seeing was a drunk Indian. His name was William Pembleton, but everyone called him Bill Uh. *Uh* means "small," because that was what he was. He was a veteran of World War I and considered himself a war hero. But here he was drunk, and it was not a big deal to Indians anymore to be a veteran of a war among white people.

I didn't know all this, of course, and I watched this little man stagger about dressed in woolen ODs (olive drabs, army color) in hot midsummer. As he got closer, I could see that he was pleading for something, maybe love, but because he was crying, he mumbled. No one seemed to pay any attention to him, which, to me, could be all the more reason to feel bad. Then, too, he was talking half Tuscarora and half English. He was saying things like, "I'm Uncle Sam's boy, he(t) g'ya(t)" *(he(t) g'ya(t),* meaning something like, "It's a fact, don't you know").

The next thing that Bill Uh did finally got Father's attention. Bill was close to us now and raised his arms skyward in a classic imploring gesture, as though to say, "All right, everybody, if you don't love me, I know somebody up there who does care."

I was transfixed by this drama, and next came a climax. Bill took sick and puked straight up. Then he lost his balance and fell over backward, banging his head on the sun-hardened earth and passing out. Flies attacked him. I just knew I had seen a man die of a broken heart. Father pulled me away and bought me some ice cream.

Autumn came and reluctantly succumbed to winter. Our sleeping arrangement was for little Freida to sleep next to the wall so she wouldn't fall out of bed, with Mother right next to her. I slept on the outside because I was the big protector in case the boogeyman came. Father slept upstairs because four in a bed is too many.

In the middle of the night, I heard a noise—CLUNK! You know how logs in a woodstove like to change position once in a while, and that's what that noise was, but it woke me up. Like the log, I changed position and started back to sleep.

I was nearly asleep when I thought I heard something else. I lay still, but I pricked up my ears. Yes, I did hear something else. Drums. Army drums. A marching unit was out there in the middle of the night drumming and marching. You know the sound, ". . . da da DUM de dum, da da DUM de dum, da da Dadada Dadada, Dadada Dadada, DUM de DUM."

The sound was not loud, but it was distinct. It was coming from the south-southwest. I thought I might be dreaming, so I waited to wake up. Didn't someone say if you pinch yourself, and it hurts, you're not dreaming? I pinched. It hurt, and now I could hear the drums a bit louder and more from the south. It was like drummers were marching along the old lane that ran east and west across the gully between us.

I didn't wake Mother. She might get scared like I was. I mean, I kind of liked the sound, but in the middle of the night? One crazy drummer, maybe, but a whole unit?

It was clear now that the night drummers were on the lane. At the end of the lane, they would come to a log house. It was old but solid. Edgar and Lulu lived in it now, but people said that it was a powder house during the American Revolution. Maybe George Washington had built it out of cherry trees.

When we had gone to bed, there had been about two inches of snow on the ground. In the morning, it was the same; no new snow had fallen. I could hardly wait to bundle up and go outside and see the tracks of the drummers. Mother made me eat breakfast first.

When I got to the lane, there was nothing. No tracks of any kind. Nothing had passed here during the night. I went home and told Mother about the drummers marching and drumming on Edgar's lane during the night, but that they left no tracks. Mother said nothing. I thought maybe she didn't believe me.

Mother said nothing, but most Indians listen to their children, even to their dogs or cats—or canaries if they have them. I'll tell you a more recent story here of an experience by a Seneca family to make my point.

This Seneca family, dog and all, were traveling in a station wagon and stopped at a commercial campsite for the night. They paid the fee, chose a site, and put up their tent. Their dog, however, refused to get out of the station wagon. Most people would have pulled the dog out and tied it to a tree, thinking, "Oh, the dog is just homesick in these unfamiliar surroundings. It'll get used to it." Instead, the Senecas listened to their dog. They took their tent down, gathered up their things, got their money back, and left. In an hour, a tornado came and wiped the whole campsite out.

When Father came home from work that evening, he had some news. Bill Uh had died early in the morning. Mother told Father of my experience of hearing what sounded like an army drum corps marching along the lane to the old log house, the old army powder house. Immediately, I heard the real news, "Uncle Sam's boy is dead."

Again.

How could he die twice?

Again.

Father looked at me. "You should have woke me up when you heard the drums," he said, "It was a warning that Bill Uh needed my help."

"How would you know that?" I asked.

Father smiled. "I have ways," was all he said.

The Way It Is

It has become fashionable in our society to use the Buddhist phrase "all is one" as a kind of benchmark way of saying, "I'm into Higher Consciousness." The children of the Six Nation Iroquois who attend the year-round ceremonies and hear the Thanksgiving Address at the beginning and end of each day's ceremony soon take for granted this oneness. Indeed, they grow up perceiving a kinship to all things. Some may go on to become Medicine people and communicate with entities, even from other galaxies.

At the time of the burning of witches at Salem, the great seers among the indigenous peoples of the eastern United States immediately "saw" this event, and all ceremony, also referred to as Medicine activity, went underground.

From here on, for simplicity, let's use the terms *white people* and *Indians*, as is the common usage within the Six Nations. So if white people were unacquainted with Indian Medicine ways before this, then it became nearly impossible to ever discover the depth of those Medicine ways.

Whether the seers sounded an all-clear or not, some of the Six Nation people gradually began practicing more openly. The Seneca, especially, became more lenient and did allow a few white writers access into the Longhouse to report what they saw. All ceremonies, however, are in the native languages, and many words—such as the Tuscarora word *Urehdeh* (the life, energy, Divine Consciousness in all things)—transcend everyday usage and defy accurate interpretation into English.

By the way, the term *Longhouse* has come to mean not only the ceremonial and sacred meeting place of the traditional people who follow the Great Law or Law of the Great Peace, but also those who follow that way of life. An Indian meeting another Indian of the Six Nations might ask, "Are you Longhouse?" and if the answer is "No," it is then understood that this person does not attend traditional ceremonies and does not follow the Great Law for whatever reason.

Also, at one time the Indians of the Six Nations lived in buildings shaped like Quonset huts with a semicircular arching roof of poles covered by elm bark. Because of their length and because they were often lengthened for additions to the family, they were called Longhouses.

The accounts written by the white writers just mentioned were, from an academic viewpoint, very good, and even some scholarly Indians who had attended schools like Carlisle Indian School reported the activities of the Longhouse people.

But where it gets a little tricky is that in crossing this line beyond what one sees from a physical consciousness, one begins to tamper with sacred laws — universal laws, not man-made.

As a lad, I was privileged to see my father gather and dispense plant Medicines or use them to cure haunted houses or change people's minds. As he did, he would be talking in Tuscarora, which is the same as praying to I didn't know what. But the thing I would hear him tell people was, "Don't let anybody see you gather this Medicine," "Don't let anybody see you taking (imbibing) this Medicine."

I questioned this supersecrecy and at the time thought it simply part of that "underground policy" in case some stray leftover witch hunter might still come snooping around.

One day a neighbor, about fifty years of age, told me about his experience with a Medicine person named Jeeeks. Having no mode of transportation and probably not knowing how to drive a car even if he had one, Jeeeks asked Basket to drive him to the Tonawanda Seneca Reservation to gather some Medicine. At a certain spot, Jeeeks told Basket to stop and let him out and to wait there for him.

Basket had brought a newspaper with him and sat in the car reading it. After nearly an hour he looked up into the woods where Jeeeks had disappeared to see if he was coming back yet. To his surprise he saw Jeeeks watching him from behind a tree. As soon as Jeeeks saw Basket look up, he pulled his head back behind the tree and hid. All this time Jeeeks had been making sure that Basket was not going to follow him and lay eyes on the Medicine.

At this point in the story I was thinking that probably Jeeeks was sorry he had asked Basket to drive him and had forgotten that Basket was an alcoholic. Jeeeks used to say that alcohol released pent-up anger and that this attitude frightened Medicine. Basket did not know this.

When Jeeeks finally came out of the woods, it was from the direction just opposite of the road where he had entered. Just to make sure.

After this I thought about and realized that on a few Medicine-gathering trips with my father, he had subtly gotten me to do something, then gone off by himself. When he returned, he would already have that certain Medicine tucked away safely out of sight in his Medicine bag. So I asked him about this secrecy, telling him about Basket's experience with Jeeeks.

"Oh, yes," he said, "You need to know about this. Certain great and powerful Medicines are very touchy. They cannot have anyone with the least bit of disbelief in them see them. Nor can you speak of them to anyone who has this disbelief. Disbelief dilutes any Medicine to the degree of the disbelief. If I should cause anyone to make fun of a Medicine, in word or thought or feeling or deed, then I would find that Medicine missing from the place where I have always gathered it. It would hide on me. Also, these Medicines know if you are bringing them a gift of Sacred Indian Tobacco or silver or not. It's a shame that many Indians have lost faith in the Indian Medicine way and will never get to see or know about these Medicines."

I then remembered Chief Beeman Logan of Tonawanda telling me about the Sacred Indian Tobacco. (He knew Medicine.) It, too, can hide. What Beeman told me was that some Indians even found out the hard way that this sacred plant would not grow for them.

"They'd come first and ask for some seed. Maybe they'd try planting seeds in two or three successive years. Then they'd ask if they could transplant some of my sprouted little Tobacco plants. Some would quit trying, but some would ask for larger plants. The Tobacco had detected some lack of reverence or some form of bad vibration in these people. The Sacred Tobacco refused to grow for them, or you could say that by dying the Tobacco disappeared on them, hid on them."

But not on my father. One time we moved from where we lived (and where I was born) at Seven Clan to a house on Dog Street, a distance of two or three miles. A week later Father said, "You know what? I left my Tobacco at our old house. I ought to go and get them and transplant them here."

The next morning he happened to look at my mother's new flower garden.

The Tobacco plants were in there with the flowers. They had moved themselves.

So, as Father was saying, "Many Indians will never get to see or know about these Medicines. Maybe they've grown too materialistic. Or could they be ashamed of themselves as Indians? Maybe seeing too many movies of the Indian as the bad guy; or hearing about fake snake-medicine hawkers.

"Last week Elton Green [a Tuscarora Chief] wasn't feeling well, so he went to gather something to cure it. When he got to the place where it grew, he found nothing. Right away he blamed Allen Jack for gathering all of it. Of course, being sick, he wasn't thinking right. After he was back home for a while, he realized something. He had not taken any Indian Tobacco with him when he went for the Medicine. So he went back a second time, this time with Tobacco. He laughed when he told me this. He said he was only halfway across the field when he could see the Medicine in a big group at the other end waiting for him.

"So maybe some people don't want to share what they know, but it's more important that we keep the Medicine happy, not dilute it. We must follow the rules.

"The amount of cure that you get from any Medicine, even a smile, is directly related to the amount of reverence that we show it. Also, we MUST talk to the Medicine."

Gradually, I began to see the Medicine way in action. In talking to the Medicine, one begins to transcend physical consciousness and expand one's belief system. Time and space fade out, and the oneness of all things becomes apparent.

Another Form of Medicine

Just below the escarpment that roughly formed the northern boundary of the Tuscarora Indian Reservation could be seen the busy Ridge Road. This road was known for a long time as "the Million-Dollar Highway." If you got on it and drove or walked westward, you'd come to the town of Lewiston, New York. At one time, the escarpment extended, unbroken, into what is now Canada.

Over the years a river now known as the Niagara River, on its way connecting Lake Erie with Lake Ontario, cut a deep swath into this escarpment. The Niagara Gorge is deep, but its width is—well, I think George Washington might barely be able to throw a silver dollar across it. From the top of the Lewiston-Queenston Bridge to the water is 252 feet.

One day when I was little, Simon Cusick (whose great-grandfather, Colonel Nicholas Cusick, was bodyguard to General Marquis de Lafayette when he was here trying to help fight some war) showed me something. Through a break in the trees on a clear day, he showed me the city of Toronto, barely visible on the horizon of Lake Ontario. Before I could make out that Toronto was a city, I thought that he was telling me that a man named Toronto could be seen walking on water.

I was just a tot full of vinegar and wanted to walk and explore farther, but Simon had walked far enough, so he said, "No. There's some bad guys out that way," pointing west.

"Really?"

"Yep. They have big stone houses like fortresses, and they might shoot you. They got fences around them houses made out of sharp iron spikes that, if you slipped trying to climb over them, they'd jab right through you. And anyway, if you got over the fence, they have wicked big dogs waiting to tear you apart." He didn't need to do any more convincing to have me turn around with him and go home.

31

After we got well on the way, maybe Simon thought he may have frightened me too much, what with all my questions.

"Well," he said, "that whole section is called Lewiston Heights. Bigwigs live there. People with money. The Niagara Country Club is there, too. But the bad guys, nobody bothers them. They are called the Mafia."

One day one of the "bad guys" came to our house. Of course, I didn't know he was one of the guys Simon was talking about. He had on a suit and vest and tie with a jewel on it and patent leather shoes. He was looking for "this Eleazer Williams that makes Medicine."

You see, even though this man could slit somebody's throat, he himself could not stomach the thought of someone else touching his skin with a knife. Not even the most sought-after surgeon in the world. This man was suffering from painful bladder stones. This case was so simple for Father that he only charged ten cents. The ten cents had to be a dime, though, because Indians had discovered that silver worked in the "balance of Medicine" if one did not have the Sacred Tobacco to use in "the Exchange." In those days a dime contained silver. The Medicine given was the roots of the great Purple Boneset.

Not long afterward, this same man came back again. He came as before, in a big shiny black limousine, driven by somebody else.

What he came for was to say that all the pain was gone now, and he was so overjoyed that he wanted to give my father a hundred dollars. Father was hoeing weeds at the far edge of our extensive vegetable garden. So happy was this dressed-to-kill man that he stepped gingerly right through the dust and dirt of the garden in them small pointed patent leather shoes. He was all smiles.

Father would not take the hundred dollars. It took quite a while to convince the man why not. "You've paid already. The Medicine is happy, but it might get mad if you disturb the balance. The stones and the pain might come back."

Finally, the man heard what Father was saying. "All right," he said, pointing a finger, "but if you ever need anything, just call the Maggadino Funeral Home and ask for Stephano." Then he recrossed the garden, tippy-toeing this time, back to the limousine and left.

A year or so later another man in another shiny car came. The car was almost as nice as Stephano's.

As soon as Chucky, our dog, began barking and we could see this car with a dusty wake appear, Father sent me off on a little job.

"Call the chickens out of the woods and give them some cracked corn. Count them. Fifteen hens. When they're all there, pull the tin trough out of the hen house and give them some laying mash. Keep the rooster out of the laying mash."

Did father suspect something?

A white man got out of the car. Father took him to a bench and sat with him in the shade. Though I listened with all my might, I couldn't make out the talk between them. I could only tell that before the man left, his voice rose ever so slightly in volume. Also, he made more dirt leaving than Stephano did. Nor was he as dressy.

What the man wanted, Father told later, was to learn the secret Medicine of a certain cure. He was willing to pay a large sum of money for the name of the remedy. Father told him that Medicine "don't work that way." You don't "buy it."

Well, wouldn't you know, in a couple of weeks that same car came back. As soon as Chucky barked, Father said, "Tomorrow your mother is going to State Fair at Syracuse. Go out to the garden and pick out a pumpkin to send with her. Pick one that will win a prize."

I went to the pumpkins, but they all looked the same to me. Two men were getting out of the car, so I kind of sidled back closer to the new arrivals in case Father needed help. Also, I had heard that when Father had attended Carlisle Indian School, he had been a good boxer. Prizefighter, they called a boxer. So I secretly wanted a ringside seat in case Father would be putting on a demonstration.

Still, Father had sent me to the garden because he must have thought some words might be spoken that shouldn't enter my ears. Maybe swearing. Such words might dilute my Medicine in case I had any.

So I didn't really get to hear much except at the last when the passenger of the car raised his voice and sounded like he was threatening my father. "Oh boy!" I thought to myself, "Here comes that fight I've been waiting for."

Instead, Father simply said something inaudible, and "zip," the men got into their car and drove off in a cloud of dust.

I rushed up to Father, who had a little bitty smirk on his face, to tell him that I couldn't find the right pumpkin. But when I got there, I said, "What did them men want?"

"I'll tell you by and by."

"Well, I can't figure out which pumpkin to get."

"Oh sure you can. That's easy. Just look at them good, and you'll know which one is the one."

I went back to the pumpkins, and sure enough, the first one I looked at looked like it wanted to go for a ride, so I took it. It was much smaller than a basketball. The next day it went to Syracuse.

By the end of the week, I thought surely the "by and by" had gone by long enough to hear, from Father, what the confrontation with the two white men was all about, so I asked him.

"Well, maybe you're old enough now to understand what them guys wanted. You see, this older fellow that came along this time owns some drug stores. He has what is called a pharmaceutical company. He wanted to pay me a lot of money to tell him about that special oo druss seh [Bracket Fungus] Medicine that doesn't even grow around here. It can hide. That means he probably could never find it anyways, let alone try to grow it. When I told him it would never work out for him, that he would come back and sue me for selling him a bill of goods, he thought I was telling lies."

"How much money was he going to give you?"

"Enough to buy two or more chicken houses."

"Heck, we don't need that, do we? I heard him raise his voice."

"Yes. When he got mad, he threatened me. He said it was very illegal to be selling Medicine in the state of New York without a license. If I sold him the Medicine secret, he wouldn't tell on me. I wouldn't have to go to jail, he said."

"What did you say to him? They left awfully quick."

"I told him that I didn't approve of what he was saying. That I knew another man that did things that I didn't approve of either. 'He made people disappear. He made double caskets and buried his enemies in the bottom compartment of those caskets in regular funerals. But I cured him of bladder stones, so he told me if I ever needed anything to call the Maggadino Funeral Home and ask for Stephano. I don't approve of your threat or what he does, but I approve of you getting in your car and leaving and never coming back.' So he did. I guess you can say I used another form of Medicine."

As we talked, we had been walking the half-mile to the mailbox on Upper Mountain Road. Now we were there, at the mailbox. The only piece of mail was a postcard from Mother. All it said was, "Pumpkin took first prize."

Uncle Charley

Uncle Charley was a nine in the Enneagram, and as you probably know, nines are wallflowerish. That also means, though, that he compulsively reacted intuitively, and that's why he did such unusual things.

When I think of Uncle Charley, I am reminded of the enlightened Chinese Zen Buddhist Empty Cloud because both of them could pass for a bum. It would seem that enlightenment is enlightenment, not A is more enlightened than B. It just may be that if what happened to Empty Cloud doesn't happen to you, then you are not yet enlightened.

Empty Cloud walked a pilgrimage of about three thousand miles, and after every third step he would bow down to the earth and touch his forehead three times. As he approached any mountain village, at about the proximity of one mile, all the bells in that town would ring by themselves. Elders of that town who knew of this phenomenon would excitedly announce that an enlightened person was approaching. People would race down the mountain path to greet the enlightened person and invariably knock Empty Cloud out of the way because his appearance was that of a bum. Like Uncle Charley looked. So don't kick an old dog; it might be the Creator in disguise.

I liked to hear Uncle Charley recite little conversations he'd had with other people because he would tell them word for word. Some people called him "Chuck."

"Hey Chuck."

"Yeah."

"How did you like the corn soup at the picnic?"

"Not bad, but I kind of like them to leave some of the bite of the ashen taste. Not wash it out so good."

"Oh. Well, uh, I made it."

Then Uncle Charley would laugh his hee-hee laugh.

Unusual things have happened to people in times of dire need, so this may be what caused Uncle Charley to be a great hunter. During the time of the Second World War, hunters could not buy ammunition to hunt with. Farmers could get a permission slip from somewhere that allowed them to purchase a box of .22 caliber bullets for varmint control, but Uncle Charley only had a little vegetable garden and didn't qualify.

One day, in desperation for food, he went rabbit hunting with nothing but a stick. Presently he came upon a rabbit that was wide-awake and looking at him with those great big eyes. Uncle Charley just KNEW that the rabbit wasn't going to just sit there and wait to be bopped on the head. But he feared that his mother might starve to death.

Desperation came. Uncle Charley pointed his pointer finger at the rabbit, and it "froze," just like a snake can charm a frog or a toad or a bird, or a spider can charm a fly. Slowly, Uncle Charley advanced on the rabbit, keeping his finger pointed like a pistol. The rabbit never moved, and Uncle Charley went right on up to it and grabbed it. Of course, the thought came that maybe the rabbit was sick or crazy, so he tried it again on the next rabbit. Same result. Then he tried a pheasant. Same result. At that time, deer were just beginning to migrate onto the Tuscarora Indian Reservation, so I don't think Uncle Charley got a chance to charm one. I wondered, though, if he did, could he hang on to it?

As the war progressed, more and more jobs needed workers as the draft board took all available men for assignment into the armed forces. Uncle Charley then found steady work and from then on had enough money to do all his hunting in the supermarket. He was too old to be drafted.

Years and years went by, and Uncle Charley retired into Social Security. He also had long retired from charming game. One day, though, he had a related recurrence.

People can be charmed. Not only by hypnotism, but in other ways, even by things. The Niagara River has that ability, especially the lower gorge section with its dark green whirlpools and eddies. The distant roar of the plunging water adds to it. Even Night Herons can be seen in the daytime staring into the majestic movement of water. Uncle Charley was one day charmed into taking a walk along its treacherous edge.

On this day Uncle Charley came upon a section where rod-and-reel fishermen were trying their luck. Whatever possessed him to do this is not known, maybe that water's magnetic charm, but he went to the dangerous edge of the river and put his pointer finger in it. A group of fish immediately gathered around his finger, some bumping their noses against it.

A nearby fisherman, seeing this, exclaimed, "Hey, that's something. I didn't know that could be done. Let me try it."

"Well," said Uncle Charley, "neither did I. I've never done it before. Go ahead," he said, stepping away. "You try it."

The fisherman put his finger in the water, and the fish scurried off into the depths. "Let me see you do that again," the disappointed fisherman said.

Uncle Charley reluctantly did as he was bid, saying, "As I said, I've never done this before."

The fish came to his finger again, and this time even bigger fish came.

"HEY, YOU GUYS!" the fisherman began shouting, "COME ON AND SEE THIS! YOU JUST GOTTA SEE THIS!"

A number of fishermen came and surrounded the scene. Soon, with shouts and gestures, the group swelled to contain all the fishermen in the area. After a while, the original witness could no longer withstand seeing all these big fish so close and yet not in his creel. "GRAB ME ONE," he implored to Uncle Charley. Everyone waited to see this.

"I can't," Uncle Charley said.

"Why not?"

The old hunter looked at the fisherman with genuine regret. "I don't have a license," he said.

One night, in the middle of his life, Uncle Charley had a dream. He dreamed he was with a small crowd of people in a small space of a building, and all seemed to be moving toward the exit of it. Directly in front of him was a woman in a black coat. He touched her on the shoulder, and she turned around. It was Doris Hudson, one of the women of the reservation, and he said to her, "How are you?"

"Not well," she answered. "I have to go to the hospital for an operation on Tuesday."

"Do you mind if I pray for you?" Uncle Charley asked in the dream.

"No," she replied.

So he did just that, prayed for her.

That was the end of the dream.

A week or so later Uncle Charley happened to be invited to the small mission church for the Wednesday night meetings that were held there. At the end of the meeting, he was walking out through the entranceway when, click, a light bulb like you see in the comics went on in his head. Here was the scene from his dream, and, sure enough, the woman in the black coat walked in front of him.

Indeed, it was Doris Hudson. He tapped her on the shoulder. The dream reenacted itself, Doris saying she needed surgery and Charley getting permission to pray for her. There, with others watching, Charley prayed in the Tuscarora language. On Tuesday the doctors could find no sign of her illness and sent her home.

From that day on Uncle Charley healed people by prayer. I once watched him do this. He faced the ill one and put his hands on their shoulders. Then he closed his eyes and cut loose a powerful supplication in Tuscarora. Tears streamed down his face.

Uncle Charley, in his later years, lived on Indian Hill near the northwest edge of the reservation. I hadn't seen him for quite some time, so I decided to see how he was. A good thing, too, for though he appeared the same as always, he died not long afterward.

We were sitting on a bench he had made, swapping tales of the past, when he said:

"Oh, you haven't seen my new friend, have you?" He began teasing, in Tuscarora, what seemed like an imaginary person. He was directing his talk to a thicket of hawthorns that surrounded the woodsy side and rear of his house.

In a minute or two, out from the bushes flew a Mockingbird and landed on the power lines so that we had to lift our heads to see it. Uncle Charley continued his teasing.

"You lazy thing! Sleeping in the bushes all day. I bet you've even forgotten some of those tricks you showed me. Come on, I have someone here to meet you."

Immediately, the bird went into a series of antics like a miniature eagle dancer. It fanned its wings upward. It shivered and turned its head backward. After it did a dozen or so song imitations of a series of other birds, it ended the songfest with cricket and tree frog songs. It then flew into the air, and I thought for a split second that it was leaving. Instead, it did a backward somersault and landed back on the wire.

Uncle Charley then let it off the hook. "OK, OK, we believe you. So then we thank you. Now then, GO ON BACK TO BED!" And off the Mockingbird flew back into the bushes.

I never saw Uncle Charley alive again. It was as though he, too, went to bed. And just like other great Medicine people who died when they were ready to, he never asked to have any Medicine person come and extend his existence. I don't know if he had ever been inside the Longhouse, but it was as though he simply became a part of the great cycle of all things.

Isaiah Joseph

First, I met Pete Joseph. It started out with just a few visits to the Tuscarora section of the Six Nation Indian Reservation, where I kept meeting more and more fascinating old folks to swap stories with. After a while, it became almost an obsession, especially after I began meeting Indians who had actually seen some of the legendary entities like the Fire Lion.

When I say I first met Pete Joseph, I mean I met him before I met his brother, Isaiah. Pete and his neighbor, Bob Mt. Pleasant, were two people who had both seen the Fire Lion, the Ga hus stee'nis.

Pete was a roly-poly Elder living in a small shack all by himself. He told me some hard-to-believe stories that often involved his brother, Isaiah. I actually stopped seeing Pete when, in his telling of his having seen the Fire Lion in action, he became so wildly animated that I labeled him a schizo. When I asked him about Medicine, though, he said, "The man you really want to see is Isaiah."

I found Isaiah, like many other powerful Medicine people, devoid of extraneous material goods. Not even a house of his own. He was living with his daughter and her family, not far from the Grand River.

When I first laid eyes on him, he gave me a little "start" because he looked like a reincarnation of someone I knew called Mocks Johnson. Both had dark skin and the boniest of faces. Both had a perpetual smile.

He immediately greeted me as though he had already known me for a long time and was expecting my arrival. I don't know why this made me laugh, but we both laughed at the same time.

When I said, "Pete sicced me on to you," he said, "Did he scare you?"

I said, "Not yet," and we laughed again.

I could tell that he was old, but he moved with such grace and ease that I knew the word *age* was not in his vocabulary. He spoke mostly Tuscarora with a bit of English mixed in.

I visited him and took notes a number of times, so it seems best to just relate some of our talks as one big interview. Indeed, I asked many questions, and he always answered so eagerly and forthrightly.

One of the very first things that impressed me about Isaiah was that he listened to me intently, as though he were the eager pupil. One day I told Isaiah about the Enneagram—how it seemed to me to be more accurate than anything I had ever come across involving human compulsions and behavior. As I began using up our time together, doing all the talking, I expected that he might become bored with my explanation; instead, he pulled his chair closer, questioning and prodding me to go on.

I was timid about this discussion because earlier, when during a reading the great seer Daisy Thomas "saw" that I was visiting Isaiah, she reacted as though I might be overstepping my bounds.

I brought my explanation of the Enneagram to a close by asking him what he thought of it.

"That," he said emphatically, "needs to be a required study in all high schools!"

So what did Isaiah and I talk about while we visited?

Oh, anything. We might get into a sort of serious silliness.

Isaiah: "Wouldn't it be something if we discovered that goodness was the same as enlightenment and that one could go there if one was good enough."

Me: "Yeah!" (Then a brief silence to think about it.) "Yeah. We could pretend to send out goodness Medicine vibes to the Universe. We could put our hands up in front of our heart as though we were holding an invisible crystal ball. In that space was the whole Universe, and we could 'zap' it with goodness."

No response from Isaiah, so I go on willy-nilly. "But what if you had to have a magic word to do this? What if you had to zap the Universe in a sort of cadence, like a chant that was in cahoots with your breath, and each time you had to say this magic word?"

Still no response from Isaiah, so I say to him, "What magic word would you use?"

Isaiah: "Zingo! . . . Zingo! . . . Zingo!" (So he was listening to my "what ifs"!) Then we both went into another laughing bout.

Another time, we were talking about any Medicine that would stop a behavior that was the cause of some illness, and this is what Isaiah DID say:

"It's like the path that you are walking is the wrong one. It takes you to your illness." After a bit, we both laughed when he said, "So to get well you have to walk backwards."

(Twenty-five or so years later, my wife, Diana, said one day that she wasn't feeling well and, though she is a great diagnostic homeopathic doctor, couldn't imagine what the cause was.

I said, "It's the path you're walking. What you have to do is walk a mile backwards."

She said, "I will if you do."

"OK."

So we both went outside and started walking backward, not saying a word. After about a half-mile of uphill backward walking, we began wondering who would give in first.

Finally, we just broke out laughing and went home. Diana said she felt better, but maybe it was just her body becoming scared that I might come up with a more arduous cure.)

Here, then, are some of the questions I asked Isaiah. (They are in italics at the beginning of each exchange.) Remember, I translated Tuscarora to English as accurately as I could.

I sometimes feel guilty that I am not following my father's Medicine way the same way as he did.

(He smiled.) "That's what I liked about what you said about the Enneagram. You are not Eleazar. All of our thoughts and beliefs and behaviors cannot be the same. It's important that you never think you are behind or ahead of anyone else in wisdom. Thoughts and feelings are extremely powerful and have a large influence on Medicine and its variable ability to manifest."

(If I asked a frivolous question, his answer would be positive but somewhat trivial and cheerful, tinged with humor.) *Why do old men walk with their hands clasped behind their back?*

"So they'll be more streamlined . . . like the shape ski jumpers assume to get more distance . . . and if they were humpbacked, why, now, wouldn't that give them lift too? Like airplane wings do [laughter]."

If a person is stuck in the physical consciousness, how would you explain "Higher Consciousness" to them?

"Depending on their priorities, that can be very difficult and maybe impossible. I mean, to get them past a mere 'head tripping' of what I say. So, first, I would say a prayer or do a little ceremony in which I would speak to the mind and spirit of the purpose of the explanation—that this person's mind can be expanded; that a light bulb go on inside their head, and they hear, 'OO RE WHEE YOOT!' (That is true!) [Maybe the reader doesn't realize that the word *purpose* can have a mind and spirit of its own.] Then I would tell incidences of experiences of examples of Higher Consciousness.

"When you humble yourself, you begin to realize that all of our family members of the Thanksgiving Address are so very alive as Medicine because they have been spoken to and spoken about so many, many times. In humbleness, we become aware that these family members are many cuts above us, especially as a group . . . greater than the sum of their parts. How much more help could we ever need?"

So what does one do?

"More people need to start to realize that by being kind and, even more so, showing reverence to our Universal Family, that we have 'pull,' help beyond our expectations. When one knows that, one needn't "blank out" in anger or panic in catastrophic situations. It's like if you were drowning and someone throws you a lifeline, and you don't see it because you're too busy panicking."

What about praying to a Higher Power?

"We can call, for simplicity, that Higher Power 'the Spirits.' When you call in the Spirits, alone or with a group, as when you sing the Spirit Calling Song, the Spirits come in and look you over. Are you in earnest? Is someone in the group harboring negative vibrations? So sometimes you may witness a weak or 'no-show' result at any given ceremony. Maybe someone in the group would as-

sume some of that power, then let it go to their head and later abuse that privilege. Higher Consciousness cannot be fooled, even innocently."

What are the most important ingredients of a successful ceremony?

"A clear, uncluttered channel to the spirit world is desirable, and the supplication ought to be as precise and to the point as possible. What, exactly, is the
problem? If a person is involved, and especially if they are not present, their exact
name or names, even nicknames, will pinpoint the afflicted one, the exact geo-
graphical spot of the person or problem. Given the time, I might purify all the
way from just washing my hands to sweating to fasting. Of course, in an emergency, if you are a compassionate person, don't worry, you'll be instantly compe-
tent. If possible, I like to do any ceremonies alone because, for instance, in a
crowd there may be a person or persons present under the influence of drugs or
alcohol. Also, depending on time and circumstances, I will smudge myself, my
implements, and, if indoors, the area of the floor that I will be using. One more
thing, the problem presented is just that, not the desires or wishes of the people
involved. Sometimes the solution is not what is expected and is oftentimes better, especially in the long run."

Why is there always war?

(Here he hesitated, and was brief, as though he disliked talking about anything negative.) "Greed—the worst of human traits, a most powerful addiction,
near impossible to overcome. [And here he ended the discussion of war by saying
something I had never heard before, and I have used it since.] But, remember, it
is impossible to make a mistake. There are only sacred lessons."

What does it seem like to you to die?

"Oh, I expect that I'll be back. I'm sure I've experienced what I was born for,
so it's a 'what's-next-in-store-for-me' feeling. Maybe, having incubated in the
fetus position, I might go in that same position, like jumping into a crystal pool
'cannonball' style with a joyful 'HIIIIIIIII!' "

(I don't know the exact circumstances of his death, but it happened too soon
for me.)

◆　◆　◆

The yin-yang. How would you explain it?

"If I were an artist, I would paint a picture of Mother Teresa standing in a sneering James Cagney pose, spraying bullets of truth from a machine gun."

Do Medicines change in strength?

"It might seem that way, but, no, you are the agent [catalyst] that does it. If you are angry or frightened or even just tired, you might not even be able to think of a Medicine. However you are, at any given moment, affects any Medicine. If you can attain a high enough degree of gratefulness, you can change ordinary things into Medicine. Let's say that one day you are looking at your food before you eat it, and you realize how important that food is to you. A gratefulness can come to you whereby you will see the food glow and have an aura. That food has become Medicine. So don't let anger or hatred get the best of you; if you do, you will sooner or later become ill."

(This answer reminded me of an incident in which my children and I saw a very good thing. We were on a vacation ride in our Volkswagon minibus to any place, and we came to the St. Regis Mohawk Reservation, where a craft show was being held. A heavy wind and rainstorm had blasted the area the night before, and everyone was scrambling about to reerect the canvas walls of the various concessions that had been blown helter-skelter. Angry words could be heard. But into all of this danced a woman of Medicine. The canvas of her booth sagged and hung down and had formed a big trough of rainwater. That day she would be demonstrating Sweetgrass basket making. She let out a big shout of joy. "Whoopee! I wondered where I was going to soak my Sweetgrass!" and with that outburst she plunged the Sweetgrass into the trough of rainwater. Anger versus gratitude.)

How did you come to learn to become invisible? (Isaiah was a master at the art of shape-shifting. He learned to shape-shift with the Four Winds.)

"I was quite young and excited over having my parents and others shape-shift into dogs and birds, and I assumed anyone could shape-shift with the Four Winds, so I tried it, and sure enough it worked."

Can floods or earthquakes or tornadoes or volcano eruptions be stopped?

"Yes, but these things we call catastrophes are part of the restoring of balance to the earth or the Universe, to a situation that is out of balance. Often, this out of balance is caused by a mass misbehavior of people so that a stoppage could be only a temporary dressing that would be only a short-term security measure. One does not do a ceremony without being asked to do so, and if the asker does not know what is really happening, it might never be known that the complete restoring to health of a given situation can only come after balance is restored."

Even as nuclear energy is being used to produce electricity, does the threat of nuclear accidents worry you?

"When you realize that you can communicate with anything, then you won't be worrying about anything. Also, any toxic elements that have been buffeted about and carried by the wind long enough will become so diluted that each tiny particle of it can become a kind of Medicine . . . similar to, say, the planting of a seed, as takes place in the workings of a vaccination . . . one might breathe in this seed and plant it."

How can the Universe be balanced when we see far more people polluting rather than purifying the earth, for example?

"Balance is not necessarily measured in terms of material size or numbers. A thousand pennies seem much more than a gemstone in the rough. The healing prayers of an enlightened person may offset the out of balance of a couple thousand ordinary greedy people."

What causes the great power of some ceremonies?

"Many ceremonies are very, very old, and the songs in them sung millions of times. The love and joy of the singers and participants goes right back into the ceremony and makes it all the more happy and powerful." (The beauty of the simple pipe-filling song still brings tears to my eyes though I have heard it many many times.)

What about the Sweat Lodge, where many songs are also sung? Does it become a more holy place?

"Yes, and not only from the songs. The ceremonies also contribute toward creating a healing vortex at such places. That good-energy spot can remain for years, and you might sometimes wonder why a group of deer or grouse will continually congregate at certain places. It will be that they have felt the good energy of old abandoned ceremonial spots."

Da ya wan du(t) [Wally Greene] said that the four things we were given, as spoken in the Prelude—good thoughts, good feelings, good words, and good deeds—are in the correct order, with good thoughts more powerful than good deeds. Is this so?

"Yes, thoughts are very powerful. Unlimited. When people do good deeds, it's always for other people, not for the stars or water, for instance."

When I touched that silky Repentance Wampum, I got a minor shock, like of electricity; or did I?

"When He a wat tut [Hiawatha] cried and cried and cried over the loss of his family, it took him to the place of enlightenment. That first Wampum that he then made was so powerful a Medicine . . . so magical . . . that it spawned all the Wampum that went into all consequent strings and belts. The one you touched has been loved and stroked by so many people that it has become so powerful that it can change a person's life."

Will there ever be a lasting world peace?

"Maybe not while the Element called People continues to exist. We are not used to thinking in terms of billions of years when worlds can come and go. But maybe we won't have to think in such lengthy terms; the bad guys seem to automatically find a way to get rid of themselves."

Now I can look back and see that the death of Isaiah Joseph was very similar in abruptness to the death of other great Medicine people. At the time I heard the news of his death, though, it felt as if I woke up with a part of me missing.

Maybe it was because the last time I went to visit him, the house where he had been living was empty. It was a house his daughter was renting on a temporary basis. I didn't know. Now they were living in Hamilton, Ontario, and if I knew the roads well enough, maybe I could be there in thirty or forty minutes.

It was about one or one-thirty on a nice afternoon when I learned of this new address. As I drove toward Hamilton, I listened to the radio. News flash. A big accident had taken place on the Queen Elizabeth Highway. Traffic was backed up for miles. I turned right around and went elsewhere. I would see him later.

Well, maybe later as in "See you later, Hale-Bopp," but not later in Hamilton. When I called to see when would be an appropriate time to visit, I was told that he was dead and buried.

He had done his cannonball jump and was once more invisible.

Ethel Wahoo

Ethel Wahoo used to be Ethel Mt. Pleasant, one of Gee'by's bunch, and although she was reclusive, as they all were, once you broke through that clannish exterior, all you did was sit and listen. I bet she was a three in the Enneagram because she could really emote. You remember how them little threes in first and second grade (teacher's pet) could not stop monkey-shining for attention. Ethel would just talk right on over you (unless you, too, were a three) if you tried to say anything. To do so was to produce melo-drama.

Her older sister, Dorothy, was famous for having lived under two separate sets of high-tension electrical lines, even though I think the second set killed her. I don't think she knew that these lines were only good for flora, not fauna, and nobody dared tell her after the first set made her so grouchy.

Her brother, Bad News, was famous for calling his .30–06 with a telescope "Medicine" after he shot the motor block of some jitney driving through and making graffiti tracks in his cornfield.

Her mother, Mu'kret Gee'by, was famous for accidentally jabbing a balloon hanging from the ceiling with the upstroke of her freshly threaded beading needle and then asking to have someone call the ambulance "because she had been shot."

Ethel herself is famous for what I am writing about here. I almost threw this chapter out because she is (was, she's dead now) the only witness to what she told me. If you think she's lying, then just rip out whichever pages don't fit your equilibrium.

Ethel married a man named Walter Zomont. He was small and said he was an Indian (from out west?), though he could have passed for white because he talked loud. He was called Wahoo, hence the name Ethel Wahoo.

Every Wednesday Wahoo and the boys went to Wednesday night prayer meeting at some church in Niagara Falls. Ethel didn't go, and when I asked, "Why not?" she said, "Because I was bad."

One evening, when the stags of the family were at church, Ethel flopped down on her bed for a rest. She fell asleep. Just as night came, she woke up. Looking past the foot of her bed, she could see through her doorway, through a hallway, and all the way to the window on the far wall. Someone was standing in the hallway silhouetted against the early night sky. Ethel froze in fear.

Now if I hadn't experienced this "freezing in fear," I might have thought (when she told me), "Oh, Ethel, you big 'fraidy cat!" except I know what that's like. I think it can happen when one is not fully awake.

What happened to me was that one night I was awakened by a noise. As I opened my eyes, I thought I was seeing a man's head in my window. The noise I was hearing sounded as though the screen of the window was being torn. I froze. Some instinctive part of me did it. It wasn't through my brain because my brain was saying, "What's this? I can't move. I can't talk. I can't holler. I can't do anything but think."

This must be what makes animals "freeze." When they are perfectly still in their surroundings and blended in by the markings and colorings that nature has given them, they are very hard to see.

In my freeze I thought to pinch myself and see if I was awake. I couldn't because I couldn't move. Finally, I came to realize what I was looking at. My cat. It had crapped on my bed and was trying to cover it up. That's what caused the "ripping the screen" noise.

So here we have Ethel Wahoo frozen in her bed and a figure in her hallway. She wasn't as lucky as I was because this "man," as she called this figure, came to her and stood near her shoulder. At this point she could only feel this presence because that part of the room was in darkness.

Next came another thing that she couldn't see but could hear and feel, like the fluttering of a moth or mothlike object. She was powerless to stop it from entering her body either through her nose or her mouth, which may have been agape. Her remembrance became sketchy because here is about where she passed out, maybe from fright because that would follow, given her melodramatic bent.

Upon her awakening and as the next few days came and went, she became increasingly plagued by catastrophic expectation. "I know the evil now in me is going to lash out one day soon. I could kill, and maybe I'll just laugh afterwards."

She said nothing to her family because of shame and because of a hope, first, that it was a dream and, later, that it might go away by itself.

It didn't go away, and soon she began fearing for her sanity. She hatched a plan. She would come to the Wednesday night prayer meeting and have an exorcism.

A traditional Indian may simply have gone to the Longhouse and gotten a Purification Ceremony. Indeed, the house they lived in would likely have "Stopper Medicine" scattered all around the building, anyway, so that any negative thing that came to Wahoo and Ethel's house would not have gotten past the Medicine.

Ethel could also have gone to Sally Dubec or Daisy Thomas, but, like many Indians, she had been unsure of the meaning of the word *heathen*. Some Christians had put out the word that heathens were in cahoots with the devil, and Ethel couldn't take a chance, especially now that maybe the devil had slipped himself into her body. She was "quite sure" that the Longhouse people were heathens.

On Wednesday night she did not go with her family to the church. She went later, by herself. Snuck in.

There had never been an exorcism performed at this little church, and many in this church believed that only Catholics "did that stuff." Still, this little church did laying on of hands, and Ethel got there late enough for them to be doing just that when she came in through the side entrance.

The suddenly turned shy Ethel went to the minister's wife and explained her worries that she might be "devil possessed," that she wanted an exorcism.

The minister's wife set Ethel straight about using the word *exorcism*, but that she would see what she could do. All this time Ethel had become very sure she was on the right track because as soon as she had entered the church, some peculiar stirrings had manifested in her tummy.

The minister, upon hearing from his wife about Ethel, became excited. Here was a chance for his small congregation to make history. They would cast out a devil.

In telling me about this part, Ethel said she didn't know what Wahoo and the boys did or said or thought about her being "healed of the devil"; she simply "played the sick patient" like she did years ago as a little girl playing hospital.

For a long time nothing happened, though as many as could fit all around Ethel were touching her and praying aloud. Then a small girl touched her. "Yeow!" it was like an electric shock, and Mrs. Wahoo went nuts. She began babbling in some foreign, unrecognizable tongue.

Now the minister got the message that he was dealing with the real thing, that he was in over his head, and that he'd better get some help. He called a halt to "tonight's healing session" and began searching through his head to see if he knew any real ringers whom he might call in. The babbling stopped.

One week later the church was jam-packed. Without question the word had gone out. Other ministers and their uncles and cousins were there. Rubberneckers were there. Ethel Wahoo was there. She was ready to babble. "Hallelujah," thought the minister, looking around.

This whole night would be dedicated to just one thing . . . the casting out of the devil! No time was wasted. Ministers from Buffalo were there; some had crossed the Lewiston-Queenston Bridge from Toronto; some wore white robes. It was like, "HEY LEADER, STRIKE UP THE BAND!" Without drum roll, though, they started in on Mrs. Wahoo. They tried and they tried and they tried, but all they did was manage to get that thing inside of Ethel's belly to wiggle. It didn't matter. The "healers" were having a ball.

Quite unnoticed was the minister's wife. She was thinking. She was thinking because she felt that she had gotten Ethel into this situation, and maybe all of it would come to naught. Then she remembered something. The little girl of last week. No one had really seen the little girl at all the week before. Was she here now? Yes, there she was with her mother.

Like the week before, the girl snuck her little hand up and touched the "sick woman." BINGO!

Ethel Wahoo threw up. Once. Twice. Three times. On the third upchuck a high-pitched squeal came out of Ethel's mouth. It was the THING. It continued this high-pitched squeal. It could be heard but not seen. That is, it could be heard by some people although the high frequency of the sound was beyond hearing range of much of the older crowd. It was hardly noticeable to half of the praying Elders, but some that had stopped when Ethel vomited, plus Ethel herself, caught this shrill almost indescribable shriek.

I think that there's more than a sixth sense, even in the seemingly nerdiest of people, that can be awakened when evil is in the acute vicinity of that person or persons, especially when it shrieks. A chilling effect.

This shrieking devil-thing darted about, momentarily seeking an exit hole between the Elders. Then it shot out into and down the aisle of the church. The very mixed congregation was much more alert, having craned and maintained a more precise fixation on the proceedings than the group surrounding Mrs. Wahoo. Even though the shrill entity could not be seen, it was immediately tracked, radarlike, by the people nearest the aisle. The scene could be likened somewhat to the running of the bulls, where the crowd noise follows the bulls along the aislelike narrow streets.

The double entrance doors to the church were closed, and here the "squeal," seeking an exit, shot about in short thrusts, creating a crowd havoc that sent the entity screeching louder than ever on a complete circle of the church aisles.

Someone hollered, "OPEN THE DOOR!" (which someone did), and the screaming meanie of evil sailed out into the night never to be heard again.

Ethel Wahoo called this incident an exorcism as though that name bestowed a more sacred ceremonial meaning than any words the little church could have come up with. She attended some of the Wednesday night meetings after that, more to have some of the atmosphere of the healing night rub off on her and thus frighten and keep her expelled boogeyman at bay. Also, she was looked at as a bit of a celebrity.

A year went by. Nothing more had happened to Ethel to scare her. She had never before been as scared as she was the night of having the exorcised entity "freeze" her. When she first married, she had lived across the road from Gee'by's (her dad's) home, the old Lyman Johnson house. One night she heard the silver in the silver drawer rattling. She got out of bed to look, but no one was in the room. That scared her but not enough to freeze her. When it happened again, she went to my father. They agreed that this was likely the ghost of Lyman or his father, Levi. In order not to offend Lyman too much, the simple Oo(t) naa wog wo(t) noo ree(t) (Ghosts-it-herds) Medicine was used. Lyman let her sleep after that.

OK, as I was saying, about a year went by. It was nearing Christmas time, and Ethel Wahoo was in town, half Christmas shopping, half window shopping. She went into a five and dime store to snoop around.

About halfway through her snooping she looked up and saw the back of a woman in a long black coat who seemed to also be snooping. For whatever reason in the world Ethel felt "I know YOU"; we will never know for sure why. But Ethel also felt compelled to get this woman's attention and say "Hi" or maybe engage in a "Have a happy Christmas time" conversation with her.

She touched the woman's shoulder. "BOOM!" This "woman" shot her elbow into Ethel, knocking her backward into a stack of tinny pots and pans that flew every which way, causing a din and racket that attracted the attention of all the shoppers. In the immediate blur of the confusion this noise caused, the "woman," never looking back, dashed from the scene and disappeared out of the store and into the streets.

Ethel Wahoo came to the conclusion that the "devil-thing," the evil that had been exorcised from her own self, had found another victim, that this "thing" feared her (Ethel Wahoo), and that she had somehow acquired a "good-over-evil power," a secret saintliness. From then on Ethel would go back to that little church periodically and make contact—"touch base," so to speak, and "feed" the saint in her just in case saints needed to be fed. After all, her grandmother, though she was a heathen, said that great Medicines needed to be fed, that a feast was a sacred thing.

So, feeling rather holy, Mrs. Wahoo expected to go on living a long and fruitful life. She didn't. She joined her long dead grandmother not long after that.

Davey Roy

There was an Indian here at Tuscarora that no one ever said anything about. I mean, like who were his parents? His name was Davey Roy.

Roy? All us Tuscaroras were tagged with white people's last names somewhere "back when." You can go to the town of Oxford, England, and you won't be able to think of a Tuscarora last name that isn't in the phone book. Roy? Maybe, but nobody else on our reservation had that surname.

Davey Roy was dark skinned and had them eyes that seem half closed like some of them Indians from up around Georgian Bay, Canada. He seemed a bit girlish to me, especially the way he threw a baseball. He was kind of shy, and you had to listen close to catch all of his soft-spoken words.

He lived in a big farmhouse near Indian Hill with a family in which Lulu Gansworth was the matriarch. She was very kind and loving, and I liked her very much for being that way. Well, maybe also because she gave me a ride to school once in a while. She may have adopted Davey. I hope she didn't steal him. Maybe she found him in a basket in some reeds. A junior Moses.

Maybe Lulu's goodness was catching. Maybe that's why Davey Roy was nice. He was older than me, but I caught up to him and passed him when he died as a young man. Almost everybody liked him. I say "almost" because somebody killed him, and we never found out who.

This place, Lulu's, had cows, and bringing them in for milking was a chore that was split between Davey Roy and Heavy-dough.

On the last day that Davey Roy ever got the cows, Heavy-dough went to get them first because it was his turn.

As Heavy neared the pasture, he happened to look down the fencerow. About halfway down stood an old large tree, or what was left of it. They're quite majestic, you know, in death, a sort of statue to themselves or to their species, the oak. You've seen them. This one was different, though.

Heavy-dough could not believe his eyes. Up on one of the bare limbs stood an angel. Angel? Well, Lulu had stood for Christian goodness, and although many Indians went to church, it hadn't been said, even in ee'yog ("they say"— that is, gossip), that anyone at Tuscarora had ever seen an angel. Especially not standing fifty feet up on a limb of a dead tree.

It is not known what Heavy would have done if the angel had just stood there or if it had disappeared. But what do you think it did? It made a motion with one of its arms to Heavy-dough, "Come to me." So because the angel did not stand motionless or disappear, we do know what Heavy did do. He made tracks, and they were far apart, as in, "I'm out of here!"

Angel or not, the cows had to be milked, so Davey Roy went after them. The angel was still there. Not only that, it was still beckoning, "Come to me."

Davey Roy went to it, but maybe he shouldn't have. His body was found the next morning. It was on the side of the road, halfway up Indian Hill. He had been bludgeoned to death.

Just the other day I found a few old notes I had squirreled away years ago in a special place so I'd "know where they were."

The notes were a sort of "who's who" among people who had passed away before my time and who had therefore receded into history as just a name. One note had been from some of old Jonesy's ramblings before he died.

It had this bit of info:

Emily Goosey—Davey Roy's grandmother, archenemy of the witch Kree gi(t) uh.

The Devil

Among the Indians of both North and South America, even the most ardent follower of traditional spirituality can never be completely free of the influences of the federal Indian schools and missionaries of various church denominations. And probably even of Santa Claus.

You will note biblical references here and there in this book. At Onondaga a verbal exchange that I found clever, on the edge of high literature, took place between Chiefs (or Faithkeepers—at any rate, between "big wheels" of the Longhouse).

A Chief became very ill, nearly died. Upon his recovery he was visited by another Chief.

"Do you know why you couldn't die?"

"No. Why?"

"There was no room at the inn."

So let me tell you about something I first heard a long time ago, in the 1930s.

The story was about a group of gamblers, card players on the Six Nation Indian Reservation in Canada. My father told it to me first. He had lived on that reservation studying Medicine under the tutelage of a Cayuga man named Juh g'wa dee. This incident may have taken place long before that.

Then, in the 1970s I heard this same thing again, this time from the Tuscarora man (also of the Six Nation Rez) whom my children had named Automatic Transmission.

He said that the incident created a big stir at the time because two of the gamblers were "church Indians" who at first asked "witnesses" to deny that the incident had taken place. People couldn't keep their mouths shut, though. It was too sensational that Indians had actually seen "the devil." The one from the Bible. It created a scandal.

Before Automatic Transmission got to telling us about this thing that took place, I had already dismissed it as a lie. Nobody sees the devil. At least, as a young know-it-all that's what I used to say to myself. "Devils and angels are just symbols of 'what we should not' or 'what we should' pattern ourselves after." But then, I had to wonder, to rethink, when Heavy-dough and Davey Roy saw an angel.

What took place at the gamblers' table was that a stranger came late to the game and asked if he could join in and play, too. Indians are normally a bit shy and distrusting when it comes to strangers, but under the influence of a bit of alcohol it was "Why not?" After all, the newcomer had on some very natty clothing, so maybe he had a bunch of money to lose. They let him play.

The rest of the evening proceeded along the lines of any con game. That is, the patsies are led to believe that they have found a soft touch. Not only does this greenhorn to poker lose every hand, but he also starts pulling out gold pieces and losing them, too. By midnight everybody had won a considerable share of gold.

But . . . here comes the big swindle.

I'm not sure just how this Six Nation card shark did his thing, but I saw a neat trick on Johnny Carson's *Tonight Show* one night. I think the card shark that night on the show was John Scarne.

What John did was seat Johnny Carson, Ed McMahon, Doc Severnson, and himself around a table and break out a new deck of cards, still in a cellophane wrapper (so there are no trick cards). Then he shuffled them, and you know how some people can shuffle . . . zip, zip zip. When I try it, quite a few end up on the floor. After the good shuffle, the cards are dealt.

So now the TV camera goes around the table showing each player's hand. Doc Severnson, four jacks and a ten. Ed McMahon, four queens and a ten. Johnny Carson, four kings and a ten. The dealer, four aces and a ten. Now, would this provoke some wicked betting or would this provoke some wicked betting?!

On that devilish night up in Canada, we don't know exactly how the "final" hand went, but it had to be something similar.

The newcomer said something like, "Whoa! It's midnight! Where did the time go? You guys have taken me to the cleaners! I gotta go. But whattya say? One more hand, no limit?"

The stranger won it all.

But how could he? He didn't know boo about betting. Just who did he think he was anyway?

The only player that didn't want to allow the stranger into the game at all was sitting next to him, scrutinizing his silken attire. What kind of shoes would he be wearing?

Heavens! There WERE no shoes! Not even any feet! Instead, the stranger had goat's feet!

The "discoverer" leaped to his feet, pointing downward. "THIS GUY'S GOT GOAT FEET! A WITCH! . . . NO! IT'S THE DEVIL!"

Zoom! The devil was on his feet . . . er, hoofs . . . and on out the door, leaving all that gold still on the table.

Did the devil get here in some shiny big limousine? The card players rushed out to see. There was nothing. A clean getaway.

Intrigued, I began asking a number of older Indians about this happening. They all knew about it. "Oh yeah, it was big news back then."

I didn't care how many times I might be told about this rare thing, the devil hanging out with Indians. So I would say, "Tell me about it." Maybe I would hear different versions. It wasn't an easy thing to believe, especially the ending.

All versions were the same.

Seeing that the devil was gone, the poker players rejoiced that the winning pile of money was still on the table. So back into the building they went to divvy up the "spoils."

What did they find on the table where the money was supposed to be? Nothing but a pile of horse shit.

Maybe the poker games were getting out of hand. Maybe the devil came to teach them a lesson. If so, isn't that quite a bit like the half-a-woman, the Ooh du(t) cheah, stopping the womanizer from depriving his family? Or what about the ice-skating-whiz entity, the Ha'jeejee, putting a stop to the going-too-far-too-late-at-night skating parties? I say this because the poker games came to a stop.

Reservation Witches

Peter Joseph, a Tuscarora at Six Nations, Canada, was walking past the local store when one of a group of men hanging around outside said, "Look! There goes a witch!"

"Why'd you say that?" Pete asked, "I'm not a witch."

One of the other men answered, "Did you ever see a Tuscarora that wasn't?"

That incidental verbal exchange, serious or not, is an excellent example of the state of affairs concerning the status of witchcraft within the Iroquois Confederacy. Most Indians use the term *witch* rather loosely; after all, it is a white man's word, not an Indian word. In the Tuscarora language the closest thing is a term used to refer to a person thought to be practicing witchcraft or a poisonous pursuit. If the person is male, we say, "ra de si yit naa ree." That translates out to, "He-poison-knows." If the referral is feminine, the first syllable *ra* is changed to *yaa* (*a* as in "as").

Maybe because the image or portrayal of a witch in children's fairytale books is that of a woman, a hag with warts on her nose, nearly all alleged witches on an Indian reservation have been women. My father was called an Indian doctor, but if he had been a woman, he may have been called a witch. Just the same, certain people were considered bona fide witches, and maybe half of the Indian population could never be convinced otherwise.

The standard "witch image" also has the hag standing over a bubbling pot of bat wings, horny toads, and so on, chanting a "bubble-trouble" chant while stirring away. Most Indians would say, "Oh, that's just the fairytale image. A real witch wouldn't be advertising like that."

Mocks Johnson had an experience, however, that was somewhat similar.

He was hunting and therefore moving along quietly. Presently he heard a swarm of bees buzzing. He stopped and listened carefully; maybe he could capture the swarm and take it home. Maybe he had found a bee tree. Yes, that might be because the sound came from a stationary place.

Now Mocks almost made a boo-boo. He pushed his way through some brush toward the sound. Just before he broke out into a clearing, he stopped. The sound wasn't quite right. Puzzled, he listened more carefully. If not bees, what could it be then?

Picking his way carefully forward, he came to a scene that made him back off. Four women were singing. They were singing to snakes. The snakes were hanging by their tails, and they didn't have any heads. The dripping blood was being caught in pots and pans.

Mocks then became a person who believed that there are bona fide witches among the Indians.

One time, Harriet Pembleton, who lived in the middle of the Tuscarora Indian Reservation, had a problem. She had a good-size tomato patch, and someone was stealing the ripening tomatoes.

The way some people might solve this would be to empty a shotgun shell of its BBs and refill the shell with rock salt. When the culprit bent over to pick whatever they were stealing, BANG! into the seat of the problem.

Harriet, though, was old and thin, and a .12-gauge shotgun might propel her backward and cripple her up long enough so that she couldn't can the tomatoes until they were rotten. So she did different. She hired a witch. She hired Helen Beaver.

Helen had a specialty. She could produce snakes. Blacksnakes. Big, long, and in great numbers.

Now let's say that you are not afraid of snakes. So you say. Then one night when you are stealing tomatoes, you feel something crawling up your pant legs. You turn the flashlight on. You find yourself surrounded by thirty or forty 8-foot blacksnakes coming toward you. Are you going to steal any more tomatoes?

After hiring Helen Beaver, Harriet had so many tomatoes that she ran out of canning jars and had to give tomatoes away.

So what else did Helen do snakewise?

Sometimes Indians of any of the Six Nations would have direct relatives on the opposite side of the international line between the United States and

Canada. Some had dual citizenship, some didn't. Property disputes occasionally came up. Helen Beaver solved one of them.

Sometime before the tomato incident, an Indian man and wife announced that they were moving from Tuscarora to Canada, to the Six Nation Reservation, because someone had died and willed a house to the wife.

Not long afterward, that couple came back to Tuscarora. Someone else, a relative too, had already taken over the house in Canada and had threatened to use a gun on the rightful owners. The "takeover" people had a long reputation of getting liquored up on weekends and exhibiting rowdy behavior, so it seemed likely that they could easily shoot to kill.

Enter Helen Beaver. It is not known how the ousted owners came to hire Helen. Possibly Helen heard about their plight. Wouldn't it be tricky if we found out that Helen had business cards that read, "HAVE SNAKES, WILL TRAVEL"?

At any rate, the disputed house was soon vacated and ready for new occupancy. The real owners of the house returned and never came back to Tuscarora. This might be how Harriet got the idea of hiring Helen because she learned, when she went to Canada, about how blacksnakes ran the rowdy people off. A huge snake was wound around the mailbox and around the post that held the mailbox, and a four-foot length of its tail trailed off on the ground. That was before Helen called her guards off and let the new people in.

Jonesy was about forty or more years older than me. He said to me (speaking of witches), "Hell, you people today never saw some of the wickedest ones."

He said that when he was a boy, one of the scariest things in the house was a contraption called a witch alarm. He was told never to touch it. Off of one side of a deer's antlers hung a silver spoon and a bag of Medicine. Just the looks of the thing had little Jonesy on edge. Then one night it went off.

"Jingling Jesus!" his father proclaimed, "Get the shotgun, Kree gi(t) uh is coming!"

The alarm was pretty trustworthy; nothing happened for a half-hour. Little Jonesy had been instructed to jerk the door open as soon as any knock sounded. His father stood at ready with the sawed-off double-barreled shotgun cradled off of his hip. The boy was shivering and his teeth chattering, even though the potbellied stove was glowing. The kerosene lamp had been blown out. There was a thin cover of snow on the ground outside.

Kree gi(t) uh was small but feared. She could make history out of people. She could do you in and get away with it because she was one of them be-in-two-places-at-once people. She would make sure that one of her would be seen at a public function miles from the scene of her mischievous other self. She was like a little Indian Mafia for hire. Jonesy's father must have been up to some no good thing himself, else why would he be expecting a retaliation of this magnitude?

There was a slight noise on the step. Here she was! Little Jonesy jerked the door open and jumped back at the first rap on the door.

With the background of white snow, any silhouette of anything would appear in the doorway. Kree gi(t) uh was small, but at first there seemed to be nothing. But there she was, on the doorstep. A black cat.

BLAM! BLAM! The shotgun spoke, and the door was slammed shut.

In the morning all they found was a set of women's size shoe prints in the snow. Running steps. Then after eighteen or twenty feet, nothing.

Jonesy, an old man now, always tried to be the tough guy as he told this story, but the tic near his eye sped up before he was done telling.

As generations came and went, the idea of hiring a witch faded out. Witches died without passing on the secrets of their trade. Science and modern living pooh-poohs the existence of witches as it does the existence of magic, hexes, and so on. Every once in a while, though, another unexplainable thing will happen.

Corbett Sundown and Beeman Logan were Chiefs on the Tonawanda Seneca Indian Reservation. Beeman's wife, Arlene, was good-looking, and Corbett was attracted to her, but what could he do about that? He was looked up to as one of the take-no-guff-from-the-government leaders, so he could not misbehave.

One Friday, at Beeman's house, the two Chiefs were discussing plans to go to the Onondaga Longhouse when Arlene came rushing into the house in a dither. The two Chiefs had been summoned to Grand Council, and there could scarcely be a situation that could stop them.

"A witch is after me!" Arlene announced, and she went on to describe how an unseen hand suddenly grasped and turned the steering wheel of her car as she drove along, heading the car toward a large tree. Her side-view mirror had been wiped off in the narrow escape. Arlene had turned right around and come directly home, too shaky to continue on.

Corbett immediately saw this as an opportunity to make points with Arlene, so he said, "Let's find out who this person is that's out to kill you. I'll make this Medicine, and you take it. Beeman and I have to go to Onondaga, but you'll be safe. Tomorrow morning this person will come here and knock on the door. They won't do anything to hurt you, especially not in front of your family; they just want to see if you're dead or not. They will probably be the first person to come to see you tomorrow, but the clue that gives them away is, they will demand something. They will say, 'I NEED such and such.' "

Corbett went on to say that when they returned from council, he would "take care of" this killer. He would "fix their clock."

So the Chiefs left, and Arlene waited anxiously for her killer to show. The killer did, and in exactly the way Corbett predicted.

The first thing in the morning there came this loud rapping on the door followed by a feminine voice demanding a cigarette. "I need a cigarette! Gimme a cigarette. I'm having a fit."

Arlene opened the door and saw her would-be killer. In a second all her fears were gone. In fact, she nearly laughed. As she went to get a cigarette, she told her guest, matter-of-factly, about her close call, then about what Corbett had said about his Medicine, how it would work, and about his threat to fix the witch's clock.

She would not be disclosing to Corbett the name of this witch. He would not be making any points after all. You see, the witch turned out to be Corbett's sister.

Meanwhile, in the Lower Cayuga section of Six Nations in Canada, another witch was at work. Chief Pat Sandy was wondering, with a certain late-night knock on the door, who could be calling instead of sleeping. When he opened the door, a smallish woman, a neighbor that he at first failed to recognize, appeared. She had drawn her shawl about her face so that, in fact, she would not be recognized. Once in the house, however, she doffed the shawl and disclosed the reason for her anonymity, her lateness, and her presence there. She was in pain.

It never crossed her mind that this sore on her back had anything to do with a witch. Proper womenfolks her age just didn't visit a bachelor without stirring up a buzz of gossip; it was just that the sore was so uncommonly painful and that no remedy produced any forthcoming relief. Maybe she hadn't attended to it soon enough, but there it was in a place she couldn't reach to get at. Also, she had put off baring her body to anyone as long as she could. Now, though, it had become too painful to perform all her daily chores.

An ordinary sore? The Chief thought otherwise. "Someone has put an object of witchcraft on this woman," Chief Sandy said to himself.

The examination was inconclusive, but the woman had come to the right place. A sacred Medicine was compressed atop the sore spot and the lady told to return on the following night.

Yes, the Chief was certain of witchcraft when she returned. Whereas on the night before, the skin had been unbroken, now a hole appeared. He removed a thorn more than an inch long.

During the previous twenty-four hours Chief Pat Sandy had been busy following his intuitions. He had brewed up a special Medicine. Now he rolled the thorn up in a strip of cloth. He then pushed this roll into a shotgun shell whose BBs had been removed. Before it went into the shell, it took a bath in the special Medicine. The point of the thorn pointed outward.

"Here," the Chief said. "Tomorrow morning, at dawn, place this shell in your gun and shoot it at a forty-five-degree angle into the east. You won't be bothered after that."

Two days went by. In the darkness of the second night there was a knock on Chief Pat Sandy's door. He knew it was the witch. And it was.

They didn't have to say anything. He nodded to her. She nodded back. Then he took the thorn out of her back.

I'm sure you've had the experience, from out of the blue, of wondering about or thinking of a remote thing or person, and a day or so later, as though these musings were dreams come true, the thing you thought about appears.

One day I was thinking about the Cattaragus Indian Reservation: How witchy was it there? Well, I wouldn't be driving up there very soon from this hidden-in-the-mountains-for-ceremonial-purposes-place in North Carolina. But maybe someday. Anyway, with the price of gasoline so prohibitive, I'd be lucky to honor my commitment to do an Elders gathering in Ohio on the very weekend of the moment.

When I got to Ohio, I ran smack into Fred Kennedy. In my mind I said, "Well, how DO you do!!! Here's Mr. Cattaragus himself." Because of my short-term memory, I had to stop him from telling too many witch stories so that I might be able to remember a couple of them and pass them on to you.

One was about a witch that the Indians called "Little Miss Lantern." Her other name was Little Rachael. It might be significant that quite a few witches were indeed little. In all of life we often see small people exhibiting a very feisty disposition from having to fight back, from having been bullied by bigger people. The much-feared Kree gi(t) uh (*uh* means "little") of Jonesy's experience was barely more than five feet tall. She came from Six Nations, Canada, and some say she crossed the border flying as a Night Heron so she didn't have to pay the toll. Anyway, back to Little Rachael.

Little Rachael was suspected of killing people. Her hatred of being so small had gotten out of hand because she couldn't stop herself. The name Little Miss Lantern came from the fact that at night she glowed with a bluish light so that she never tripped in the dark. For her, there was no dark. The reason I say that she couldn't stop herself is that she went on killing after she had been accosted and warned.

Too many people came up missing. Rachael had the habit of breathing on her windows and steaming them up so people couldn't see what went on inside her house. Nevertheless, with so many cases of missing people, two and two could be put together, and the sum pointed to Little Miss Lantern.

By now, of course, everyone was afraid of her, and no single person dared do anything about the killing. A posse of people was consequently formed. One night Rachael came glowing down the road and walked right into their ambush. They yelled at her. They threatened her. But of course the witch played the part of the great innocent one: "Who, ME? Why I NEV-er!" and so on, and so forth.

Did this stop the witch? Yes, for a while. But then her kill-oriented addiction overtook her. She steamed up her windows and killed again. One of the trade-marks of the Lantern's kills was that the victim's body was never found. ZIP, gone. When she took her next victim, however, she miscalculated the amount of rage that her act would provoke. She killed a baby.

This time the posse would not threaten; it would avenge. It did. Little Miss Lantern was shot. It is not known if any bullets or any of the shots used contained any silver, but at any rate the witch was never seen at Cattaragus again. She did bleed. The blood trail was followed, but just like the case of a big wounded buck that can heal, the trail became fainter and fainter until it disappeared altogether. But just like all those victims had disappeared, so did the witch. Forever. That's why Fred and I dare to tell on her.

Now, before we all get any witchier, I'm going to tell you about a borderline activity among Indians that Fred reminded me of. Shape-shifting. Before Henry Ford and even later, among Indians who couldn't even afford a horse to ride, it was fashionable to shape-shift into a dog or crow so that one could travel to a destination instead of walking as a person, then, just before arriving, to become a person again.

Every now and then, though, some people would be caught cruising about as, for instance, a pig. One man, a Tuscarora named Li fee'yette, took the shortcut from Blacknose Spring Road to Tom Reed's Trailer Court. On the way he saw a wild turkey roosting on a rail fence. This was early morning, not fully light yet. He snuck up on the turkey and swung at its neck with his cane. There were no wild turkeys yet living as far north as Tuscarora, so this would be a prize, a first. "Don't hit me!" the turkey yelled. It yelled because it was a man, a Tuscarora, shape-shifting.

So it may be that shape-shifters were not necessarily witches, but most of them got tagged as such. Fred tells of such an incident that took place in Mohawk territory near Hogansburg, New York, on Cook Road.

Clyde Cole as a boy was sent to the store for some bread. Now you know that at night, if there are no clouds, the sky is light enough to serve as background for silhouettes to appear.

Clyde had had to do this before, so a nighttime errand was not such a big deal. This time, however, Clyde heard a scuffing sound coming in the dark, and it was quite close to him. Now Clyde did get scared. He bent down and felt around on the ground for a stone or stick to protect himself with. What his hand found was a brick-sized stone.

Darned if this thing, which was now directly opposite him on Plank Road, didn't grunt like a pig. Kneeling low, Clyde saw in the sky, indeed, the outline of a big pig.

Clyde slammed the rock into the middle of the piggy-looking thing.

"Aw 'gay!" it said (which I think is "ouch" in Mohawk).

Clyde ran home without the bread. But he didn't jump in bed and cover up his head. Instead, he told his mother what had happened.

"You stay here," his mother directed, "Don't go outside."

She went outside and over to the neighbors' house. There, she found the matriarch of the house lying down with three broken ribs. Maybe Clyde's mother was a discreet person and simply initiated some nice pie-in-the-sky crabgrass talk.

Back to Cattaragus.

Lilah Jimerson was a looker, a woman who bugged men's eyes out. But she was also a witch.

If you have ever wondered if witches can fall in love, they can. Lilah was in love with some man. I don't know but what this man may have been an unsuspecting white man, but he endeared himself by being a good painter—the Rembrandt type, not a house painter. The fly in the ointment, in this case, was that the painter man was already married.

"Not to worry," was the witch's outlook; after all, a little love Medicine would suck the man right out of his wife's arms. Lilah, though, had bigger and, in her mind, better plans. She would eliminate the negative. She would make her lover a legal, single man.

Somewhere in the picture of the painter, his wife, and their house lived a girl who could not speak. She was "dumb," as in the unfortunate who end up in institutions because, if their family is rich, they are sometimes secreted to a "better-off" place to be spoken of as little as possible. As if they were of no use, except to besmirch the family name. The witch, though, saw the dumb girl as indispensable.

So what did pretty Lilah do? She witched the child. She put it in the girl's head to kill the painter's wife. The dumb girl waited at the bottom of the stairs with a hammer in her hand, and when the wife came down, she was "Lizzy Bordened," whacked to death.

Now for the part where the witch and the painter lived happily ever after. Not so. I'm not sure exactly what happened next as I wasn't listening to Fred carefully enough. But it doesn't matter how this next short-lived "justice triumphs" part happened. Maybe the painter loved his wife, and when his witch lover told him how she had set him free, he panicked and testified against her. At any rate the witch went to jail.

If the painter did, in fact, squeal on the witch, and if he didn't want to follow his wife to never-never land, then it was clear that he had better pack up his oils and brushes and light out for Kokomo because jails don't hold witches very well.

Of all the trickier tricks I have ever heard of a witch pulling, Lilah Jimerson pulled the best one. She made herself pregnant, then charmed the judge into letting her go bye-bye. It just wouldn't be ethically kosher, now would it, to have the whole town speculating on which elected official was "the father."

Had she simply shape-shifted into a mouse or hummingbird and flown the coop, she would be absent without leave and have to be on the lam for who knows how long.

Bally Huff says he once heard her say, "I may be good-looking, but I ain't dumb."

When I asked Isaiah Joseph what he thought about his brother being called a witch (remember the comment, "Ever see a Tuscarora that wasn't?"), he smiled.

"The Tuscaroras never got the message," he said, "In the sixteen hundreds, when the Five Nations held Grand Council and reported that certain of their great seers had 'seen' the burning of witches at Salem and that their Medicine people were to go 'underground,' the Tuscaroras were still in North Carolina. Down there, they even held yearly exhibitions or contests of power. So when they came up here, they were all pretty loose, not realizing that shape-shifting and Medicine tricks could get them in trouble. Especially with church." He then told me about Black Betchry, a Tuscarora witch who lived near the Grande River, not far from Bob Mt. Pleasant's place.

Black Betchry had most everyone's total respect. She had a seemingly endless repertoire of feats of power, but as long as she was left alone, so did she keep her tricks to herself.

One day a nine-year-old girl threw a stone at Black Betchry. What the witch did was sic a large bee after the girl. How big? Three inches long. The girl went running and screaming all the way home. By the time she got there, she was in hysterics. The girl's mother tried to calm her so that the girl's blubberings could be understood. Why it was so hard to find out what was wrong was that the bee was invisible to all but the girl. The girl kept on screaming and swatting at "nothing."

What a night that household spent. Who could have slept a wink? The next morning mother and daughter high-tailed it off to the school clinic. How embarrassing to parade a daughter who was clearly "out of her tree" into the hub of the day. To sit there among the other Indian mothers and their children with this big nine-year-old screaming about an invisible bee and flailing away at it while waiting for the white doctor to arrive.

It was only a few minutes, but it seemed like forever before the clinic opened. Through the open door the Indian mothers listened carefully for the verdict. It didn't have to be said. The girl was pronounced crazy. What the doctor said was, "I'm very very sorry, but I can do nothing. I'm afraid you'll just have to have her put away."

The hearts of the Indian mothers were very sad, and one of them was driven to do some shrewd thinking. When the mother and raving daughter walked past on the way to the door, the thinker said, "If I were you, I'd take your daughter and a ten-dollar bill and go and see Black Betchry. She might be able to help."

Of course, the girl was cured. Cured not only of the bee attack, but also of throwing stones.

The next thing that happened was that two small girls badmouthed the witch. What would be the penalty this time? Silence. The girls were struck mute. One thing different, though, from the screaming "bee girl" case was that the family of the mute girls slept the night through.

The next day was like in the other case, though. The mother and her daughters sat with other mothers and children waiting to see the white doctor at the school clinic, but it was a much calmer scene. Just the same, the other waiting mothers were in great sympathy for the two silent children and their mother. When the three went in to see the doctor, it was but a few moments before the waiting women put their hands over their mouths to keep from laughing too loudly.

You see, a certain item of interesting news must have gotten back to the clinic because through the open door the white doctor was heard to say, "Why don't you take ten dollars and go and see Black Betchry?"

When the mother and the two cured children got back home and the father heard the tinkling voices of his two little daughters again, he broke out into a huge grin. After he heard the whole story, his big smile took on a naughty little twist. Then he winked at his wife and said, "Maybe the doc and the witch are in cahoots."

Another Spooky Place

We used to refer to the Allegheny Seneca Indian Reservation as Redhouse. I took my mother, Amelia, down there to visit another Amelia, Amelia Henry, who had moved to Redhouse from Tuscarora after her husband, Eli Henry, died.

. I'm not really sure that we could remember just how to get to Mrs. Henry's house; we planned to take Lillian Fish with us as a guide.

As I drove from Rochester, New York, to Tuscarora, a sparrow flew directly into the windshield of my car, as though it came to meet me with some news. So directly was it flying into my face that I unconsciously ducked as it killed itself on the glass. The "news" was that Lillian Fish had died during the previous night. So it was bad news that we took to Redhouse.

Here, at Redhouse, is where I met Amelia Henry's brother. Amelia's maiden name must have been Pierce because her brother's name was Holly Pierce.

Holly and I began swapping stories, and I happened to tell him about the place we call the Commons, the woods adjacent to Blacknose Spring Road that played tricks on people. Holly then told me about a road that he was scared to walk on or even to drive on, especially at night.

What happened on that road was that three Seneca men, speeding recklessly in the wee hours on their way home from a drinking bout, smashed their vehicle into a tree and were killed. This occurrence alone might make Holly detour that spot at night, but an incident took place later that, for sure, kept him off that road.

One night after that fateful accident, another carload of drunks came motoring along the same road on their way home. At the very spot of the accident one of the rear tires blew out.

The driver, none too steady on his feet, assessed the situation. Try as he may, he could not even come close to getting a rise out of the passed-out passengers in the car. Perplexed, he nonetheless set about replacing the flat with a spare. The footing for the jack was poor, and just as he got the flat tire off, the jack slipped and "clickety thump," down came the whole works. Still, even then, the drunken passengers did not stir. Now there was no way the driver could get the jack back under the collapsed vehicle.

Finally, just as the driver had given up all hope of rectifying the situation and was about to walk off in despair, lo and behold, help arrived. Three men approached, and one of them said, "Need some help?"

The driver acknowledged that, indeed, he needed help, but that the situation seemed hopeless.

"Grab the spare," the spokesman of the trio said, "We'll lift the car up, and you slip the spare on."

Sure enough the three men grabbed the bumper and raised the car high enough to get the spare on and loosely bolted.

There was only a sliver of a moon and some stars to cast any light, but the driver, try as he might, could not see any feet or even dark shapes of any feet on the three lifters. Though this gave him an eerie feeling, he was able to rationalize that it was, indeed, the middle of the night. Still, he fumbled a bit getting the needed nuts on. At the "OK" word, the car lifters let the car back down.

"How can I ever thank you?" the driver asked.

"You got anything to drink?" came the reply.

"Well, I think there might be a few swigs left in the jug. Let's take a look."

The driver opened the car door to grab the jug and check it out. The dome light came on, and, yes, there was the jug with some booze left over.

As the driver handed over the jug, he saw in the light the faces of the three Samaritans for the first time. He froze in terror. They were, all three faces, skeleton skulls. One of them was smashed in or grated off.

All the poor driver could do was watch, transfixed, unable to move a hair, as the ghosts of the three dead men of the earlier accident emptied the jug and drifted off.

Nobody knows how long it was before the driver "recovered" and spun the wheels out of there, never to pass that way again.

Holly Pierce never ever did trespass on that road, and he never ever will, because Holly, like the three skeletons, is dead now, too.

I'sic oi(t), Asa, and Dug dih HANa'ree

The word *oi(t)* (Tuscarora) means "big," and I'sic oi(t) WAS big. He loved to eat, and when he began thinking of himself as having reaching "freak" proportions, he vowed to cut back on pigging out. No dice. He gave up. He let himself catch himself cheating on himself. That is, until he fell in love. This can cause willy-nillyness.

To this day, no one has ever found out who this woman was that I'sic oi(t) became gaga over. Even on his own deathbed, he would not reveal this woman's name. He did, however, spill the beans on himself, hoping that a confession would save him from hell. If he hadn't, we would only have known what Dug dih HANa'ree knew.

Dug dih HANa'ree lived with his brother, Asa, down the hill just west of where Deadman's Road meets Chew Road. Asa was just a kind, quiet homebody of a man, probably a nine in the Enneagram because he abhorred the rippling of any human waters. His brother, though, who didn't care who punched who, was also a very good Indian doctor and quite often away from home.

There is an herb that is locally called "Heal-all" (there must be ten plants with that name), whose botanical name is *Prunella vulgaris*. So well did this herb work for Dug dih HANa'ree that he put it in with every other concoction for any illness. So successful was he that all the other Indian herbalists began calling *Prunella vulgaris* by the name "Dug dih HANa'ree g'yeh ho(t)," meaning "Dug dih HANa'ree's species," somewhat like the practice of naming a plant after its discoverer. (Except Indians would only do this to be funny. Attaching one's name to anything in the naming of it would be to exercise the universal law that says that this practice automatically dilutes the Medicine, akin to a person calling themselves a Medicine man or Medicine woman.)

One day Asa, being nice to everybody, inadvertently spoke to I'sic oi(t)'s secret love. Big I'sic went into a secret rage. Asa had committed the biggest no-no of his life—of his shortened life—because love has no bounds. I'sic oi(t) killed him.

This act took place at what I'sic oi(t) considered the most opportune time—when Asa was home alone, his brother off on another trip to who knows where.

What I'sic oi(t) did was concoct a great "can't refuse" offer to cut wood on shares. Normally, this is a fifty/fifty deal in which a good woodsman offers to cut and haul your firewood to you if you let him have half of it. Old folks who owned timber were only too glad to let this happen.

What I'sic proposed was a seventy-five/twenty-five deal: Asa to get seventy-five percent because he would be helping "down the trees" and because he was told, "I'm fat and warm-blooded and don't need as much wood as you do." Of course, it was not mentioned that Asa would not be needing ANY wood.

The cutting of wood did not last long. Two trees. Just enough to supply the right amount of trimmed-off limbs and branches to cover Asa's body once his head had been chopped off.

Now I'm sure that you have known that everyone's family tree bears some nuts. Asa and Dug dih HANa'ree and his girlfriend, Heeengs, were not the nutti-est family tree members that I had, but Williams was their last name. Asa, Dan (Dug dih HANa'ree), and Cathrine Williams. Cathrine—or Heeengs, as most people knew her—was considered a strong witch, with Dan not far behind.

Ee'yog, gossip, said, "Guy yaa dee'sy'yit naa ree" (They know poison).

Dug dih HANa'ree, as soon as he got home and being who he was, picked up immediately that something was drastically wrong, not just ordinary wrong. He made the Jeh nih, ah gut guh too (t) Medicine and spoke to it, asking, "Where in tarnation is Asa?"

To use this Medicine, one talks to it constantly (like a pep talk) and, when it is ready, pours it into a wooden bowl, then covers one's head with a shawl or some sacred thing like a deer or bear or buffalo hide, something like those old photographers used to have to do. But instead of looking out through the camera, one looks down into the bowl.

Dan Williams saw Asa Williams, with no head on, under a brush pile. He re-trieved the body, arranged the funeral, and had Asa properly buried.

I'sic oi(t), meanwhile, was brought to some of his senses with the speed with which his wicked deed had been discovered. Knowing Dug dih HANa'ree's repu-tation, he panicked and fled to Swaa gi(t) (the Six Nations Reservation in Canada) to escape extradition.

Dug dih HANa'ree, of course, using Medicine (probably the same way he discovered the exact location of Asa's body) knew who the killer was. There was no hurry, no thought of revenge. The balancing laws of the Universe would take care of that. There would be no escape.

Nevertheless, as the tidbits of the situation leaked out into the Tuscarora grapevine, ee'yog, many even pitied I'sic oi(t) knowing that Dug dih HANa'ree could "zap" him anytime he wanted to and was free to dream up atrocious "pay-backs," which he did.

I'sic oi(t) went crazy. He didn't live long after that. In his craziness he craved and demanded food! food! food! It had always been his drug, but now it became a permanent anodyne, and it killed him.

When he died, he garnered a pedestal in the history of all Indian-dom. He had eaten so much that he had become a hippopotamus clone. He is the only In-dian ever to be buried in a piano box.

How We Have Lived, Small Incidences

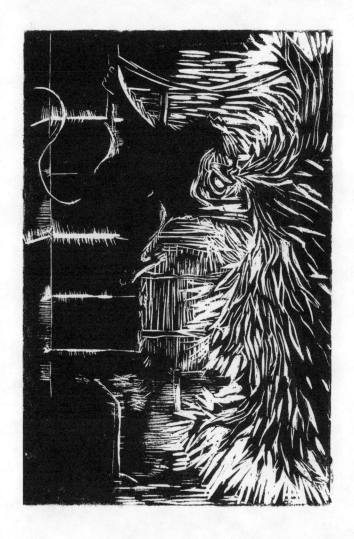

Overleaf: The Fire Monkey; see "The Fire Monkey," pp. 152–54.
Woodcut by Rhiannon Miles Osborne.

Relativity

A good example of the treatment of "things" as though everything is alive and could talk to us came up one day when I was visiting Isaiah Joseph. Actually, he stole the direction of the conversation, and now I think he put a clearer angle to it.

I wanted to see what he would have to say about relativity, and I was thinking in terms of movement, different rates or speeds of movement, and no movement.

Isaiah said, "Yeah . . . all things are relative . . . time, for instance. What about insects? The ones that might only have a life span of two days. One lady insect might be talking over the back fence to her neighbor, 'Look at my daughter . . . buzzing about already . . . how time flies! . . . she's twenty seconds old already!'

"Then at the same time some mountain might be saying to another mountain, 'My son wants to get married!'

"And the other mountain says, 'OH NO! He's nowhere near ready! He's only two thousand years old!' "

Ee'see

Ee'see Mt. Pleasant liked corn. So although he was an ironworker, each spring after work he would find time to work up a plot of land and plant some corn. This he did back of his house, quite a ways — that is, quite a ways from Dog Street.

One springtime he had no more than gotten this plot ready for planting when someone, young people with a jalopy probably, spun some figure-eights in the dirt.

Ee'see told his corn seeds not to worry about such shenanigans, that he would think about a cure. He said this because he went right on ahead and planted the field full of corn. The access to this cornfield was old Saphronie's Lane.

When the corn got to be about six inches tall, Ee'see heard the sound of a vehicle on Saphronie's Lane. It sounded like maybe a motor with quite a bit of horsepower; and maybe it had a four-barrel carburetor, too.

Ee'see grabbed his "thought-up" Medicine and ran to the cornfield. His Medicine was a high-powered rifle with an eight-powered telescope on it, plus some armor-piercing bullets.

At the cornfield Ee'see could see through the 'scope, with the aid of a small moon and some starlight, a vehicle, a jalopy, starting into the cornfield.

Two explosions and some fire belched forth from the high-powered rifle. Then silence. He had killed the intruder, the jalopy. In the morning the abandoned old Oldsmobile showed two bullet holes through its engine block.

The driver, or drivers, of this vehicle never were identified by Ee'see, who, by the way, was not called Ee'see anymore. It is truly amazing how quickly everyone gets to know all about "tricky events" that never make the newspapers. Ee'see became "BADnews."

BADnews left the dead car in the cornfield as a "scarecrow" to warn other would-be "ram-around" jalopies. It didn't matter who the driver of the dead car was because "the Medicine" had worked. Nobody used Saphronie's Lane anymore.

Who Did What?

At the risk of putting too many of my own experiences in this book, as though I were "crowing," I'll let you decide if this story belongs in here or not. Maybe you have had a similar experience.

I used to shoot archery at the professional level. I lived in Rochester, New York, at the time, and two other guys, members of the Professional Archery Association (PAA) often traveled with me to various big shoots around the country (the United States).

In the wintertime we northerners often found practice facilities hard to find. We discovered that there was a church basement some thirty miles into the countryside where local bow hunters practiced.

Some tournaments were indoors, and the PAA had set up an official "indoor round." In this type of tournament the distance to the special target was sixty feet, the same as the lane of a bowling alley. The target was a twelve-inch square of cardboard with a bull's-eye in the center that was about the size of the bottom of a regular glass in your cupboard that you drank out of. A "hit" in this circle scored five points. Hitting another bigger circle outside of that scored three points.

After five arrows (called an "end") had been shot, the total score of these five arrows was recorded on a score sheet (a possible twenty-five points per end). A total "round" consisted of twelve ends. A perfect score, all bull's-eyes, added up to a score of three hundred.

My two pro archery companions stopped going to that church basement to practice because of local archers' habit of shooting there. About eight guys would line up, and each one would have four to six arrows, all mismatched wooden arrows, some of them crooked, and they would "fling" them at the target (pinned in the middle of three straw bales banded three-high). Bing, bing, bing, bing, bing. Then they would all stand there waiting for us "pros" to shoot one arrow.

I didn't mind. They shot so fast, there was only a small wait. (I'd motion them to "go get your arrows," a goodly number of which would not even be in the cardboard targets).

But I'm telling this part of the story because one night when I arrived a bit late, I had to laugh inside of myself at what one of them said quietly (I pretended I didn't hear). Most of my arrows, after a lengthy aim, would land in the bull's-eye or very close to it. I assume this is why, when I entered, one of them said to the other, "Here comes Monotonous."

A pro tournament (indoor) came up to be held at St. Clair Shores, Michigan. We three from Rochester decided to go. Taking the shortcut to the Detroit Tunnel through Canada, we ran into a nasty snowstorm. In fact, snow blowing in on the motor killed it, and we came to a stop. In desperation we ripped out the shelving (some kind of fiberboard material) underneath the back window of our car, to cover the air intake of the front of the hood to keep out the snow. The heat of the motor dried the wet motor enough to get us going again. So we arrived having survived these trying circumstances—not the easiest way to get ready to perform our best.

I started shooting, and what do you think happened? When I went to pull those first five arrows out, the "group hole" that they had made (all bunched together) could be covered by a penny. This hole was just slightly above "dead center" of the bull's-eye. "Wow!" I said to myself, "How often does THIS happen?"

None of us shooters ever pay much attention to one another. None of my buddies were next to me in the lineup, and we all just kept shooting. But by the third end I began wondering what was going on! That little hole into which all my arrows were landing (fifteen now) had only expanded to where it took a nickel now to cover it.

I had to have gone into some other conscious state because I didn't seem to allow that supernatural precision to "psyche" me out. "Zip . . . tink" was the sound as arrow after arrow clipped another arrow in that group. This had never happened before, but, hey, if it wants to happen, let it. Once in a while I thought I had "flinched" a bit on release, but nothing seemed to matter. The arrows kept on going into that little hole. Maybe Robin Hood or William Tell or Cupid was shooting FOR me, but "something else" had to be involved.

Now you would think that after seven ends (thirty-five arrows), I would freak out, or SOMETHING would happen. Well, it did. As I was walking back to the "shoot-from" line, I saw a crowd of spectators awaiting me.

As I drew up to shoot the next arrow, I could feel my blood crawling up both sides of my face. "Plunk." That next arrow went high, barely out of the bull's-eye but nevertheless, out of it. In one shot I went back to my regular self. Some of the crowd of spectators, sensing that they had spooked me, moved on. I still peppered the bull's-eye pretty good, but even after the whole crowd moved away, I still never resumed zeroing in on that little hole.

I won that tournament handily, but whoever or whatever shot those first thirty-five arrows for me never came back to my rescue, and though I did have some hot streaks later, never again at subsequent tournaments did I have a thirty-five-in-a-row bull's-eye performance.

This happened when I was in my thirties, when I wasn't, what you might say, spiritually hip.

The main thing that separates this tiny "grouping" of thirty-five arrows from, say, this same thing being done with a pistol is something that ought to be pointed out. A bullet "disappears" into the hole it makes in a target. An arrow in the bull's-eye gets right in the way of the next arrow being shot. It can deflect that next arrow right out of the bull's-eye. When four arrows of an "end" (five arrows) are bunched tightly in a group, that fifth arrow has all the more chance of being deflected.

That's why thirty-five arrows "in the same hole" were so phenomenal. That's why I wondered if someone else, maybe the ghost of Robin Hood, was shooting those first thirty-five arrows. That's why the question, who did what?

Adolphus Martin

There used to be a legless man named Adolphus Martin at Swaa gi(t) (the Tuscarora name for the Six Nations Rez in Canada) who could "tell fortune."

Unerringly.

People went to him if they lost something or maybe just to see into the future. Everybody knew about Adolphus, so now wouldn't you think that no thieves would be in existence around Osweken?

But maybe others have had the same thing happen to them that I had happen to me. I lost my new posthole digger and accused "somebody" (?) of stealing it. I told people to keep an eye out for it. A digger with a splash of light blue paint on the handle. Well, one day I found my posthole digger. I had used it to put in a new clothesline pole and had left it in the tall grass. Now, if somebody steals from me, I won't say anything because maybe my own self, with a memory like a colander, just misplaced it. Thieves could thrive on this lesson.

Yes, and there WAS a thief near Adolphus. Stanley Buck had his new axe stolen, so he went to the seer to see where it was. The thief was "told on."

When Stanley confronted the thief, the thief said, "It's mine. I bought it last month at So-and-So's store."

At the store, the storekeeper said, "No. That guy hasn't bought anything here in a year or more; and furthermore I don't want him here at all. He steals."

Stanley went back and stole his axe back. Right in front of the thief.

It wouldn't have been good to say, "Adolphus says you stole my axe," because then the thief might harm the fortune-teller, who couldn't very well get out of harm's way. Remember? Adolphus didn't have any legs.

Love Power

There must be something in the power of love or compassion that, if directed toward a manifestation, can bring about what we might consider "magic."

Some small children, either at Onondaga or Tonawanda, were given some very young puppies. The children were wild with excitement about these little dogs and played with them all day. That night they put these puppies in a cardboard box with a soft cloth at the bottom and "put them to bed" down in the basement of the house.

That night a cold snap came, bringing record low temperatures. Even canned fruit jars on a shelf turned to ice, and the jars burst. In the morning the baby dogs were dead. Frozen.

Of course, now, the children's grief knew no bounds. The father had to rush off to work, and so didn't have time to bury the puppies. Besides, the children wouldn't have let that happen so quickly. It would have been just too much to have such happiness end so abruptly—the disappearance of bundles of love.

So the children carried the little frozen bodies upstairs and sobbed over them and hugged and petted them to the highest degree.

How high? Very high. High enough to bring the baby dogs back to life.

Stanley Buck

It seems to me that when Stanley Buck (originally from Six Nations, Canada, but now residing in Onondaga Territory) told me about this little imp that was an ice-skating whiz, and in the back of my head I had a memory of having heard of such a thing. I think it was called the Ha'jeejee.

We had a small ice-skating pond in the gully near our house, but because a high bank of tall trees surrounded the south side of it, it was extra dark down there at night. I thought maybe the Ha'jeejee used it after sundown, so I only went there during the day. This was the "good skater" that Stanley Buck was referring to, and Stanley don't tell lies.

He said that one time in his early days on the rez in Canada, the young folks got to having ice-skating parties. The menfolk of them would drag logs and limbs of wood and make a big fire by the ice. The young ladies would bring cocoa and other drinks and maybe sandwiches.

This skate-party thing got to be such a popular activity as to become addictive. It was like they couldn't stop it from happening EVERY night and ending it later and later.

One night one of the Elders of the area came to the party. He said, "It is all well and good to have fun, but it could get out of hand. If it does, the way that you will know is that something will tell you. It can't talk, but it can skate. I mean REALLY skate. It is very small, but it will skate rings around you."

Of course, the feeling within the skaters was, "All old fuddy-duddies say these things."

Yeah, but on the very next night the little demon skate whiz came.

At a "coffee break" they noticed, from the light of the bonfire, something fooling around out on the ice. It was the Ha'jeejee zipping all over the pond on skates and doing triple jumps and pirouettes with ease.

Among the men were hockey players who got an idea. "Let's catch it. Let's form a line and surround it."

This they did. Now they had the Ha'jeejee cornered. Or did they?

At the edge of the pond a farmer had chopped a big hole in the ice for his herd of cattle to drink there. Suddenly the ice whiz leaped high into the air and dove into the icy water of the cattle hole.

Disappeared.

YAW WEEE! (The Tuscarora word that means "that's BONE CHILLING!")

And so did the skate parties disappear.

Tongue Not in Cheek

One early evening four young guys from Tuscarora were out cruising in one guy's car. They were of the age where "mischievousness could walk upon the scene." They were J. J., Boozer, Smokin' Joe, and Yogi. They were, like, prowling.

Presently, they came to someplace along Hyde Park Boulevard where a young man and woman were leaning against a fence.

"Let's see if we can talk that gal away from that guy."

They stopped, but they didn't have to talk. The girl pranced right out toward the car. Then she stopped and stuck out her tongue. And out. And out . . . until the driver spun the wheels out of there.

Yogi was sitting in the back corner of the back seat. He was, for the moment, "not with it," and he "missed the show."

"What? What? What happened?!"

"Didn't you see THAT?"

"No. Turn around! Let's go back, I wanna see what you saw!"

Now Yogi all the more DID want to see. He pestered the driver. Well, the overall thought was, "Did we really see what we thought we saw?"

The driver turned around and went back.

Joe called out to the couple, "Are you devil worshippers or what?"

When the answer came back, "Oh, you are believers, too?" the prowlers stopped prowling, like dogs with their tails between their legs.

Their attitude was more like, "Maybe we should go and get some ice cream. If we can eat it."

Even today, years later, if any of the three who saw that long, long pointed tongue should retell of that eerie incident, it is with increasing animation and emotion.

Emerson Waterman

This guy, Emerson Waterman, maybe he was a Faithkeeper or a Chief or a Speaker or a whatever. He was a guy who could really manipulate the Onondaga language into beautiful oratory (at the Onondaga Longhouse). This ability to captivate listeners is the essence of the oral tradition at any traditional ceremony at any Longhouse.

One day in a ceremony I happened to be sitting next to him as he was standing and reeling off one of his speeches.

All of a sudden, in a low, almost inaudible voice, he said in English, "Oh hell, I don't know what I'm talking about," and he sat down.

So classic was this act to have been a witness to that I shouted, "N'YAHH!" (Like "BRAVO!" or "OLÉ!")

This response caused everyone else to echo that cheer, "N'YAHH!"—thinking I was cheering the speech.

Had photography been allowed in the Longhouse, a photo of Emerson would have shown the grin of a true imp.

Allen Jack

Allen Jack knew that some people thought he was crazy, and he liked them to think that. He's the one that some people said, "He studied too hard." Others said, "He jumped too high playing basketball and hit his head on the backboard."

Whatever, he could expound philosophically to a degree that reflected his having attended two different universities. I liked having him do that, and maybe I would subconsciously bait him.

One time I said to him, "Very few people can understand the Longhouse premise that Grandfather Thunder, when he speaks, is scolding the evil forces that are getting too close to us, back to where they came from or into the earth."

"That's only because textbooks don't verify that," he said right away, "and that's because it isn't known yet exactly what all the effects are that lightning can have on various subatomic particles. Maybe Grandfather didn't want crime to become too rampant when we all became too exposed to an overabundance of positive ions at full moon."

When I didn't say anything, he baited me to see where I stood on the subject. He said, ". . . and the nightshade continues to grow along the fence."

I said, "That was beautiful." It was the same as saying, "Craziness is in the mind of the beholder."

Ducky Anderson

Ducky Anderson saw a nice thing one night. He saw a light about the size of a glowing ping-pong ball. It was playing on the stairway in the old but now gone house where he was born. The lit ball bounced up and down the stairs.

This was the same house in which he had lost a very rare coin. He found this coin at Old Saw Mill in the cherry orchards on the boarder of the Tuscarora Reservation. It was an old French coin. It had a picture of a plowshare on it. Also, some really old date.

Well, this was his prize thing. Maybe he prized it too much. I bet he said, "Ha ha! I got something that nobody else has got!" But he lost it.

How can you just drop something and lose it? Well, we know it happens because we've all done it. Well, he went wild looking for it and never ever saw it again. And I know Duck; he's the kind of a guy who would pry every board up until he wrecked the whole floor. The whole house.

Two Suns?

When I was in Australia, I couldn't get used to the sun being in the north. Well, one day something happened to me, here in North Carolina, that reminded me of that northern sun.

Sometimes when people are looking for a certain herb or tree bark but can't find it in their area, they will ask me if I know of its source. One day a man in Florida said his wife was ill and needed some Shagbark Hickory bark but couldn't find it in Florida. If I could find any, would I send some to them?

"Sure," I said, "I know where there is some."

There were three large such trees only twenty minutes walk from where I lived at that time.

It was, timewise, high noon when I left the cabin. I'd walked this old logging road twelve or fifteen times before, and because I've always had a good sense of direction, I didn't need the sun to tell me at noon which direction was south. For twenty minutes, as I walked, the sun hovered off to the left side.

This logging road followed the bottom of an east-west long, low ridge. This ridge, about the height of a one and a half story house, stayed, all twenty minutes, to the right side of me.

When I came to the area of the three big hickory nut trees, I turned and climbed over this small ridge.

All of this area, except for the road itself, was wooded, and it was a welcome sight as I reached the downhill side of the ridge to see the three hickory trees appear as if on cue.

But . . . try to imagine this . . . here, in the sky, shining in my face, was the sun. It was like being back in Australia and being disoriented by my compass.

(This otherworldliness was not as bad as that incident when the spooky Commons Woods at Tuscarora reversed east and west directions on four of us teenagers. See "Energy Places" later in the book.)

Maybe you know of somewhere like the Promiseland Road place near
Olean, New York, where you can appear to be traveling downhill in your car but
not be. If you stop, put the shift into neutral and let off the brakes, you will back
up. This can be an optical illusion, but it would give you, at first, a feeling of dis-
orientation. If there is water in the ditch at Promiseland Road's edge, it will appear to be flowing uphill.

So at the hickory trees I quickly left some Tobacco, said "Thanks," and gathered some strips of bark. When I got back over the ridge, I followed my "tracks"
in a sort of "I'm-out-of-here!" mode, and sure enough . . . here was the (other?)
sun, the regular one, in the south, waiting for me.

Maybe the "suns" were telling me "wrong Medicine." The man's wife did
not recover and died.

Big Dog

In a casual conversation I was having with Doris Printup Hudson, she happened to say to me, "One day a big black dog ran across the road in front of me as I was driving along. I told my mother [Harriett Pembleton] about it, and she said, 'OH MY! THAT IS VERY BAD LUCK!' And sure enough, that very next day my husband [Clifford Printup] flipped his jitney over on Greene Road, and it landed on top of him and killed him."

She used the word *jitney* to refer to what quite a few Indians did to a car. They would use an acetylene torch and cut off the roof and body of a car and with wooden planking make a small truck out of it with which to haul firewood.

To myself I said, "Heh . . . I've seen lots of big black dogs, but nothing happened afterwards."

Then I asked her, "How big was the dog?"

She said, "As big as a horse."

"Oh," I said back to myself, "That WAS a BIG dog!"

O. J.

O. J. Simpson ran through football players at a high speed. O. J. Johnson ran to school when she was late. She was a good friend of my sister Free, when we lived on Dog Street. O. J. married Jumbo.

I don't know when she did what I'm going to tell you about—not recently because she's dead. What she did was take a walk in back of her house toward Saunders Settlement Road. Of course, you don't go too far before you run into this big ol' swamp. So what is tricky is, Who would ever build a house back there? Nevertheless, O. J. came to a house.

She went into it. On a table in that house was a pile of pictures. She stole one of them pictures, a picture of that very same house, and took it back home.

When she showed the picture to her parents, they said, "Hmmmmm. There's no house back there."

So a bunch of them went back there to make sure they weren't lying, and sure enough, they weren't. There WAS no house back there even though they had a picture of it.

So it must be that a material thing can materialize from nothing. SO THERE!

Abraham geh he(t)
(Abraham Dead and Gone)

We take things in our lives for granted. Those of us who are not blind take for granted that when we awaken tomorrow morning, we will open our eyes and see what there is to see. We will take for granted that daylight will replace the darkness. What we observe that takes place on a regular basis can even be a crude clock that also becomes taken for granted. The school bus. The mailman.

Wesley Hoi(t) and Jonesy were chatting at the end of Wesley's lane at Upper Mountain Road one day when the mailman came through. East of there, about 150 yards, there lived a man named Abraham Printup. Abe had an alcohol problem, but, like all alcoholics think, he thought nobody knew it. On a certain day of the month a check would arrive for him. Maybe it was his U.S. Navy retirement check, or maybe it was Social Security or even a welfare check, but whatever it was, it came on a certain day. Abe would be waiting. Like clockwork he would come out of his house, get the check, then drive to a bank and cash it. Wherever he went after that was to get into the sauce and stay until he closed some tavern before coming home. He always made it back, though he would be quite polluted. Clockwork.

Abe ought to have known that in every small community in the world, everybody knows what everybody else does, but of course, as in every alcoholic's case, he considered himself ultradiscreet and therefore exempt from ee'yog ("they say" or, more crassly put, "just plain gossip").

So, as in knowing the sun will rise, both Wes and Jonesy looked up to watch Abraham Printup go to the mailbox. They were not disappointed. They saw the figure of Abe do his thing. But it was not Abe. It was the ghost of Abe. They saw the ghost of Abe come out and get his check and go back into the house.

Now, this is the crux of this episode. Can it be that sometimes the power of expectation or of take-it-for-grantedness is so strong as to manifest our expectation? Or could it be in this case that Wesley and Jonesy had enough "seer" power to make what they saw happen? Jonesy had quite a bit, and Abe was a brother to Wesley's wife, Alta. But why do we have to know why?

How do we know that it was a ghost that went to the mailbox? Clockwork. Jonesy and Wes waited for the next thing that was supposed to happen—that is, to see Abe drive out of his driveway on his way to the bank. When an alcoholic doesn't drink, something is wrong. It was as if today the sun didn't come up.

Fifteen minutes was much too long for no car to come out of Abe's driveway. Twenty minutes was the limit of discretion. The two men went to investigate.

Jonesy's apprehension spoke. "I knew something was wrong when we were less than halfway to the house. I could feel it. I could hear Abe's little dog yapping with fear in its voice. Then when we got there, I got the chills. That little dog would run full tilt to the end of its chain and be snapped into a somersault. Over and over, like it wanted to run away and never come back."

The door was unlocked. The men went in. They found Abe bent over, dead. He'd been dead long enough to stink.

Giveaway

Wherever Red Earth Woman (the great Ute Medicine person) goes, she leaves a trail of goodness. Like the dust of little stars trailing behind the Ga hus stee'nis (the Fire Lion). Or those little pale blue butterflies that act like a living jubilation of confetti.

She taught me Giveaway and then went on to help me see it come alive before my very eyes.

I went to a Peace Elder gathering in Australia and arrived a couple of days late. In order to catch up to "schedule," I was driven to Ulladulla Bay by motorcar. Display booths had been erected, and a good variety of aboriginal arts and crafts were on display and for sale.

A sizeable crowd was milling about, and I quickly "lost" myself in it lest some organizers of the Elders program spot me and drag me off to a "meet the dignitaries" cocktail party or some such silly equivalent. I wanted to "Simple Simon it" and sample the wares being offered.

Right off the bat, don't I see something that I can't afford? A boomerang with some grabby dreamtime art on it. It was forty-five dollars, but I had already spent seven hundred getting from New York to Los Angeles, where a ticket to Sydney awaited me. I was promised a rebate but hadn't gotten it yet. (And let me tell you something: if you become an Elder and someone says, "I'll give you a rebate," just laugh and pretend you're deaf. I never got mine.)

Now tell me this, how many times have we liked or wanted something and decided against buying it? Five minutes later we change our minds, run back, and find it already sold. One-of-a-kind item gone. I bought the boomerang.

The seller smiled and tried to find a bag big enough to put it in, but failed. One-third of it stuck out of the biggest bag available, but I didn't mind. I was like a kid with a "see-what-I-got" toy. I walked around whistling some tune I never heard of.

I was still whistling when I ran smack into an Elder. Of all the Elders in the world, who do you think it was?

Yep. Ms. Red "Giveaway" Earth Woman. And she was looking at one-third of My New Toy. There was JUST NO WAY I could not give it to her. I gave it to her.

The rest of the conference was like most other enjoyable conferences I had been to, and soon it was over. My plane wouldn't be leaving for a day or so yet, and I received, from an unexpected source, an offer I couldn't refuse. From an Aborigine. A nice didgeridoo-playing Aborigine who wanted to take me into his country and show me some power sites. I couldn't refuse.

He showed me the Blue Mountains and the legendary Three Sisters. Some red parrots landed on us. We saw the laughing Kookaburra and the rare "witchy" bird, the Pied Currawong.

Right in the middle of my having a nice time, I had to go and think, "Do you realize that this exotic Heyoka-like sun-in-the-north trip is about over?" Probably with all the pleasure I was enjoying, I had gracefully slipped into a "five" of the Enneagram (the Observer). My newfound friend would be driving me directly to the airport in his rattletrap tomorrow. I had planned to bring some Australian Christmas presents back with me for my children. Why hadn't I thought of using my charge card to shop in Sydney while I had the time?

Now we came to the home of a large family of Aborigine friends of my companion. They were all smiles and laughter when I began showing them the dances and songs that we did at our socials. They encouraged me to go on and on. We finally had to tell them that we simply had to start back, that we had a long drive yet.

As we started to leave, they handed me a package. A gift. The package was quite heavy. I opened it. It was quite heavy because it contained ten boomerangs. They were all painted exquisitely in dreamtime.

I had gotten tenfold for tithing the one boomerang to Red "Giveaway" Earth Woman.

A year or so went by before I ever saw Red Earth Woman again. When I did, she told me a little story.

"Remember when you give me the boomerang at Ulladulla Bay in Australia? Well, this is what really happened. I saw that boomerang before you did. I planned on buying it. I said to myself, 'I'll just take a swing around and see what else there is. Maybe I'll like something else even better!' I didn't see anything I liked. When I got back to buy the boomerang, it was gone. I got mad at myself, but you taught me not to do that because when I ran into you, not only did I get my boomerang, I got it free, with love."

I told her my side of the story. She beamed. But then she is always beaming. She knew how the story would end because she teaches the rules of Giveaway. She knew I would receive tenfold for making her happy with only one boomerang.

Duke

I grew up with Duke Jacobs. He was in the Eighty-second Airborne with a number of us from Tuscarora when he defied death a couple of times. He came home on leave one time driving a U.S. Army jeep, so we were not too sure how legal this leave was. The army is not in the habit of providing transportation for people like Duke, especially considering that he held the lowest rank there was.

Sometimes Duke made his life more interesting by screwing up. This time what he did was flip the jeep over on its top, even though it had no top. One of the clues that Duke may have illegally borrowed this jeep was that there was a large field radio, about three foot tall, attached to the back seat.

When the jeep was upside down, someone looking at it would be inclined to say, "The driver must have been thrown clear out because there's no room for anything to be under there."

Just the same, the first ones arriving at the scene of the accident called out his name, "Duke!"

From under that no-room-for-anything place came Duke's reply, "What?"

The next close call was VERY close. We were putting on a free-fall jump exhibition at Myrtle Beach, South Carolina. When Duke took his turn, he did a "delay" to thrill the crowd, especially the women. When the form of his downward hurtling body disappeared behind the treetops of a small woods, women screamed and fainted.

We rushed around the woods to find Duke rolling up his parachute. Maybe he held the record for "closest to the ground opening" because he said, "As soon as I got my opening shock, I found myself sitting on the ground."

Some say he timed the pulling of the ripcord by counting off the seconds of descent, ". . . five thousand, six thousand, seven thousand. . . ," but that the "delay" was actually too delayed because Duke had a speech problem: he stuttered.

So maybe some kind of higher power was protecting Duke so that he could show others not to be afraid of anything. I know he wasn't afraid of ghosts.

Everybody, though, has a chink in their armor, and so did Duke. He was afraid, but only when he was among his Indian pals, that he might not be believed because he knew that some of his experiences were beyond belief.

He was part of a gang of four who were also members of the Seven Clan Archery Club. We referred to this group of four as the "Flu-Flu Boys." That was because whenever these four went bow hunting, they always carried a bunch of flu-flu arrows with them.

Flu-flu arrows are homemade arrows that are hard to lose. Instead of the regular feather vanes of regular arrows, flu-flus have a big "wad" of feathers, usually brightly colored for easy tracking, that slows the arrow rapidly. This "wad" is made by stripping one side of a large feather (pulling it, skinning it, off the quill) then wrapping and gluing it, spiralwise, around the feather end of the shaft. The finished product looks like a little porcupine or hedgehog "en garde." One could shoot a flu-flu at, say, a squirrel in a tree, but if one missed, the arrow would "parachute" itself back down. It made a "swooosh" noise as it left the bow. Its purpose was to "force" the archer to have fun.

One time the flu-flu boys invited me to go bow hunting in the Adirondack Mountains. The other three flu-flu boys, besides Duke, were Fill and Kenny Rickard and Erwin Printup. We went for bear.

Now I was familiar with the Speculator area, but these guys, having to be different, more daring, took me to a place that none of us had ever been to. Maybe somewhat nearer the area of Mount Marcy. Of course, it would be unmanly to have a map of the area. Bears don't have maps.

In the afternoon of the first day of hunting I found an old trail that looked man-made and inviting. From where I stood before taking it, I could see a lake and our camp on the other side of it, so I knew, pretty much, where I was. The wilds of the Adirondacks enchant one to the Nth degree, and I followed the "come-into-my-parlor" lure until I had a feeling it would be dark before I got back.

With overcast sky, darkness trapped me. When I finally got back to the lake, I let out a loud war whoop to let everybody know that I was OK, not lost, and would soon be in camp.

No answer.

I was imagining the other hunters to be worried about me out there in the dark.

Wrong.

There wasn't anybody in camp when I got there. They were all still "hunting." During the night they came straggling in.

Hardly did first light appear but Duke roused us all.

"YOU GUYS! YOU GOTTA COME WITH ME! WE BETTER GET GOING RIGHT NOW! I SEEN THE BIGGEST BUCK DEER ALIVE! He's got a herd of ten does with him, and I know where they're all bedded down. Let's go and surround them."

We all reluctantly woke up, got ready, and followed Duke into the woods.

On and on we went until we began suspecting that Duke was lost. He tried to assure us that he knew what he was doing, but long after we knew that the deer would be up and gone, members of our group peeled off one by one and went on their own.

Finally, and now it was way past noon, I was the only one left with Duke. I tried to think of a gentle, maybe a "legit" reason to leave him, too. In the distance ahead I now occasionally caught snatches of the sound of running water, maybe a small stream.

I stopped. "Duke," I said, "When you were at the place of the deer, could you hear running water?"

Now here is where fear came to Duke. He panicked. He didn't want EVERYbody to leave him, to think he lied.

He stuttered his answer. "D-d-d-damn near."

Later, I told on him because of the classic nature of his statement, and for quite a while we referred to him by the Indian name "Damn-near-can-hear" instead of by "Duke."

Now why did I let myself ramble into an area that has nothing to do with Medicine? Maybe fear. Maybe I had a fear that I couldn't come up with enough words for this book. Just the same, it was the ONLY thing that I could come up with regarding fear in Duke. For sure, he was not afraid of ghosts.

For a while Duke lived in a house that was on the west side of Garlow Road. It is now the site of a dike.

One of his friends was a young man of the reservation, one of the Art Davis boys, who died in a motorcycle accident. A week later, after the burial, Duke was looking out over the hayfields behind the house. He was sitting with his legs hanging out, off the ledge of a second-story window.

In the distance and getting closer came a motorcycle through the field. It was the ghost of the dead man, doing about sixty, on the death motorcycle. As it came into Duke's yard, it came to a stop.

"Hey," Duke yelled, "Come in and tell me about your accident."

Up came the ghost, looking every bit like a living version of the dead person, even to being without one of his legs that he had lost in the accident. Of course, living people don't generally float upward if you ask them to visit on the second floor simply because that's where you happen to be. So it's not likely that Duke had any illusions that his visitor was alive. Duke climbed back in and off the window ledge to let the ghost in. And in it came, sporting one missing leg.

A half-hour conversation ensued, after which the ghost decided to leave. Out the window he went, landing on the bike and starting it.

"Your engine's missing!" Duke called down over the noise.

"I know it," came the answer, "I gotta get some new plugs." And away he/it went on across the field toward the cemetery.

Duke had so many experiences with ghosts of various kinds that they would fill a volume by themselves. One such experience occurred when he was walking north on Walmore Road, only about a hundred yards from where Walmore ended at Upper Mountain Road. Just then the shaggiest, raggediest big old dog he'd ever seen came around the corner, off Upper Mountain, toward him. It seemed slow and harmless, but just to be sure Duke went to the opposite side of the road. As soon as he did, the dog ambled over to that side, too. Back went Duke to the opposite side. Back came the dog.

By now the dog was close enough for Duke to see how truly seedy it looked. Along with extralong mangy hair, it also had extralong toenails, maybe four inches long. They could be heard scraping the pavement, ". . . grawgs, grawgs, grawgs, grawgs."

Now Duke hatched a plan. Never did the dog cross the road quickly, so he let it stay coming toward him on his side of the road. When it got near enough, Duke planned on leaping out of the way.

Sure enough, the dog was not quick, and when Duke jumped, it continued moseying on past. But Duke had more plans. Realizing that this was not a real dog, he gave it a swift kick into its "center" to see what would happen.

"POOF" . . . his foot went right through the dog, and a small cloudlike form of feathery particles floated temporarily up and above the dog, following it briefly over the dog, at the dog's speed, then settling back down into place. Then the ghost dog continued south while Duke continued on northerly.

Maybe when this dog died, it had a dog girlfriend that it was so in love with that its soul would not "give up the ghost"; and maybe its hair and its fingernails (pawnails?) refused to accept that the rest of the dog had died. Anyways, this was Duke's explanation of why this dog's ghost refused to go to wherever other dogs' essences went to after they died.

I'm sure that lots of people couldn't take Duke seriously, believing him to be a "dreamer," maybe even half a bubble off. It took him a while to pick up on this view, but when he did, he began keeping his experiences to himself, except for his family and trusted friends.

One day a friend of mine, Quinny Printup, who lived directly across the road from Duke, said, "I think Duke has lost it."

"Why do you say that?"

"Yesterday he told me he has a new refrigerator. But then he said it was out in the woods."

The next time I saw Duke I asked him about it. He became animated. "Come on," he said, "Let me show it to you. You'll like it."

Not far from his place was an old homestead we used to call, "Raa juh g'yeh gih he(t)." It is a saying used at Tuscarora to mark a certain area that a certain person, now deceased, used to own and where they had lived. "Raa juh" was just the Indian version of "Rachael." Rachael Mt. Pleasant. Before that it was "Helen Beaver g'yeh gih he(t)." A Catholic church came to be built there, from the old barn.

A small creek went through the property. Much of it was quite concealed by thicket. Here, in a hidden portion of that creek, in the middle of it, Duke had dug out and formed a small pond. It was banked and had screened-off pipe at each end of it so the water could flow on through. In the pond, lazily working their gills, were five rainbow trout.

Propriety and Derangement

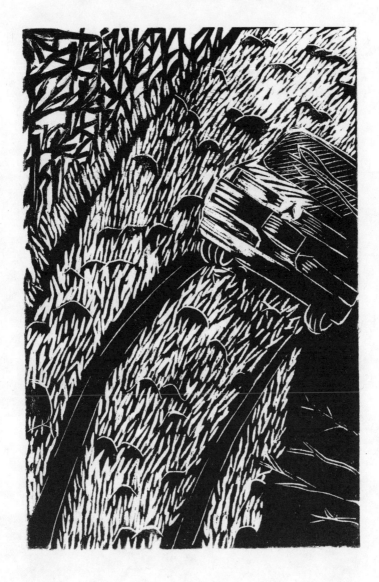

Overleaf: Ted sings a sacred song and rolls the Mercedes down the mountainside; see "Songs of Power," pp. 200–205. Woodcut by Rhiannon Miles Osborne.

Don't Hunt Too Early

Eleazer Williams was an Indian doctor. He was also Senior Chief of the (Snapping) Turtle Clan of the Tuscarora Indian Reservation, New York State. The title of this position is Sa qwa ree(t) thre(t). It means, "Dragging a Lance." He was my father, and several times he said to me (regarding the hunting of deer), "Don't hunt too early. September is too early; the fawns still need their parents." One year in the middle of September, though, Big Sy's kids said to me, "Let's go look for deer on Garlow Road."

Big Sy's kids were a little bit like he was. You might say he was an Indian con man, so then his kids were little con kids. For instance, Big Sy sold a load of firewood to someone who lived off the reservation. The wood was Basswood—a soft wood that burns quickly, like a matchstick, and nothing anyone would want in winter because one would have to get up every two hours to refeed the stove.

The buyer asked, "What kind of wood is it?"

"It's not hardwood," Big Sy said. The way he said it, it sounded like "Knot Hardwood," then he took the money and drove away.

The kids liked to tell lies, and sometimes they stole. Also they were the worst shots with a gun on the whole reservation, maybe even in the whole Northern Hemisphere. That's why I was often invited to hunt with them. I shared with them whatever I shot. That's why they never stole from me.

"No," I said. "It's too early to hunt yet. The fawns aren't ready to be on their own yet."

"Yeah, but we can shoot a buck. The does will take care of the fawns."

"But the deer haven't mated yet."

"Oh, that don't matter. How can we kill all the bucks if we just hunt this once? It only takes one buck to make all the does pregnant on the whole reservation."

"Who told you that?"

"Grandpa Ole Sy. He was a snare drummer in the army."

(Boy! THAT made sense.) "I don't have any bullets anyway."

"We'll give you some. Come on . . . we'll just split up and look around. Check the fields. We won't be long. We'll pick you up late this afternoon, that's when the deer come out. Oh, you know."

I gave in. "OK . . . I'll take my twelve" (meaning my .12-gauge shotgun).

This shotgun had a clip that held three slugs (or bird shot shells). I could also put one in the chamber.

There is now a reservoir or dike at the area on Garlow Road where we parked Big Sy's beat-up old truck. On either side of the road were hay fields surrounded by bushlines of Nu hee(t) (a shrub). We spread out in four directions to sneak through these bushlines and see if any deer were grazing in the fields. Everett went northeast. John-hoodoo went southeast. Alfie went southwest. I went northwest. I was loaned four slugs. When I got out to a safe distance, I loaded the clip and put the fourth slug into the chamber.

In the area that I hunted I could see a long ways. There were no bush lines until I circled back. It would be two hours before darkness came, so I took my time.

When I did come to a bush line, I realized that there would be no field on the other side of it. Big Sy's kids had sort of conned me. They had taken the best hunt areas. Ahead of me I could see a roadway through the bush line—on the other side was Gibbon's pear orchard. The pear orchard was right behind Ethel Wahoo's house. I went toward the opening. If I didn't see a deer, maybe I'd see some pears. With that thought I walked a bit faster, right on through the opening. But then I put on the brakes.

There standing in the freshly cultivated earth of the orchard stood one of the finest ten-point bucks any hunter would be thrilled to see.

The distance was about twenty-five yards. I could hit a tomato-paste can at this distance. The deer was broadside to me. I aimed carefully and shot it.

The deer leaped into the bushes of the bush line. I ran back through the opening to see the deer run out into the field and fall dead. Nothing happened. "Good shot," I thought to myself, "The deer died before it even made it through the bush line." There was not a sound to be heard, not even of an insect.

I hurried back to the place in the bush line where the deer had plunged. I picked my way carefully through the bush Line. I retraced my steps, looking carefully from side to side. Nothing.

You have looked for something like your car keys. Back and forth, over and over, you look in all the likely places. After a while you start all over again, picking up and looking under the same things you've already looked under twice. It's maddening.

Now I began to look for blood, traversing the ground at first, then carefully checking small limbs and leaves for any sign. Nothing.

At this point now in the search of your car keys, you might sit down and rub what might be the first tiny beads of sweat from your forehead. "This is ridiculous," you hear yourself say.

I stopped looking. Big Sy's kids would now be back at the truck wondering where I was. The sun was very low now in the sky.

In a sort of fog of resignation I walked back out to where the deer had been standing when I shot it. The earth was soft and inviting to my feet. I was making clear footprints. There were no deer hoof prints anywhere.

What did Father say? "Don't hunt too early."

I started back toward the truck. I could hurry along. There was actually a tractor-width path in the hay that I could follow. Though I hurried along, something nagged at my brain about what had just happened. Yes, yes. It was something more that Father had said. "If you do, one day you'll see a ghost deer."

Don't forget, at the time of this incident I was about in my middle teens, close to the time when one knows everything. I didn't want to accept the facts. I had hunted too early. I had seen a ghost deer. I had been told that this might happen.

Maybe I needed a little more convincing. Maybe the Universe knew this. If so, this is what happened next.

As I came within a hundred yards or so of the truck and the other hunters who sat waiting on the tailgate, I proceeded to unload my gun. I would return to them the remaining three slugs that I hadn't used.

I opened the breech. There was nothing in the gun. Nothing in the clip. No three slugs left over to return. I stopped and looked about on the ground and on the path behind me. Maybe somehow three slugs jumped up out of the gun by themselves.

Now, this bothered me the most of all. In a couple of minutes I was going to be made into a liar.

Guess what. I needn't have fretted. Big Sy's kids expected everybody in the world to act the same "normal" way they did. My cock-and-bull story was the same cock-and-bull story that all people tell so they can steal four slugs. They simply started talking about other things. Things equal to the price of tea in China.

The good name I thought I had meant diddly. I was angry and doubly so because I could do nothing about it. The Universe knew this and wanted it that way. I would not forget this lesson. Thus ends the story of this incident, doesn't it? I mean, the moral of it is, "Don't hunt too early." And furthermore, if you persist, the Universe will rub it in, and then you WON'T forget.

Well, I don't care if I ruin the ending of the story of this incident by adding a weak postscript. I was bothered so much by what had happened that I made one more feeble attempt to clear my name to myself or make more sense of the whole thing or maybe even find the deer and missing slugs and show them to Big Sy's kids and say, "SEE! I WAS telling you the truth. Here's your three slugs, and when I get to town and buy some, I'll give you back the fourth one!"

Like, "SO THERE!"

I seethed all night. The next morning, Saturday morning, I jumped on my bike and went to Garlow Road and went all over that path and place with a fine-toothed comb. At the spot where I'd stood and fired that one shot, I especially looked about with care. A last-ditch theory of mine was that maybe I wasn't as cool a cucumber under fire as I thought I was. Maybe for the first time in my life I had experienced "buck fever" and emptied the gun into the sky. No such luck, though I did immediately find the one empty shell right where it "ought" to be.

But I have failed to mention that there IS one more thing I got out of all this. It is the same thing that Perry Hoi(t) got one time.

Howard Hill tells of this incident. He told me that Perry Hoi(t) was down at Old Sawmill with a metal detector looking for gold.

I asked, "Did he get anything?"

"Oh yes," Howard said, ". . . exercise."

Mike Jacobs and Stan Hill were sitting in the shade because it was August. Dog days. Mike said, "I'm dry." Stan says, "You shouldn't have said that." It was akin to fasting all week and dancing in the hot sun at Sundance and having the Heyoka clown come dancing in backward and pouring dippersfull of water on the ground in front of the dancers. In the two men's heads, visions of frosted steins of cold beer danced just out of reach.

"I'm broke," Mike said.

"Me too," Stan replied quickly lest Mike think he was holding out on him.

"Dinato's was the last place that would let us run up a bar bill."

"Yeah, but now we're barred from there, too, and we weren't even in the fight that got us barred."

"Let's change the subject."

Both quit talking. Both tried to think of something else. It was no use.

"I know!" Stan exclaimed, "I know it's only August, but we can jacklight a deer and sell it at what-you-may-call-its on Ontario Avenue."

"I hate for you to have such a good idea. Let's not wait till night. We ain't got no light anyways. Let's go now. There's always a bunch of deer hanging around the edge of the swamp back of Ham's" (referring to Hamilton Mt. Pleasant's place).

Slowly they got up and dumped the lawn mower gas into the cut-down (cutting-torched) Ford jitney. They got their guns, both .30–30 high-powered rifles, some ammo, and off they went down Dog Street.

The walk into the swamp was murder. Cicadas screeching made it seem worse. Maybe this wasn't such a good idea after all. "You think we'll have to gut the deer, or will they take it as is?" Mike was having second thoughts, especially any thoughts that suggested effort of any kind. The deer would not walk out by itself; someone would have to drag it. He never had noticed until now that a .30–30 rifle could become heavier in direct proportion to an increase in the temperature of the sun. He ought to have been a physicist.

Before Ham switched to oil, he used to cross the creek at an opening that led out onto a wee meadow when he was hauling firewood. I say "opening" because the creek was lined with trees and brush except for this abandoned roadway. The creek bed was dry, but some mosquitoes whined about seeking victims. But here was shade. The two men stopped for a breather and a cooler despite the tiny flying bloodsuckers.

Mike was about to say something when Stan tapped him on the shoulder. Mike looked at Stan, who gave a small jerk of his head toward the wee meadow.

Six adult deer were moseying into view. They were heading for the wee meadow. Once in a while one of them would flick a tail or maybe an ear at a circling deer fly.

Providence! A magical reward for ontological need! The miseries of the day disappeared.

Stan gave the orders in a whispery voice. "OK, this is the plan. You can hear that phoebe out there flicking its tail. Time it. When it sings, flip off the safety on your gun. We're gonna get two deer. You take that one on the far left. I'll take that big one in the middle. On the count of three, fire."

Both men, both hunters, made no quick or jerky movements. Both came to the ready smoothly. Both aimed carefully.

One . . . two . . . KA-BOOM! As one, the two high-powered rifles broke the sound barrier of the quiet of the day.

The phoebe flew off, but the six deer, who by now had started nibbling the tops of Thoo ro(t) na gi(t), continued to nibble.

Incredible. Or incredible luck. Six deer at forty yards can stir any hunter's sensibility beyond sense. "Shoot again!" Stan says.

Both men aimed and shot two more times before they stopped.

Stan looked at Mike. Mike's face had a grin on it that was half imp and half embarrassment, as though to say, "I should have known after the first two shots." Aloud, he said, "Oo(t) naa wog" (ghosts).

The two men looked back at the deer. They weren't there anymore. The phoebe was gone. Even the cicadas were quiet.

They would not be going to Ontario Avenue or to Dinatos. Or after any more deer. They would not be downing beer from frosted steins. That barrage of crashing bangs had told all the real deer to exit the scene.

The insidious craving came back.

In the insanity of alcoholism and with the craving unbearable, they automatically drifted toward even the remotest possibility of some alcohol. They drifted toward Ham's house. Maybe he was one of them secret drinkers like Abraham Printup.

It is amazing how, within the connive-ability of an alcoholic, no stones are left unturned in the tiniest possibility of a plan to reach a drink that will eventually kill the drinker. In this instance, wouldn't it be just devastating if they discovered that Ham indeed had a secret cache of beer, but that the sight of two men carrying high-powered rifles caused him to think that they had come to rob him at gunpoint? They hid their guns.

Ham greeted them with the "open arms" enthusiasm of a lonely person who seldom had visitors stop in. He opened up with an outpouring of crabgrass talk that made the hunters squirm in their chairs, especially during the part about the hot weather. Of course, the alcoholic is not to be put off by ANY kind of talk.

With crafty "cutting ins" on Ham's ramblings, and with cleverly laced innuendoes regarding the kind of drink that Ham ought to "come clean about" and reward them with, they soon realized that Ham was clean. Even the feeble thought that he might have gotten the wrong hint faded when he brought them two glasses of water.

Ham could play classical piano, and no guest was immune from being "treated" to his talent. Mike and Stan feared this would happen. They allowed Ham to sail into one of Schubert's concertos because, after all, he had been so gracious as a host.

In the interim between the first and second movements of the concerto, Ham paused for effect. The pause was short, but it was too long. The hunters, still slightly tone-deaf from the three-gun salute that they had given the oo(t) naa wog, and not knowing Schubert from Adam, took this pause to be a clue to a reprieving chance to flee. With the least amount of rudeness that hunters possess, they excused themselves, and using the law "when in doubt, mumble," they mumbled some excuse as to why.

Ham tried gracefully to stop them. Using panic as the mother of invention, his mind raced searchingly for any topic of conversation that would grab and hold them.

"I heard some very loud shooting not long before you came in. It was very upsetting. What do you think was going on?"

Stan and Mike were already going through the doorway. "Kids," Mike said, continuing on out. "You know how they like to shoot at nothing."

Juuh ne(t) raath

One day Father and I went for a walk down the path that led into the wooded place where we drew our drinking water from a spring. The area being virgin forest, huge trees, mostly Sugar Maples, surrounded us. We stopped near a very large old tree. I was five years old. Father was eleven times my age, and although I never told him this, I secretly knew that I was smarter than he was.

"When I was your age, I never could go any farther than this," he said. "This is where my father would stop the horses, and I would get off the wagon, and he would go on to down some trees for firewood for winter. He was afraid I might get in the way or be hurt by the falling trees, but he'd say, 'Stay right here, and you'll get some playmates.' As soon as the horses went out of sight, Little People would come out of this tree and play with me all day long." He indicated the large tree nearby.

"When we could hear the jingling of the harness of the horses coming back," he continued, "the Little People would jump back into that tree."

To myself, I said, "Yep. And so did the Tooth Fairy and the Easter Bunny."

Thirty-five years went by, and I was working at the Eastman Kodak Company in Rochester, New York. Word came that my friend Mad Bear had had a heart attack at his home on the reservation. On Saturday, I drove to his house to see if this was so. No sooner had I gotten into his house than we heard another car pull into his graveled driveway. Bear looked out the window and got all excited. "It's Beeman Logan!" he said, "I don't feel anything wrong with me; it's a nice day, let's take Chief Beeman to Seven Clan and show him the Medicines your father planted there."

After greeting the Chief, we all agreed that Bear's suggestion of a walk on such a fine day was a nice idea, so we drove to Seven Clan and did just that. If

Bear had had a heart attack, he certainly didn't show it. He was in his element and couldn't stop talking as we walked single file along the path, Mad Bear leading the way.

After a while I noticed that Beeman wasn't with us. I stopped and looked back. Beeman was standing some twenty-five yards behind us. "What's the matter?" I called to him.

"It feels like the Little People are here," he answered.

"Where?"

"Right here in this tree," he said. He was pointing to the same tree that thirty-five years earlier my father said that the Little People had come out of to play with him.

I made a note right then and there that if ever I had a question that I couldn't answer, here was the man to come to.

The years went by, and indeed I visited Beeman, sometimes with a question and sometimes just to visit. I wanted my children to meet him, so one day the occasion of an opportunity arose. We'd started out to look for an unusual plant whose roots were used by alcoholics. Two of my sons, Bob and Mike, were with me as we drove along on the New York Thruway nearing the Tonawanda Indian Reservation. But let me tell you a bit about this Medicine first.

We called this Medicine Juuh ne(t) raath, which means, "long root," and it was used in two different ways. When alcoholics got together, some came and went, but others just stayed and drank until they began hallucinating because the supply never stopped as the newcomers brought more alcohol.

They gave names to two hallucinations that often then occurred, the Bees and the Snakes. In these hallucinations an unbearable panic would set in whereby the sufferer would begin begging for help. If the supplication was directed, either by a pureness of will or by a high level of panic, to a Divine Higher Consciousness, that person would be led, staggering and falling and hollering for help, into the woods and directly to this Medicine. One bite of the root and the hallucinations would leave. Sometimes the alcoholic would leave the habit from that day on, but at the least he would abstain for a long period. It is very interesting that this plant hid from those who didn't really need it, as though one had to suffer and experience a deep need first.

The second use for this Medicine was more drastic. The alcoholic had to be willing to risk death in this form of cure. It was akin to making a vow to the Creator: "I vow not to allow another drop of alcohol to enter my body or you can take me." Whoever had that strong a conviction would go to a Medicine person and ask for the cure. A piece of this root would then be placed in a secure container such as a small piece of metal tubing with the ends pinched and brazed or welded shut and attached similarly by chain around the vower's neck. If that person drank alcohol or took the Medicine off, they would die.

Isaiah Joseph told me the names of two people who had died when they took this cure as a mockery to prove that it was just a hoax. After that, so few dared to try it that it generally fell into disuse. Also, the knowledge of this Medicine became lost, and it didn't help that the Medicine was so rare. I was told by Mocks Johnson that in 1970 this Medicine plant had been extinct for about twenty years, and that if it were found, it would be a dangerous thing because young people wouldn't believe it would kill them.

I could believe Mocks. I'm skeptical and found it hard to believe many of the things about Medicine that the Elders told me. When I was supposed to be asleep as a schoolboy, I would often put my ear to the heat register on the floor of my upstairs bedroom and listen to visiting Medicine people swapping stories and information with my father. Skeptical or not, though, I sure was intrigued by the Juuh ne(t) raath. This then was the Medicine that I continued to keep my eye out for on any Medicine-gathering trip.

Bob and Mike went with me on this particular trip. I drove off the New York Thruway and said, "I want you to meet someone special, Chief Beeman Logan."

We drove into Beeman's driveway, and here were five or six other cars parked every which way, like Indians do. "Oh," I said, "We better not bother him, he has all these visitors, maybe it's a Chiefs' meeting."

I started backing out, but Beeman came hurrying out, waving us toward him. I told him that we didn't want to bother him, and he said, "Well, I thought you were joining us. Big caravan of Indians coming from California and picking up more along the way. We're meeting up with them tomorrow morning, and then we'll go on to help the Penobscots up in Maine. So what are you guys up to then?"

"I just wanted my children to meet you. We were just bumming around looking for Medicine, but I've been told that it's been extinct for about twenty years."

"Oh, no such a thing!" Beeman said loudly. "But you came at the right time. We're having a sweat tonight. You take the sweat and don't towel off. I'll do a purification on you, and you'll be able to find that Medicine anytime you want to."

We drove back in and parked. This was even better. These were the things I wanted my children to see.

At the Sweat Ceremony Bob and Mike acted as doorkeepers, opening and closing the door between rounds.

After the sweat Beeman took an eagle feather and made brushing motions over me with it, doing the Four Directions. He spoke in Seneca while doing so. It seemed like such a short little ceremony, and I wondered if I may have gone into a conscious state that transcended time. (Many years later I was still wondering about the time span, so I called Bob by phone and asked him to recall that purification and, if he could, how long he thought it took Beeman to do it. "About three minutes," he said.)

Being as Beeman would be doing a Tobacco-Burning Ceremony the next morning for the success of their venture, we stayed and slept on the lawn under a Cucumber tree. I wanted Bob and Mike to see this, too.

In the morning, as soon as the Burning was over, we took off in the Volkswagon bus for Tuscarora. We drove directly to this creepy old woods off Black-nose Spring Road called the Commons. Here was where the Medicine had last been seen.

As soon as we parked and got out of the bus, I saw on the ground the biggest set of a deer tracks I have ever seen. "MAN!" I said to myself, "A MOOSE IS LOOSE!" Then to the children, "Be quiet. Maybe you'll see the biggest deer you'll ever see."

So we tippy-toed into the woods following the giant deer as it wandered around boggy places. After about two hundred yards the tracks went into a wide circle.

"Forget it," I said, "He's too wise for us. He has our scent blowing toward him right now. He's gone."

I looked up from the tracks that I had been intently studying, and what do you think I saw? All around us Juuh ne(t) raath. The Medicine.

And I have seen it ever since. (Even growing along the side of the road here in North Carolina. Anytime.)

One evening I was speaking to a group of young folks at the Indian Center in Rochester, New York. I was talking about the insanity of drugs and alcohol. I happened to tell about the Juuh ne(t) raath, its cure of alcohol hallucinations, and the deadly necklace cure.

"MAKE ME ONE! MAKE ME ONE!" one brash young man shouted to me, "Make me one of them necklaces."

Soon a few more were asking me if I would make them a necklace. I had to do some serious thinking. Finally, I said, "OK. I'll make some, but I'll make them loose so you can take them off. I'll run them all through a ceremony with that stipulation — that you won't be harmed if you take it off. This is a very very serious thing you'll be doing."

I made five large beads out of the root of the Medicine. I strung them on necklaces of eighty-pound test monofilament fishing line. A week later I passed them out to the five who asked for them, the first one going to the young man who asked first. For the sake of his anonymity I'll call him Jim.

A year later, at the Indian Center, someone asked me, "Did you hear what happened to Jim?"

"No, tell me."

"He got a high-paying job as an ironworker, and he got married. His wife, Marie, was a dental assistant, and together they made good money. They bought a new Chevy Blazer, big wide oval tires. One night they went to a party. On the way Marie, knowing that there would be liquor there, said, 'Hey! Jim! You got that thing around your neck?'

"Jim took it off and hung it on the rearview mirror. Marie said, 'Don't you think we ought to take it home?'

" 'Oh no,' he said, 'It'll be all right.'

"They hadn't gone another block when both brand-new front tires had blowouts. BAM BAM!

"I don't know if Jim ever drank anything since you gave him that necklace, but I do know this. Jim and Marie never went to that party, and they haven't touched a drop since."

◆　◆　◆

A bunch of years went by, and now I was retired and living in the mountains of North Carolina, about fifty-five miles from the Cherokee Reservation.

One day I got a call from Cherokee asking if I would run a Sweat Lodge there.

"No," I said, "I don't run Sweat Lodges."

"Oh, but this is different," came the reply. "About twelve Indians want to get sober, and they're saying that they think you can help them."

"Yes, that IS different," I said, "I'll do it, just give me the date." We then arranged the time.

Before the time came, an anonymous caller tipped me off. "Guess what? Someone put it on the Internet that you were running a sweat, and a hundred and fifty more people are coming to the sweat."

"No!"

What I did then was boil up a gallon of the Juuh ne(t) raath and take it with me. When I got there, sure enough here were about 165 people waiting to sweat. Only about fourteen were Indians.

I told them to gather around me and be very quiet. Then I told them about the Medicine, naming the names that Isaiah Joseph had told me of people who had died when they tried to expose the Juuh ne(t) raath as a fake. I showed them the gallon of the Medicine, telling them that THIS is what would be creating the steam, that the decision to go into that Sweat Lodge would be the most vital decision they could ever make.

When the line formed to go into that lodge, there were only thirteen, and only six of them were Indians. But I'm sure that there are thirteen more alcohol-free people in the world now.

OO naa g'yeh

OO naa g'yeh is how you say "alcoholic beverage" in the Tuscarora language. It has been the most visible of several influences that are strongly responsible for Indians' straying from their traditional spiritual way of life. Less visible but equally responsible are the U.S. government's Indian schools and what Indians call the white man's religion.

It has been said that there is both positive and negative in all things, as in the concept of the yin-yang in Chinese cosmology. So let me tell you about my bout with OO naa g'yeh and whether or not, for me, any significant benefit came from it.

When I was fifteen years old, I became president of the Baptist Young People's Union (BYPU). Why? A good-looking girl named Dolores House took my eye in church, so I did whatever might impress her. We became girlfriend and boyfriend.

That summer on Jonas Hasley's muck farm I made a dollar a day weeding. Argys' Bus Lines sent a bus every Saturday through the reservation around noontime for anyone wishing to go into the U.S. side of the city of Niagara Falls. It would leave the South End terminal at 11:00 P.M. In order to spend my dollar-a-day money, I got on that bus.

On the way home, nearing the witching hour, I heard laughing and singing at the back of the bus, so I went back there to investigate. Bottles of beer were being (discreetly?) passed around, so I took a drink, and just like every alcoholic says in defense of their morality as they tell on themselves at their first Alcoholics Anonymous meeting, "My first taste of beer was yucky!"

So from then on, for that summer, on Saturday nights I slipped into bed very tipsy and giggled to myself over the tales I'd heard on the bus that were laced with some naughty language. On Sunday night Dolores and I would run the

BYPU meeting at the Baptist church and do a bit of preaching. So here in my life, you might say, was born a mild form of the yin-yang.

In June 1948 I graduated from LaSalle High School in Niagara Falls. The talk among the Indian boys of my age at that time centered quite often on some rumors that we could be drafted into the U.S. Army in the near future. The Korean conflict was festering. Several of us said, "Why wait and be drafted and stuck into some straight-leg outfit? Let's sign up and have more of a choice." So we did, and following the derring-do of high-climbing steelworkers, we signed up as those Indians before us had done: we signed up to be paratroopers.

Lest the reader see these forays of mine into areas leading away from the title of this book, let me say that the boogeyman of science, ESP, seems to be attracted to Indians and doesn't stay on the Indian reservations only. On my second assignment (the first was for jump school) to Fort Benning, Georgia, for parachute riggers training, I experienced a reminding incident.

In order to qualify for extra "hazardous pay" (at that time about fifty dollars more a month), all airborne personnel had to jump a minimum of once every three months. My name appeared on a roster of who would be jumping the next day.

After class I walked to the PX store, which was about a mile away. By going through thick woods, I could take a shortcut. I did. At the PX I came to an unexpected thing. A large, mangy dog stood growling and showing its teeth, as if daring me to take another step forward. Well, it didn't know that I had lived on Dog Street on the reservation and had waded through much fiercer adversaries, so it backed off and ran the other way.

Darkness came about the same time that I left the PX. I went through the woods again, having walked through many woods at night because I often went too far. When I got to the middle of the woods, the most unusual thought came into my head.

Many Indians on the Tuscarora Indian Reservation told of having heard the holler of the Oos skit ra ree. This is a special entity, a special skeleton that warned of death. It could be seen or heard, and then someone would die. I never heard it, so I would ask those who had, "What does it sound like?"

One might say, "Oh, it sounds like when you blow across the open mouth of a gallon jug."

Another might say, "It sounds like a sick, dying cow bellowing."

Another might say, "It sounds like a big man hollering from fright."

Why now, in the middle of these woods, did I suddenly think about that sound? Not only that, but I got a strong urge to see if I could imitate it. I mean strong. So strong that before I could stop myself, out of my mouth came this "big man fright holler."

Lordy Lord! I froze, having scared my own little self. After a while, though, I laughed and went on. But why in the Sam Hill did I do that?

Wait, there's more. Back at the barracks, the outside light was on. And who do you think was there to greet me? Mr. Mangy Dog again, growling and menacing. Why?

I stoned it, and it ran off.

Inside the barracks, at the pool table, an 8-ball game was on. "Next!" I yelled. The game I got into progressed rapidly, and now all I had to do was sink the 13 ball with enough zip and topspin to come all the way back down the table. I lined up and "wham!" The 13 ball broke into three pieces.

I have never seen a billiard ball break before or since. I don't have triskaidekaphobia (fear of the number 13), but, hey, I was to jump the next day. I thought, "Maybe I should keep an itchy trigger finger on the reserve parachute handle, eh?"

Usually, when I jump, I don't bother to check my chute as we're supposed to. Being a seven in the Enneagram and wearing perpetual rose-colored glasses, I see these precautions as things that belong in books. This time, though, when I jumped, I followed the book.

After the opening shock, which I wasn't too sure if I would get one or not, I reached up and pulled on the risers and looked upward into the canopy. One panel was beautiful because it wasn't there, just a long triangular sliver of blue sky.

What to do? Should I panic? After all, panic may be the true mother of invention. I looked at the other guys floating down. It looked like someone had swished a white-headed dandelion through the air, and the seedlings were little paratroopers in a long line. I felt part of it. I couldn't see that I was coming down any faster than anyone else, so I just rode it on in. I even feel sorry now not to be able to bring this story to a more smashing ending. It's just that the cruddy dog, the 13 ball, and the Oos skit ra ree, all manifesting on one day, were more than a coincidence, even if they just were meant to tell me I'd be seeing a blown panel on a parachute.

About four of us Tuscaroras ended up in the 82nd Airborne at Fort Bragg, North Carolina. Two or three others went to the 101st in Kentucky. It wasn't all that easy for the four of us at Bragg to keep in touch with each other, but when we did, we'd get drunk. We'd signed up for three years, but the Korean War extended our stay for nine more months. In all that time, I didn't get into the OO naa g'yeh all that much, but looking back now, I see that a symptom of alcoholism was there. I had no preferences; any brand of beer, wine, whiskey, vodka, or champagne—it was all the same to me, all OO naa g'yeh. All good.

The service hitch over, it was home again, home again, jiggedy jig. I looked forward to playing sports again: lacrosse, baseball, basketball, whatever there was. But then came a phone call from Milwaukee, Wisconsin.

It was Duke Garland. At Bragg we had become jazz fans. Before Bragg, I used to listen on a small radio to Oscar Peterson on piano in Montreal and to Maynard Ferguson at Crystal Beach, Ontario. Maynard's ultrahigh scream trumpet astounded me so much that I bought a trumpet and took it to Bragg, though I took no formal lessons. Over the phone Duke said, "Hey, man, dig this. There's a jazz school in Chicago. They're accepting enrollment of GIs and having the GI Bill pay for it. Grab your ax [trumpet] and meet me at the Blue Note in the Loop [Chicago] on Saturday night about seven."

Duke was the only man in our company at Bragg to wear a "duck's ass" hairstyle. He kept it trimmed to within a hair over the edge of the rules. After hours he turned up the back of his collar. He was "in the know." I said, "OK, I'll be there."

Chicago was fun, and in eighteen months I was jamming at jam sessions. The world was my oyster, and I walked around in a euphoric state all the time. It seemed like I didn't need much sleep. I'd be up half the night doing an arrangement, trying to get those Stan Kenton flatted ninth and raised eleventh sounds from a trio. After a while, though, the guys at the school got after me. "Loosen up!" "Live a little!" What they meant was, "You're missing the real fun. Drink up.

Take a drag on a joint. Snort some coke." I inherently knew this was not for me. OO naa g'yeh, yes, but not drugs, too.

I had recently been to a small jazz joint called the Beehive. The Bird (Charley Parker), the great alto man, was doing a one-night show. I went early and got a seat. Then I waited. We all waited and waited. Finally, half or more of the crowd went home. I should have, too, but I had gone past that line where an alcoholic can't stop.

Somebody whistled. Out from the curtain on the stage came the Bird. Stoned out of his tree. We erupted. He put the alto to his lips and cut loose with "Ornithology." Oh man! Too much! He soloed for an hour straight, then went back out of sight. Forever.

"Forever" because I never saw him again. In a week or so he was dead. Heroin. I couldn't believe it. I wanted out of Chicago, but I was hooked on the jazz scene. What to do?

A woman did it. Sue, I'll call her. She had started coming to the lacrosse games and cheered me on before I left for Chicago. A fan. I liked her. She was not from the reservation.

What happened was, Sue, out of the blue, blew into the Windy City shortly after I had announced my dilemma to myself. She knocked on my door. She visited a day or so, then was gone, back to Niagara Falls, New York, where she lived along the river.

A month went by. I got a letter. In essence, "I'm pregnant. We must be married."

Sevens in the Enneagram have been described as having a "butterfly mind." Not only in thought do they go from flower to flower, but even in action they go from project to project. Overnight I was married and living along the upper Niagara River, eight miles or so from the Tuscarora Indian Reservation. The wedding was quick but quite large. A "six-toaster," giftwise, wedding.

Daddy-in-law was a bulldozer operator, an old-time, well-known member of the local Operating Engineers Union. He was also an alcoholic. He said to me, "Say! While you're waiting to write some famous song or something, why don't I just get you into the union with me?"

"Sounds good to me," I said, not knowing one way or the other.

Now, some might say opportunity came knocking. Some might say fate. The state of New York was financing the huge Niagara Power Project (that is, they floated bonds). It would take six to eight years to complete. Soon I was making more money than I ought to. Soon every weekend was party time at Ted's-on-the-river. Entrance fee . . . a six-pack of OO naa g'yeh. I learned to drink.

I had never encountered such awesome capacities to drink as among construction workers. For me, the experience was like a high school football player jumping directly into the pros. On his first play he is left lying on the ground with a busted head and the air knocked out of him. Someone running past says, "Welcome to the NFL!"

At lunchtime I went into a bar with six ditch diggers. We sat at the bar. Before I could say boo, there were seven big steins of beer in front of us. I didn't know the rules. Everyone buys a round. Lunch is thirty minutes long.

If we can say that we have a guardian angel within or an inborn warning system or ESP to varying degrees, whatever, I had them and was using them.

I'll give you a few instances. If, in my sobriety today, I refuse to touch any form of alcohol, including cough medicine, mouthwash, or any form of alcohol, it's like I'm saying, "Alcohol is only negative to me," yet this happened before I quit.

So one weekend my son Tom and I were to go fishing. He forgot about it, and when I got to his house with two bottles of wino wine, he wasn't home. I called his friend's house. A strange voice said, "Billy doesn't live here anymore. I think he moved to North Tonawanda or Tonawanda."

Down the road I cruised in my Volkswagon bus in disappointment. I picked up one of the wine bottles and said to it, "Take me to Tom." Then I drank it.

After a while the street began to weave back and forth in front of me. Soon a police car with two policemen in it pulled me over. One of them opened my door and said, "Get over!" I slid over. He drove me to a parking lot and said, "Sleep it off. Don't let me see you driving again tonight!" (Well, how often does this happen?)

After a bit I got out and started walking toward a streetlight in the distance. A large apartment building stood at the end of the street I was on. As I neared it, I saw a man with his head stuck out of a top-floor window. His was the only room with a light on. It was late. "Hi there," he said as I approached, "Come on up. I'll give you a beer. I've got a bad case of asthma. I'm just getting some air."

"I'll come up and chat with you," I said. "I know a plant medicine that might help you, so I'll walk down to the streetlight first. It might just be growing there."

I got about halfway to the light when, from the other portion of the building that now came into view, came a voice, son Tom's, "Dad!"

I turned to see him grinning and waving from another window on the other angle of the same building.

So maybe there is a yin-yang in all things, even in the Wild Irish Rose wine. (Don't tell anybody if there is.)

Incidentally, the asthma medicine was indeed under the streetlight, another big "now what are the odds of that!"

OO naa g'yeh. Now it was running my life. On a Wednesday the job I was on finished up. Back to the union hall the next day? Not me. I declared Indian Holiday for myself. But when I mentioned my layoff to my friends, they said, "Oh, you lucky dog! Don't you know the bow-hunting season is open in Pennsylvania? Get down there and get the camp ready. We'll be there on Saturday."

"Heavens to Betsy! Hold me back! Where have I been? Bow season? I'm gone!" That was the one thing I couldn't miss after waiting a whole year.

The next day, after a slow start, I found myself, about one o'clock in the afternoon, at a crossing in the road near a place called Butter Creek. The roads were dirt, and as I drove through the intersection, I couldn't help but notice the shape of a small mountain to my right. The mountain seemed to be made to order for that spot, like one corner of a pyramid. You know, like a ridge ran from the road level straight up to the peak. This ridge was perfect except for one small glitch.

Let's say this mountain was made out of cheese. Then say a big big big rat came and took a nibble out of the middle of that ridge. That's what this ding in the ridge looked like.

"Hmmm," I said in my thoughts, "I bet the deer cross there. I bet they have a trail that crosses that bite mark."

I parked the car and climbed to that spot with my trusty little bow and arrows. To be tricky I circled and came down from above. I was right. As soon as I got there, ZING! a nice-looking buck shot through that opening.

◆ ◆ ◆

Do you know how fast a deer runs? I mean in miles per hour? And I mean top speed. Sports magazines say forty. Well, they lie. Know how I know? I chased one. In a Volkswagon Bug, though someone else was driving.

It was like this. Cal Loomis, forty-second cousin to my wife, said to me one night, "Wanna see a big deer?"

"Sure."

We got into his Bug, and when we got to a certain clover field, he drove into it with no lights on. It's uneasy to ride with no lights on, and just when I was at my uneasiest, he put the headlights on. About a hundred yards away, chewing cud (if deer chew cud), lay this huge buck. It could have had its picture in a magazine what with its rocking-chair-size antlers.

To the deer, we were just two small lights putt-putting along in the clover. He took his time getting up, and when we got close enough, he went into that classic graceful bounding run, faster than he had ever run, as long as he could remember.

Good. I'd seen deer like this at Montezuma Swamp, so now it was OK to go on back home. Cal, though, thought I wanted a closer look. He floored the gas pedal. Well, how much guts does a Volkswagon Bug have in a clover field? Not much, but after a while we came up behind the deer. I looked at the speedometer. Forty miles per hour like the books say. (I think these experts just copycat one another.)

As the Bug began to feel its oats, it gained on the deer until I thought Cal was thinking of running over it. Now this regal animal looked back and saw this puny little car, far far beneath its dignity, stepping way beyond its bounds.

You could almost hear the deer say, "Get thee behind me." It left. It went into scamper mode, the same gear it used years ago as a fawn to keep up with its mother. It left us like we were standing still. Then, to add insult to injury, it shot off into the darkness with a sharp left turn, never to be seen again. Well, Cal tried to turn, too, but at that speed clover becomes a bit slippery, so we went home with our tails between our legs.

Back to the gap in the ridge. When I got to it, a deer, a nice buck, had gone ZINGO through it. In bow hunting one can never be too ready. I was ready, but not ready enough apparently. I raised the bow and drew at the same time. Things happened so fast. The hand was quicker than the eye, and the eye was quicker than the mind. The mind, if it could talk, would have at that moment said, "OH NUTS!" I only got about one-fourth of a draw on the arrow before it slipped out of my fingers! I could have shot one of my toes off! But wait! Here came another deer!

Sure enough, here was another deer on the trail of the first one. It was looking in the direction of where the first deer had gone. By lowering to one knee, I fancied myself hidden. I called to the deer with a low soft blat.

The deer said to itself, "Unbelievable. What a pitiful imitation." The next thing I saw, instead of its head, was its tail. The big white part. The part that says, "Ta-ta."

I stood up with that "Well, I'm glad nobody saw that bungle in the jungle" feeling, and I looked on the ground in front of me, expecting to see my arrow stuck there and protruding. Well, maybe I did manage to shoot it a little farther out after all. Maybe it's even stuck under the leaves. But wasn't that a beautiful and exciting moment? Worth an arrow any day. Even two arrows. "I'll walk out to the deer trail," I thought to myself. "If I don't see my arrow, it's not my arrow anymore. The woods are the new owner."

I could see the deer trail before I got to it. It disappeared around a thicket, which is where the streaking deer also disappeared. At this point I no longer looked for an arrow. I was thirty or more yards from my debacle. That arrow would never have reached this far. I started stepping right along. Good-bye arrow. I'll just cross the deer trail and go on down to the car.

I started across the trail but then FROZE in midstride. There, upside down, dead, was that streaking buck. It was caught in the narrowness of the path through the thicket.

I got the shivers. I got the willies. I got the heebie-jeebies. I just KNEW, before I even checked its warm body, that this was the deer I shot at. At? That's why I was freaking.

I looked around. Someone was playing tricks on me. I saw no one, but I did see another unbelievable thing. There, on the ground, a short ways back, was my arrow, all bloody. No. Arrows don't just go through the lower lungs, the top of the heart, and the rib cage, then conveniently fall to the ground. ESPECIALLY not from a bow that was only very partially drawn back.

These thoughts went through my head over and over as I cleaned the deer. I took lots of time. Sometimes I'd just stop and look at the deer to see if it was real. Feel it. Maybe it was a dream.

The rest of the day and into the night was dilly-dally. Going through the motions. I tagged the deer and hung it under the bridge over cool water to chill it. I went to a bar and ate. No OO naa g'yeh. Well, that was strange.

It was as though I knew what I was going to do all along. I continued to go through the motions. I drove back to the deer, loaded it, and drove north. Someone on the reservation would get this deer. I seemed unaware of the distance of the drive.

So it was midnight before I got there. I said, "Whoever still has a light burning gets the deer."

I drove around and came to the house of Chief Tracy Johnson. His light was on. He was the Subchief of the same clan as my father. Turtle.

He laughed and shook his head, but said "Yes" when I asked if he wanted this deer.

I might hunt New York State, but no more Pennsylvania. Too eerie down there.

Fifteen years went by, along with the easy money of the Niagara Power Project. Everybody's uncle and cousin had come from Ohio and Pennsylvania and joined the local unions as though work here would be never ending. Overnight it did end; you could buy the union business agent a case of booze or subsist for twenty-six weeks on unemployment checks. So I went to work for the Eastman Kodak Company at Rochester, New York, some seventy miles or so from the Tuscarora Indian Reservation.

I was cocky and spoiled. As a union member, I was used to waltzing into the union hall when I needed a job and pretending I could do ANYTHING. For example, a union business agent (BA) comes out of his office:

BA: "Anyone here know anything about a Herman-Nelson heater?"

Me: (loudly, with upraised hand) "That's all I've ever done."

BA: "Well, go on down to the Merritt Chapman job site and report in."

At Kodak, when I went there on a Monday morning for a job interview, I was sent to the office of the Crane Department. The crane boss and his superior were sitting there waiting. Unbeknownst to me, two days earlier, on Saturday, a Kodak crane operator had tipped a crane over on a busy adjacent city street, blocking traffic for hours. The two bosses were there, not so much for me, but meeting to discuss the punishment to dish out to the "tip-over" crane operator. They considered themselves rough-and-tumble bosses from the old school. They believed in scaring the worker.

As soon as I walked in, one of them bellowed, "WHAT WOULD YOU DO IF YOU TIPPED A CRANE OVER?"

I said, "I'd grease the bottom of it."

Well, this set the two bosses off in a fit of guffawing like you never heard. No more questions. End of interview. I had a job. It lasted twenty-four years.

Having said earlier that "fifteen years went by," I meant from the time of the deer incident in Pennsylvania. Every year, when the deer-hunting season rolled around, I'd be haunted again by the thoughts of that incident. No matter how I carefully pieced it together again, it remained an eerie mystery. Sometimes I thought, "Maybe it didn't happen." Maybe I just "thought" it did. Dreamed it. Made it up so I could use it as a boogeyman story to tell my grandchildren. A great idea. A concept. Yeah, a conception. I called it "the Immaculate Conception" and left it at that.

Meanwhile, I continued my love affair with OO naa g'yeh. Like so many unrecovering alcoholics, I KNEW I wasn't an alcoholic because I worked every day. I'd had this good old WASP "work hard and you'll be respected" ethic handed down to me by my father, who had gotten it from Carlisle Indian School. This life of denial threads its way through all the "war" stories told by recovering alcoholics. Smashed cars, divorce, jail, fights in bars, "I couldn't remember where I left my car (what bar), ha ha," and so on. I wound my way through this same path of denial. Along with this denial, then, was an unawareness of the insidious progressiveness of the disease of alcoholism. It didn't matter that I wasn't an everyday drinker. I was at my worst near closing time at a bar or party. Stolen drinks. Loud, four-letter words. Two cigarettes lit at once. But, no, I wasn't an alcoholic.

Then there was the good guy "put-on" part of me. I knew herbal plants and healing-with-hands, and I helped many people. I didn't charge (but took donations—some were big ones). I gave hitchhikers rides; whatever made me look good. People like me went to heaven, you know.

At the end of the fifteen years, the charade was over. The OO naa g'yeh in me went too far.

I no longer drank people under the table. I had acquired "alcoholic thinking." I was superclever, and I secretly enjoyed knowing that other people didn't know this. More and more symptoms of this type of insanity were accumulating in me, but of course I had this great thing called denial that I didn't even know about.

I began enjoying wicked thoughts. I secretly wanted to show what a super intelligence I had acquired. With it, I could kill someone and get away with it. I could eat them. Then I'd know if it were true what I'd heard about the consuming of human flesh, that it was addictive. I could make a drum using the leather of human skin. I could do anything I wanted to.

I had a cabin in the woods near Naples, New York. It was so isolated that it was difficult to get to. I took a week's vacation starting on Monday.

I don't know how it is for other people, but I can tell you how it is to be a seven in the Enneagram. If I get free of everything, I get euphoric. Too euphoric. I might even be dangerous.

Instead of leaving immediately for the camp, I stopped at a bar first. I had one screwdriver. As I was having it, a friend, Oss, came in and said he was pissed that I had checkmated him the last time we played chess, just one move before he could checkmate me. Would I please give him another chance?

At his house we got into a six-pack of Canadian beer. That one screwdriver was my limit. Three Molson beers later I shouldn't have driven, but I did. Under a streetlight I recognized someone walking who in the past had lied to me.

Whoa! There was the perfect person to kill! A walking motive!

Not only that, here on the seat of my Volkswagon bus was an almost perfectly round, grapefruit-size stone. I'd seen it in a creek bed and liked it, but now, in my drunken stupor, it became a symbol. It was a Divine message, that, yes, THIS WAS THE MOMENT for its existence! The culmination of all my clever plans for the perfect crime!

I stopped the bus and started to back up, but here was a better place, darker, away from the streetlight. "Want a ride?" I called out.

When the person approached the bus, I pointed into the window and said, "Look what I've got!" Then the stone came down, boom, on the person's head.

At this moment the grand plan fizzled. I was dumbfounded.

Under the influence of OO naa g'yeh I was not coordinated. Nor did I understand the law of inertia. That stone needed to accelerate. With a yelp my victim was gone, and a few moments later so was I.

It's amazing how fast the smoke cleared as soon as I realized I had been caught with my hand in the cookie jar. All the exciting esteem I had for myself and my perfect plan went up in that smoke. Something like superfear took its place, thanks to my adrenal gland, and I drove straight for that camp in the wilderness where nobody could find me. But I was two miles away before I realized that I still gripped that nice round stone in one of my hands.

Inside of us all is a tapable energy much greater than ourselves—a connection to a Higher Consciousness, a Higher Consciousness that can be summoned if the need is dire enough.

Isaiah Joseph taught me this, and of all the great human beings I have known, for me, he was THE MAN. He was the first to elucidate to me the Law of the Great Peace, the history of the formation of this great Indian confederacy.

When he came to the confrontation between evil and good, between the evil Tadadaho and the Peacemaker, I could feel pins and needles all over my body. I asked, "Was the Peacemaker scared?"

"Naww," Isaiah said, "He knew that for every degree of evil that a person or a thing has, so does it have that capacity for good. It was simple to the Peacemaker that here was only one unit of evil. The Peacemaker was one unit of good. He a wat tut [Hiawatha] was one unit of good. If everyone brought gifts to the evil one, they would be one unit of good. There were all kinds of goodness units. The song "The Hi HI." A feast. The Thanksgiving Address. The poor man didn't have a chance. The evil Tadadaho would be bombarded with love. What chance did he have? Not only that, if he had all that much evil, his capacity for good was tremendous. Why do you think, then, when they combed the snakes out of his hair, when they got his flip side, he was chosen to be the head honcho of the Law of the Great Peace?"

I was crying. This history lesson was TOO MUCH! I thought I knew what healing was. I thought I knew Medicine. Now a voice was saying, "Hey, man, you wanna talk MEDICINE?" I knew that I had just heard an example of the epitome of Medicine. The living embodiment.

The evil Tadadaho had been a cannibal. I had wanted to kill and taste human flesh.

As I ran away, as I drove to this hidden camp, I felt that everything had gone wrong. I had made the biggest mistake of my life.

Isaiah Joseph had told me, "It's impossible to make a mistake. There are only sacred lessons." Isaiah had passed to spirit twelve years earlier.

As I drove away from reality, I didn't know that I had already consumed the last drop of OO naa g'yeh that I ever would. I didn't know that my life would never again be the same. It was time to have the masks of protection made that Daisy Thomas said I needed. It was time to enter the Longhouse.

I reached camp hideaway well after midnight, but in the morning I realized that by hiding, I could only multiply my troubles. I called a counselor I knew. He asked, "Were you drinking?"

"Yes."

"Well, get yourself into an alcohol treatment center as fast as you can. Maybe the law will go easier on you." I drove to a well-known treatment center and was told, "We don't just take bums off the street. Get sobered up first." Apparently, in my desperate attempt to evade the law, I made up too wild a reason to be accepted. Only a drunk spoke like that.

But it was impossible to make a mistake.

I went next to Strong Memorial Hospital of Rochester, New York, and told them that I was insane and dangerous. They put me in R-wing. Apparently, my story was not that of a sane person. But because it was impossible to make a mistake, when I called Kodak and told them where I was calling from and why, they canceled my vacation time and put me on sick leave. Here I was now, getting paid to be crazy.

Isn't it ostensibly to be cute when we say, "There's a madness to my method," and everybody's supposed to laugh?

It's hard to say just when I sensed any kind of a turnaround in my life. If indeed I did. At night, among the other crazies, I would vacillate in my conversations with myself:

"Hey, it's not so bad in here, maybe I ought to consider living my life out in here."

"Wadaya NUTS?"

"No, seriously, it's free, Blue Cross and Blue Shield is paying for it."

"Wait a minute! What about the fun you're missing? No more sports. No more hiking through the woods. No more taking your children to Six Nations to hear the ghost stories."

After three days I capitulated and called the John Morris Alcohol Treatment Center and told them I'd been in Strong Memorial for three days sobering up and that I was now ready to become one of their success stories. They took me.

Now I called my lawyer. He said, like Mae West, "Why don't you come up and see me?"

I told him I was locked into a thirty-day in-patient program, but he said, "Oh, they'll let you out [like I was already in jail]. Call me in a couple of days. I think I have a solution to your problem."

He was right. I was allowed to see my attorney. We set a date.

When I got there, he first saw me alone. Speaking softly, he said, "You have two options. For seven hundred dollars, I'll do whatever I can do. But you also have the choice of a sure thing. I'm going to introduce you to So-and-So [I can't think of the name now, maybe Alfonso Something or Other], who is the best criminal attorney around. He has PULL, believe me. For another twelve hundred dollars he'll get you off scot-free."

Welcome to the NFL! So this is where Rolls-Royces are sold. I told him I'd see this best criminal lawyer, but that I'd already made up my mind. "I'll take the lesser of two evils."

He gave me his best-hurt smile and led me into another room.

Alfonso was dressed well enough to eat at the Waldorf—though, of course not at my expense.

The meeting was short and sweet. No matter what he said, I said, "No." I told him that I was in the AA program and that it advocated honesty.

"But this way, you're clean. No criminal record." He was becoming more and more put out that he had wasted his time on me. Finally, I wore him out.

When a person goes to the flip side, a new release of energy takes place, the threads or symptoms of which reach into that place of Higher Consciousness. Of course, the average person, compared to whom the beginning recovered is even more average, would just say such symptoms are a piece of good luck. "What a coincidence." Angels and plant divas and Divine little entities such as the Little

People (Eh gwess hi yih) are drawn to such places, though not all people can see them.

So at this time a new symptom appeared.

I showed my lawyer, Bruce, my checkbook and gave him one of them for fifty dollars, saying, "The rest of the agreed upon fee comes as soon as you do your homework."

He laughed, but he actually did something. He found out that the police were looking for me and that my victim was out to sue me for, as he said, "Twelve K." He phoned my victim, ostensibly to see if he "needed an attorney," and this was the beginning of the good part, the symptom. The victim's attorney was Bruce's best buddy.

But more. My victim had a sizeable police record that could be exploited.

And it was. I got probation.

Meanwhile, back at the ranch. The rules at the John Norris Treatment Center were reasonably lenient. I could, if I watched my Ps and Qs for a certain time, have the weekend off. Just be back on Monday morning.

Alcohol treatment places have inmates that are leery of being on their own on weekends. A perfect setup for a slip. Also, a kind of brotherhood or family atmosphere develops among the serious of us. So, after the Friday evening meal one weekend, instead of zooming off like I could have, I sat on the outdoor steps and chatted with some of the leery ones. It was the time of the equinox of June 1980.

A big, white, immaculate Cadillac convertible pulled into the parking lot. The driver was all by himself. He got out of his Caddy with grace, and we all kind of looked at each other to see who of us knew this sharply dressed person. He was all in white, including the Stetson on his head. He looked like he may have come directly from the country club. Not a word came out of any of our lips from the moment we heard the sound of his tires turning in on gravel. That meant that none of us knew him.

You ever get the feeling that someone is looking at you? You turn around, and, sure enough, someone is staring. I didn't even have to turn around. This man was looking at me. All the way. He didn't scare me, but he was such an imposing figure, I kind of wondered why not. Still with his eyes locked on to me, he stopped when he got to within ten feet of me. His soft, suntanned face hinted a smile. I liked him immediately. He pointed his finger at me and in a strong voice said, "I DON'T GIVE A GOOD GODDAMN WHAT YOU SAY! I'M GONNA BE YOUR SPONSOR, AND YOU'RE GONNA GET SOBER!"

I thought, "What a charmingly wicked thing to say to an Indian." I needed to joust with him. "Cool!" I said.

"DO YOU PRAY?"

"I pray all the time. Nothing happens."

"I'LL BET YOU DON'T EVEN [louder] GET ON YOUR KNEES WHEN YOU PRAY! [normal loud] PROMISE ME ONE THING. TONIGHT, GET ON YOUR KNEES AND SAY THAT YOU DON'T KNOW DIDDLY ABOUT PRAYER, THAT YOU NEED TO BE SHOWN."

I said, "Yessir."

We smiled at each other, and he walked off, got into the Caddy, and drove away.

Everybody started talking at once. He had impressed us all. We talked until near dark, when everyone, except me, left for the dayroom to see the movie *Jaws*.

I went to my bed and kneeled, trying to assume the humblest prayer position that I could. Not a soul was anywhere near me. It was like the time to gather Medicine, the time to drink the Medicine.

I'll not tell you what I said. ("Don't let anyone see you.")

When I finished, I wiped my eyes and lay down for just a few minutes. But then I fell deeply asleep.

About 3:00 A.M. I woke up because I hadn't covered myself. I was cold. Then it dawned on me, I didn't have to be here! If I leave here now, I'll get to Tuscarora in time to see the dawn break at Seven Clan.

The dawn breaking at Seven Clan is special. Not just visually special. Add to that audibly special. A variety of great songbirds are there. And they let you know WHY they are called great songbirds. It was also June.

So on this day of the Equinox, I was there on a bedroll, propped against one of the wheels of the Volkswagon bus, facing east. The birds were playing a day gig. NO ONE must come and disturb us.

But a car came. It made bumpity-bump noises.

When the driver saw me, he drove his front tire very close to my foot just to tease me. In the bumpity-bump car was the Chief that I had given the Pennsylvania "spook" deer to fifteen years earlier. He rolled down his window.

He said, "I've been wanting and wanting to tell you this. Remember when you brought me the deer? Well, we were starving. Norma came to me about one o'clock in the afternoon [the same time as I had climbed the pyramid mountain]. She was crying. 'Tray,' she said, 'There's nothing in the house to eat. What are we going to do?'

"I have asthma, as I did then. I couldn't work anymore. I hugged her, and I whispered in her ear. 'There's only one thing left to do. Let's get on our knees and pray.' So we got on our knees, and we prayed. Every hour we got on our knees and prayed.

"At midnight I said, 'I guess we're not going to have our prayers answered. But before we go to bed, let's get on our knees once more and pray.'

"We were on our knees when you knocked on the door."

One Time This Happened

One time when I was still living on Hillside Avenue in Rochester, New York, I saw an ad in the city newspaper that said that the local food co-op was into holistic things and that a Dr. Ash was coming from London, England, to teach "radiasthesia." There was a phone number to call, and, wanting to know what radiasthesia was, I called. This word *radiasthesia* was not in my dictionary, and I pictured it as some far-out thing that I ought to know about.

I was about thirty-eight years old and wanting to know everything and was head-tripping all that stuff from Big Sur and Esalen: Fritz Pearls, Alan Watts, Maslow, "Games People Play," "In and Out this Garbage Pail," "What do you say after you say hello," whatever. It turns out that radiasthesia probably came out of Dr. Ash's head because all it meant was "healing with the hands." Still, it was another thing to know about. This was not something my father did, and so maybe I could sort of catch up to him some if I learned it.

"How much does it cost?"

"Thirty-five dollars for laymen and seventy-five for professionals."

"Do you have a place for Dr. Ash to stay yet?"

"No."

"Well, send him to my place. I'll take him."

The arrangements were made. Dr. Ash would be coming in on a Friday evening from Texas. Somehow I pictured him as looking like Michelangelo's God on the Sistine Chapel ceiling.

Friday arrival time came. I heard the dog bark. A Volkswagon bus with a Texas license plate and poor muffler chugged into the driveway. A nice-looking young lady stepped out, followed by a nice-looking young man. Next came the driver, a thin regular-looking young lady. They all then helped out a sixtyish-looking man out, and darned if he didn't look like he may have emerged from the ceiling of the Sistine Chapel. Dr. Ash.

Somewhere I had heard that if vegetarians were healthier than carnivores, then fruitarians were even healthier. Adele Davis? I brought them in and hugged them all properly and set a big bowl of fruit in the middle of the living-room floor and told them to go at it. They did.

I then let them know that no one had mentioned that anyone else would be with Dr. Ash and that three of them would have to sleep on the porch. Maybe they thought I was kidding because they laughed.

Classes would start on Monday. I announced that I would be taking Dr. Ash the next day to the Tuscarora Indian Reservation to meet my uncle Charley and then take him to my cousin Minnie Murdock, who was a seer. This was to find out if he was a fake or not. They knew I was kidding about why we would see Minnie, and we all laughed quite hard.

The next day Dr. Ash and I left the others to fend for themselves, and I drove him to Tuscarora. At Uncle Charley's place we were told that he could be anywhere, maybe in the woods someplace.

Down the road we went, and I was not sure where to. Dr. Ash pulled out a pendulum, a poor man's radar. The pendulum bob was teardrop in shape and was made from the fossil resin amber. I liked it because a big housefly was mummified in the middle of it.

In most places on earth a Tuscarora chauffeuring a man who looked like the face of God and who was guiding the car with a pendulum may have turned heads, but not here. We had lots of unusual people running around loose, people like Allen Jack, who wore a Medicine hat consisting of two hats. I was told that before my time I had an uncle so crazy that he traipsed about in his Carlisle uniform saluting people and that sometimes people saluted him back.

We'd gone only about three-quarters of a mile when Dr. Ash said, "Slow down." As we approached Short-Shot Patterson's house, he said, "Turn into this driveway."

We did. There sat Uncle Charley drinking tea and chatting with Short. I said, "We don't need to go and see Minnie." The face of God smiled.

I knew that I would have to tear Uncle Charley and Dr. Ash apart because they would hit it off perfectly. I also knew, too, though, that Dr. Ash wanted to meet Minnie Murdock, maybe to see if *she* was a fake or not. I couldn't have been more in my element.

Minnie did not disappoint Dr. Ash. Among the things she said to him was, "You are going to New York City from here, aren't you?"

"Yes."

"When you do your thing there, you will be asked to do another. If you take this second job, don't take the route directions you will be given. I see you in a bad accident there. You may be asked to do other jobs, but the one of danger is one you can avoid. The clue will be that the person asking you to do this will be the only one to use these words, ' . . . and while you're there you can also do such and such.' "

Before we left the reservation, I told Dr. Ash that I needed to stop off at a friend's house and offer my condolences. Paul Bissell's wife had died not long before that, and I had been unable to attend the funeral.

Paul came on strong when he saw me.

"TEDDY! You're just the man I want to see! Somebody's witching me." Paul had big eyes, but today they were bigger.

"I just came to tell you how sorry I am about your wife's passing away. What does this witch do to you?"

"It's like somebody's under the house hitting the bottom side of the floor with a heavy hammer. They do it at night so I can't sleep."

"Wait a minute. I got somebody in the car outside that might like to know about this. Let's find out."

I went to the car and told Dr. Ash about Paul's problem, and he got right up and came out of the car, saying, "My, isn't life interesting."

He asked Paul if he had things that, if anyone came to my house and asked for them, I never would have had. He asked for copper wire, brazing rods, and a piece of one-inch pipe. Paul had all that and more. He was a construction worker, a Jack-of-all-trades, a dynamite man, and maybe suffering from a bit of kleptomania.

Paul did as he was told. When he finished, a copper wire had been strung from pipe to pipe encircling his house. The wire was attached to brazing rods inside each pipe. Like better grounding to the earth. This little fencelike wire was only about a foot off the ground. I say it circled the house, but actually we ran out of wire, which left an eight-foot gap, but then it seemed right to let Paul go in and out of his house without tripping. Plus, Dr. Ash proclaimed it was adequate. We shook Paul's hand and left.

• • •

On Monday evening the radiasthesia class for laymen took place. I was one of the pupils.

Dr. Ash had a setup that consisted of a gadget that produced radiations of some sort, and these radiations were aimed at another gadget that "caught" them and relayed this amount to a round dial with a needle that hovered around the number twenty. I'm not trying to belittle these instruments, which likely were somewhat expensive, by calling them gadgets, but if they had fancier names, it doesn't matter because they did what they were meant to do.

First, Dr. Ash poured water through the beam of radiation, and the number of digits of radiation on the dial went from twenty to seventeen. Next Dr. Ash put a potted geranium plant in the middle of the beam. The needle came down to fifteen. Now Dr. Ash held his hands out, palms facing each other, one hand on either side of the radiation beam, bringing the needle on the dial steadily downward until it came to fourteen. Then he had the whole class of twelve or fourteen students give it a go to prove to ourselves that we could really emanate a force or beam of our own from our hands.

Oh, I liked this. I told the person next to me, "When you go up there for your turn, wait just a bit. Watch the dial. I'm going to try to move it from here."

When he came back, he said, "Well, you jiggled it."

When I went up for my turn, I tried to block out all of the radiation. I tried to picture a solid block of the metal, lead, between my hands. The needle came down to thirteen, one more than the teacher's number.

Dr. Ash laughed. "You don't need to be here," he teased.

One girl said, "That ain't fair! You're an Indian."

The rest of the teaching went from placing the hands about five or six inches above a person's injury or burn or ill spot to placing the hands on an ill person's picture to using the hands for diagnosis.

As a seven in the Enneagram, I wanted more fun and excitement. I took to charging up round or oval stones full of energy, then placing them on the ill spot of a picture of an ill person. I lost interest in diagnosis because I thought, "If we can heal ANYTHING, then what does it matter what is wrong?"

When Dr. Ash finished teaching and left, I never saw him again. He did call once to tell me that Minnie's prediction of someone saying, ". . . and when you come here, you can do this other thing" came true.

Before we go on to bigger things, let me tell you what happened to Paul Bissell and Dr. Ash's one-strand spiderweb of wire.

What the wire did was it quieted the hammer noise down enough for Paul to sleep. Nevertheless, it sort of bugged Paul to know that something was still there.

One day Paul happened to be at Six Nations, so he decided to see what Daisy Thomas might have to say. Daisy had never been to Paul's house, but she could see it. She could see a small brush pile east of his house near his garden. Something not good was in that brush pile. Paul knew what she was talking about.

She told Paul to sneak up on this small brush pile, douse it with a coffee can of kerosene, and set it afire immediately. Then if he wished to see who was responsible for his lack of sleep, he should duck into the bushes and note who was the first to pass on the road and look at the fire.

Paul went home and followed her instructions. After he lit the fire, he hid and watched the road. In a little while Mad Bear came cruising past. He was eyeing the fire.

All went well for a while. Paul removed the wire. But now something else started up. Voices. Two people talking under Paul's bedroom window at night. It was hot that summer, so the window had to be left open. Paul would suddenly shine a light on the voices. No one would be there.

Back to Daisy Thomas sped Paul. He was losing much sleep.

"Oh, this one's simple," Daisy said, "Just throw a glass of whiskey on them voices. They'll shut up."

Paul did as Daisy told him to. In fact, he threw two glasses of whiskey. The voices left and never came back.

Paul slept for a month before anything else came. This time three glowing balls came bouncing around in the air outside of his windows. That is, they would go to whatever window Paul could see them from, and they would glow bright enough to get his attention. They were red, white, and blue.

About this time some ee'yog (gossip) went around, and it wound up in Paul's ears. He and his neighbor, Big Sy, had been having an ongoing boundary dispute. The ee'yog was that Big Sy had hired a witch to scare Paul into moving off the property.

Paul dug in his heels. He went to Daisy again.

"Oh, that's nothing. All you need is a gun and a silver bullet."

"SILVER BULLET? Where am I gonna get a silver bullet?"

"Oh, that's nothing." Daisy went into the next room and came back with some old Canadian dimes. "I'll sell you ten dimes. When them lights come looking in at you, you just let them see you cut these dimes up with a tin snips. Then dump the BBs out of a shotgun shell and fill the shell with them silver clippings. If the lights are still there, blast them."

This procedure tickled Paul. He could hardly wait. When the lights came, Paul showed them the dimes. Maybe Paul was too anxious, and this showed. Maybe his big eyes gave it all away. Whatever. As soon as he pulled out the tin snips, the lights split the scene and never came back. Paul never got to use his itchy trigger finger. I could see part of the shotgun stock protruding from between the wall and his refrigerator.

As I was leaving, Paul showed me his big-eyed grin. He pointed to the full-of-silver shotgun shell on the top of the fridge. "Sometimes I even oversleep now," he said.

What came next is in another part of this book, my overcoming of OO naa g'yeh (alcohol). Sometimes though, the connectedness of all things would make an unending story, maybe a huge cycle that would include reincarnation.

We can roughly say that in my case the period of the turnaround from alcoholic to recovering alcoholic was one month. The term *cycle* is significant. In the study of alcoholism recovery it has been discovered that the thirtieth day following the complete stoppage of alcohol intake by an alcoholic whose intention is never to drink again is when a strong and subtle urge hits again. If the alcoholic survives this sneaky compulsion, thirty days later this urge returns.

Thirty days later it's back again. This cycle may even vary enough to trick the "informed" alcoholic by a day or so in a sneak attack. There are also bound to be enough inexplicable individuals who have been unaffected by this cycle, who can then pooh-pooh such a phenomenon to the detriment of some other poor recoverer, who then succumbs to the "no such thing."

Ninety days of what had now become overconfidence: gone.

On day ninety this is what happened to me.

I was in the woods at the hideaway cabin with my wife. In fifteen minutes we were leaving to attend a birthday party. Alcohol there? I'll never know. If some benevolent Higher Consciousness, being, or protector did see an alcoholic catastrophe awaiting me, and if it stepped in to save me, it chose an alarming but sure-fire way to do it.

The view from the cabin was striking. The open porch looked into a lush deep valley that opened into rolling hills below. There was only one small thing. A tall eighteen-inch-diameter Chestnut Oak leaned out smack dab into the middle of the view of the rolling hills. No problem. With my big new chainsaw, I could drop that tree before we left for the party.

Did I talk to the tree and give it some Sacred Tobacco as I did to any other tree before I felled it? No. Is wanting a better view that was already spectacular a good reason to kill a sixty-year-old tree? Maybe that is why I said nothing.

A leaning tree is a potentially dangerous thing to fell. I didn't notch it properly, not deep enough. Before I was a little more than halfway through the tree, it started to go down.

Now let's see if I can tell this part right. The tree split its trunk upward from the depth of the cut of the saw blade. I continued cutting in an attempt to nearly sever it. A leaning tree falls fast. The one-third of the tree still part of the stump became a huge springy sliver, like a diving board. This took place in about two seconds.

From this moment on it was as though the tree became more animal than vegetable. As I started to run from the tree, the situation still seemed like "Oh this could be dangerous, I better make tracks." Quick acceleration on the side of a hill was not as forthcoming as I hoped in this circumstance, although two steps from the stump seemed to express the feeling "Whew! That was close!"

Where do you think the tree was at that moment? It was eight or nine feet directly over my head and moving in the same direction as I was moving. Maybe its shadow alerted me. I stopped and started back toward the stump.

Now this tree, which I say had become an animal, chased me. When I stopped, so did the oak. It stopped because it had slammed into a sturdy young maple, which springboarded it back at me. It had flown over my head in the first place because the big springboarded sliver of itself on the stump had propelled it with such tremendous force.

Down I went with the tree on me. I was half twisted with my face looking at the earth. The tree was on the small of my back. My legs were twisted up with the chainsaw, which, however miraculous anything like this could be, was shut off. I would not be attending any birthday party. I would not be threatened by alcohol. Death maybe, but not alcohol.

The pain in my back was barely bearable. I had screamed on impact, so it was only minutes before my wife was on her way to the nearest phone.

I imagine all people know when they are near death. I knew I was. Not the cocky, flippant me with the rose-colored glasses; another me knew. Also, with the swelling came the real pain. I think I went half crazy. I measured the tree with my one free hand. Eighteen inches. Sixty growth rings. I felt like hollering. My teeth were chattering.

The rescue squad came in about forty-five minutes. I begged the four men and one woman for some painkillers.

"Sorry. We are not allowed to dispense them. We'll get you to a hospital as fast as we can."

Everything took forever. Getting the tree off. Carefully and slowly straightening me out and slipping this special stretcher under me. Getting me up the steep bank to the rescue vehicle. The slow ride down the bumpy road and on to the hospital at Canandaigua, New York.

When we got to the hospital, that little voice inside of myself that was telling me I could die began to fade. It knew the extent of my injury, but now we had come to a place of doctors whose purpose in life was to fix people.

The first fix was the best. Demerol. The pain subsided. I don't know how long I spent in this hospital because as soon as the X rays were looked at, the word was, "We can do nothing. The third lumbar is split, and the fourth is in six pieces. Take him to Strong Memorial in Rochester. They have neurosurgeons there. Maybe they can do something. Whatever you do, drive with extreme care. No jerking."

On the road again, the little "you could die" voice came back. Just a month earlier I had seen a man die, and it had happened not far from the very place of my accident, making the hideaway camp area seem a bit jinxy. As I rode slowly toward Rochester, this "see death come" scene returned to me.

I had been on my way into the town of Naples, about five miles from camp. From the higher elevation near camp I could see a string of aircraft of some type coming in the distant valley toward Naples. I thought maybe they were gliders, and because they were a long ways off yet, I didn't get a much better look before the foliage of trees blocked my vision. I drove a good ways before another opening allowed a momentary view of the valley. In that flash view I saw, or thought I saw, what could only be the red of some aircraft falling straight downward.

If my eyes didn't deceive me, maybe someone had indeed crashed. I heard a police car siren coming from Naples. Yes, one of these small aircraft called an ultralite had crashed behind a local fruit stand.

Maybe I could help. I went to see. A small crowd stood near the pilot, who was sitting up on the ground. The ambulance and rescue people had not arrived yet.

The pilot was talking. He was telling what had happened. A gap in the ridge to his left had allowed a rush of wind to nearly bring his ultralite (which is not much more than a wing with a lawn mower motor for a prop drive) to a near stop or stall. He then stepped on the throttle. Up went the nose of the ultralite, to a vertical stop, then down it came backward to crash. This is what I had seen coming down.

The pilot was talking matter-of-factly. I stood only a couple of steps away listening. In midsentence he stopped talking. I was looking into his eyes. I saw death come into them.

This is something that I had witnessed before, but not in a human being. In the beginning of my bow-and-arrow hunting days I had shot a young buck from a tree at Montezuma Swamp. I was up too high, or at least I hadn't learned yet to aim lower. The arrow struck too high, or so I thought. The deer went down immediately. I slid down and approached it. We went eye to eye. At first contact the deer looked into my eyes. Then, as death came, it looked right through me, right past me. One little razor insert of the arrowhead had caused this. It just happened to fit between two vertebrae.

When the pilot's eyes did the same as the deer's eyes, I said, "He's dead."

I doubt anyone believed me. I heard a weak, "No."

So here I was in a rescue vehicle on my way to better experts with an inner voice telling me, "Be careful. A jagged piece of your broken spine might do to you what the razor insert did to the deer."

At Strong Memorial the story was the same. "We can do nothing. When the swelling goes down, we'll put a full cast on you. Maybe after six or eight weeks, we can go into your back. Maybe then there'll be something to fuse the bones to."

In a day or so I got the full cast. I was a bit silly on Demerol (Meperidine). With lots of time on my hands, I asked for some marking pencils and drew a full skeleton on the cast. Between the ribs, in color, were the heart, lungs, guts, and so on. The nurse said, "Morbid."

Next to me was a man named Merton Millspaw. I think he was Amish or Mennonite from McKean, Pennsylvania. He'd just received a new stainless steel ball joint in his hip. Maybe he was forbidden by his peers to use drugs because he kept groaning in pain. I told him, "If I could get over there, I'd do a healing on you to shut you up. All I can suggest is that tomorrow you order some orange juice, and I'll fill it full of healing."

I lay there thinking, "Wait a minute! WHOA! What's the matter with me? Why don't I heal myself???"

My arms were down at my sides. I bent them upward at the elbows. I cupped my hands slightly and aimed them about thirty degrees "above the horizon." I closed my eyes and started "zapping" the Universe with a solid beam of healing. "Whatever gets in the way gets healed," I said. Don't forget I was still on Demerol.

Expecting a response from a law that might not even be a law, I was thinking, "What you give is what you get."

After a while my palms began to tingle. "Oh, getting stronger, eh?" I said to the beam. "Good! Go to it!"

Soon my palms were really tingling. In fact, they were getting to a place of discomfort. I was just about ready to put the beams on my spine when the beams began pushing against my palms. In a short time the pressure from them was enough to start pushing my hands backward. I turned my hands downward and aimed the beams at my spine.

"YEOW!" The pain was too much. I aimed the beams up at the ceiling, but I didn't want to waste that energy. Seeing that I had a half-cup of grape juice on my stand, I put it on my cast and shot it full of healing.

After a while I lifted the paper cup and juice in a half salute toward Millspaw's bed. "That's too strong for him," I said with my mind and then drank it myself.

Blue Cross and Blue Shield don't like to pay for too many days in a hospital, so I got sent home. Even with two TVs and a radio going on Sunday to catch all the football games, life was still boring, especially for a seven in the Enneagram.

I began to wiggle and tense myself in my cast so as not to start wasting away. I was off the Demerol, and I felt no pain. I began thinking I might be healed. I began calling Dr. Chan, the neurosurgeon, and telling him so.

At first he just said, "No. No."

I persisted. Stubbornly.

Finally he got angry. "All right," he said, "I'm sending an ambulance after you, and I'll show you that you're not healed."

The X-ray technicians laid me out and ran this big picture taker over me. Then I had to wait.

While I was waiting, I heard Dr. Chan chewing out the X-ray technician for bringing the wrong pictures. More words followed. Then I heard Dr. Chan say, "I'll take the picture."

He did, and apparently the results were the same. The X rays showed a complete healing. The third lumbar had closed up. The fourth showed all six pieces back in place.

I'm sure that what made Dr. Chan so disbelieving is that there wasn't even a mark on either vertebra to show that there was ever a break.

The cast was removed. Earlier, when I still had it on, Mad Bear had sent me some bark from three trees: Wild Cherry, Sumac, and Prickly Ash. Using them would prevent rheumatism from setting into the injured area.

A week later I was asked back into the hospital. Dr. Chan had assembled a group of doctors to witness the miraculous cure. (That he had affected?) When I came in, he said, "Mr. Williams, how do you feel?"

I went into a wicked shimmy dance like a go-go dancer. "Doctor," I said, grinning, "I can boogie all night."

Afraid that I might fly into pieces like a smitten china doll, he rushed up and grabbed me. "No. No. No," he chastised.

When the other doctors had left, he took me into his office. "There's just one thing," he said, "I want to warn you. You may have an attack of rheumatism in your lower back one day."

"Too late. I have already taken some Indian Medicine for that."

A trace of a smile played upon his lips. He shook his head slowly from side to side. Then he made a little sweeping motion with his fingers at me. I haven't seen him since.

The Fire Monkey

Willie Chew lived on Chew Road near a place called Stateditch. It was an area of the reservation where people have seen unusual things.

Ducky Anderson was driving along one day when he saw a nice deer. Well, I call it nice because he could see right through it.

Just south of the ditch, on the east side of the road, the roadside is lined with small trees. Not so many that you can't see through them, and this particular year someone had a cornfield planted behind the trees. The strip of trees slants upward away from the road a bit, and the deer was walking along between the trees and the corn. Ducky said he could see right through the deer. He could see the leaves of the cornstalks on the other side of the deer. They were waving in the breeze.

Another time, Clem Hill and a friend hiked into this area, walking toward the Muck farms. Here, in a field, they saw, moving parallel to them, a roll of thick fog, like a giant caterpillar. They stopped to look at it. It stopped, too. They began to move again. So did the caterpillar.

At the end of the field was a dirt lane. They hurried toward it, the fog caterpillar keeping pace but still on a parallel course. When they reached the lane, they began to run, but then, not being able to see what happened to the big caterpillar, they went back for a look. They shouldn't have. It had turned and was coming toward them. This time when they ran, it was not down the lane. It was toward home. Home is the safest place, you know. You know how if you keep shooting at a fox, each time you shoot, it finds a faster gear? It was the same case here. The caterpillar was quite fast, but not as fast as fear. The boys left it behind them someplace.

People hearing about this said it was an omen to Clem to "thot ne heh west" (behave yourself) because shortly after that he went to jail for being naughty.

. . .

152

Another time Duke Jacobs was telling his fellow construction workers about all the ghosty phenomena he had seen. Nobody believed him, and one of them said, "Hey, Duke, why don't you show us some of this stuff?"

Duke was quiet for a moment, and they thought they had trapped him. Instead, Duke was running through an imaginary calendar in his head. "How about Thursday evening?" he said. "Come to my place on Chew Road."

On Thursday evening, only two fellow workers showed up, and they were carrying .12-gauge shotguns.

"What you got them guns for?" Duke asked. "You can't shoot a ghost with a gun. And besides, I don't see things every day; we probably won't see anything."

This calmed the two gun toters down some, but not enough for them to let go of their guns. So down the road the trio went.

"We didn't go far," Duke was to say later. "Maybe a couple hundred yards shy of Stateditch. On the right-hand side of the road was a bushy tree with a trunk about six inches in diameter. We were about fifty yards away from it when damned if it didn't start shaking. I mean really shaking. I was fascinated by it. I couldn't take my eyes off it. Behind me I could hear the footsteps of the guys running to their car, 'be(t)be(t)be(t) be(t) be(t) be(t).' They didn't even drive back down Chew Road. They took Deadman's Road even if it took them away from where they lived."

But back to Willie Chew.

Willie had a barn and a stable that was like another small barn because it had hay in it and a horse or two.

One day Horatio Jones, who was fresh back from Carlisle Indian School, came over to visit. Willie and Jonesy happened to go into the stable, and lo and behold, what did they see in there but a monkey. It looked just like any other zoo-type monkey, and that's probably what Willie thought, "A monkey escaped from a zoo."

Jonesy, though, had been around more in the world, and he glanced around thinking that an organ grinder might be asleep in the hay. Willie, being cool, merely watched the small animal with interest, but devilish Jonesy couldn't leave it alone. I say "devilish" because after a bit Jonesy got to chasing the monkey around with a pitchfork. The monkey was tremendously agile, but Jonesy had letters in all sports and was highly competitive, so he couldn't believe that a monkey could make a monkey out of him. It refused to leave the barn. Now, after he had bragged to Willie of his sports feats, Jonesy's ego was at stake. He jabbed the monkey in the butt with the pitchfork. He shouldn't have. The little monkey let out a screech and to both men's astonishment and consternation emitted flames from its nostrils or mouth and set the hay on fire.

With nothing but the old hand pump, which had to be primed for water, extinguishing the fire was a lost cause. To make it more impossible, Jonesy, in his avid desire to make amends, broke the cast-iron pump handle jerking it too hard.

As they watched the stable burn, Willie turned philosophical. He did not have a great command of the English language, and he disliked, as a Chief, having to go to Washington to speak for his nation, but he was more intelligent than most people thought.

He spoke of the Tuscarora name for monkey, *ga jeeg nogs* (it-lice-eats), and how we must walk the thin line between "making fun of" and "laughing with the truth when it is funny." He spoke of the power of the clowns in the Longhouse and the strong Medicine of the Heyokas, who personified the last lines of a poem by Lao-tzu: "When the Fool learns The Way, / he only laughs at it / Yet, if he did not laugh at it / It would not be The Way."

As though enticed by the dying embers, Jonesy exited the scene. There was no indication in Willie's measured words that he now spoke only to the Elements.

"Mocks Johnson used to tell of the Fire Monkey, but I never believed him. Maybe you wouldn't have either, but if you ask me, I don't think we ought to kick an old dog. It might be the devil or the Creator in disguise."

Deer

In the Thanksgiving Address, when we speak of the Element that includes all creaturehood, including those creatures of the sea as well as of the land, the deer is named as the principal one among them.

When a Chief is raised (ordained) in the Condolence Ceremony of the Six Nations Iroquois Confederacy, he will be told that, symbolically, deer antlers have been placed upon his head. The purpose of these sensory organs is to act as antennas to keep the Chief alerted to the direction of either danger or peace and safety, day and night.

The deer have Elders among them. They are not seen very often. I think that one time I may have been at the wrong place at the wrong time. I was up in a tree trunk at Montezuma Swamp. This very large tree had fallen and become wedged between some other trees at a spot about twenty feet off the ground. A deer trail crossed underneath the fallen tree.

I was drowsily gazing toward the trail south when I heard something. I looked north. Here came five magnificent stags trotting abreast. Elders. Ten points each or more.

I was well hidden in bunches of leaves. No matter. At about fifty yards, as though commanded by an officer, they all slammed on the brakes and ran back to where they came from. I automatically turned to see what had scared them, maybe someone walking on the ground. NO. At the very area I had just been watching were five Elder deer, an inkblot of the five I had just seen fleeing. They were slamming on brakes, too. Then they were gone.

In ten seconds I had seen more grand Elders of stags than I had seen in ten years. I think they were planning an Elders conference, and I screwed it up.

Deer make many sounds. You probably have heard them snort. It has a sort of swooshy sound to it. I get the feeling they are saying, "Just WHAT are you doing in my territory?!!"

They can bark. I once crept up on what I thought was a fox. I wanted to see what it was barking at. It was not a fox; it was two small deer.

Another time, in the late afternoon, I sat on a sparsely wooded hillside. This hillside was part of a bowl-shaped area that broke downward into a valley. It was perhaps three hundred yards across the "bowl." I expected to see groups of deer meander out of the surrounding woods to feed on the grassy patches within the bowl. Down at the bottom of the hillside of my side of the bowl grew a quarter-acre patch of scrub brush that looked impenetrable.

At just about the time that I was getting the feeling that maybe I ought to be starting the long walk back to my vehicle, a chorus of rapid grunt sounds came issuing from the thicket. Pigs could not have imitated themselves more perfectly. I thought, "Some farmer has turned his pigs loose up here; no wonder the deer are disassociating themselves from this place."

Next, there was the sound of the rustling of leaves as a sleek-looking doe came prancing out of the thicket. She was followed by five bucks wearing antlers in the six- and eight-point range. They began fighting each other for rights to the favors of the doe. They charged one another with lowered heads. One of the bucks, dashing from the group for distance to make a wicked charge into his adversaries, spotted me. An imperceptible order was given, and instantly all the deer were in flight. The jousting party was over. A human being, me, apparently cannot be tolerated under any deer circumstances, even for an evening of romance with a doe.

Automatic Transmission told me as much. We were walking in a place where Swamp Marigold grew. He said that some Medicine people used to eat this plant. Then they would throw up. Four times they would eat the Swamp Marigold, then throw up. They would become superpurified, could detect the most delicate of substances by smell. Of all smells among living things, it was reported, the human smell was the worst.

Communication between many living things must certainly be acute to instantly promote the greatest chance for survival. Witness the oneness of quick evasive movements of flocks of birds or schools of fish.

What does a snake say to a bird or toad when it zaps it and charms it? GOTCHA! As when Uncle Charley charmed or hypnotized a rabbit by pointing at it? Whatever a snake says to charm a bird out of the air has to be quick. Not "and now . . . you are gently going to go . . . into a deep . . . relaxed . . . peaceful . . . place" as a hypnotist might lull one into a hypnotic state.

So then there must be other and many forms of communication. The Venus Fly-trap luring its victims. Some exotic fish developing a part of themselves to look like enticing bait.

In the incident where a large deer had left an acquaintance and me, who were chasing it in a Volkswagon Bug, by accelerating from forty miles per hour to sixty-five or so, it was simply saying, "Good-bye."

The ghost deer that I had wasted a slug on was simply reiterating my father's dictation, "Don't hunt deer too early."

The deer that had participated in an "impossible" kill in Pennsylvania—the one who ended up as food for Chief Tracy Johnson and his family, who were at home starving and praying for food—gave them the message, "Prayer can be powerful."

The white deer that told me I didn't have to do a Sundance spoke not a word, but I got the message clearly.

One day, here in North Carolina, I saw a jet black deer. Our drive-in lane wends on past our house on down to an old Tobacco-drying "minibarn" and on past to a small bog pond. It's about fifty-five yards from the house to the barn.

On this day of misty rain I opened the door and started to step out toward the barn. The lane is woodsy on each side, making it a somewhat darkened passageway anytime, but even more so on this darkened day. So when I noticed what I thought were two stray hunting dogs not far up from the barn, I didn't pay much attention. Many hunters here own large bear-hunting hound dogs, and these dogs are forever getting lost, so we quite often see them. One of what I was paying scant attention to was tan, the other black. The rickety screen door I pushed open creaked, and the two "dogs' " heads stood up on long necks, and the two animals became two beautiful deer. They'd been grazing on grass.

I called to my wife, Diana, and together we—that is, humans and deer—formed two twosomes studying each other. This, of course, is always the time when the daughter has borrowed the camera. After some three to four minutes the deer unhurriedly turned and left. I realized then that I had never heard of anyone having seen a jet black deer.

The next day I was reflecting absentmindedly on the possible meaning of seeing a black deer. The phone rang. It was a message from Tuscarora that my cousin, Doc Patterson, had died. He had been an ironworker foreman for Red Dog. He had overseen the rebuilding of the Tuscarora Baptist church after it had burned down.

This church burning has nothing to do with deer, but because I may never get to tell you about it otherwise, with my memory in such shape that I can hide my own Easter eggs, I'll slip it in now.

The burning of any church in an isolated instance is nothing. Such things are bound to happen. But then, within a few days, the Medina Baptist church at Six Nations Reservation burned, too. Still maybe nothing, a mere coincidence. Just the same, both churches had lasted a very long time. The members of both churches visited each other's services from time to time.

Years ago Mocks Johnson told me about an entity whose Tuscarora name I have forgotten. It was a long name that meant "It-rumbles-along-under-the-ground." He said that when a family got to arguing and fighting in an overly spiteful manner, and if this caused a deep enough rift, this rumbling entity might pass under their house. In those times this entity was well known and greatly feared because if the rift wasn't mended, the house would burn down. I forgot that Mocks had said this.

Enter Tootsie the Liar. I was sitting at the counter of my mother's minirestaurant having a tea when Tootsie came in for coffee. I said, "Tell me something tricky."

"Like what?"

"Oh, tell me something unusual that ever happened to you."

He must have taken me seriously because he actually thought for a while. Then he chuckled, as was one of his identifying idiosyncrasies.

"Here's one," he said. "One night I got a flat tire near the Baptist church. It musta been a Wednesday. Wednesday night prayer meeting night. All of a sudden I heard a noise on the side of the road. On the church side. By jeez, it sounded like it was in the ground and getting louder and moving. Well, it was moving. It crossed the road right in front of me. You should have been there. The ground was shaking. I mean it. But then it kept on going. I was half scairt to keep going, but then Paul Bissell came by and lent me his jack."

"Did you tell Paul?"

"Yeah."

"What did he say?"

"He asked me what I'd been drinking."

Tootsie's brother, Mooh'mooh, said, "Oh, he's just a big baby. He only lies about half the time, but he went and gave himself a bad rep. He's a regular Ripley's."

"But one thing, he's a real Dunninger for finding deer. A real Daisy Thomas."

That was true enough, but his reputation for finding deer came much more slowly than his reputation for fibbing. It started in the Adirondack Mountains. Wherever he went, there would often be the only deer seen that day. He himself was not the best hunter or best shot, and he was quite lazy. But if a deer was gotten, you could bet Tootsie had been somewhere in the vicinity.

A bunch of hunters "drove" the Commons Woods (walked abreast to push deer to the watchers). That was the time Gary Patterson saw the ghost deer and shot at it. Then, being too embarrassed, he said, "My gun went off accidentally."

It was also the same hunt in which, after shooting at nothing, the witchy Commons got him so disoriented that he never finished the drive. Instead, he went straight home because he would have been so late arriving at the "watcher's line" that no one would have been there, or if they were, they would have teased him: "The great hunter got lost, didn't you? Look at them scratches on your face. Your hair's all messed up. You been running, haven't you!"

When the drivers did finish the drive, the feeling, because no deer were seen, was, "Well, we tried, but that's it for me. I'm too tired to try anything more."

So what did Tootsie say? He hadn't walked. He was on "watch" closest to the main road and to the vehicles. "I think there's some deer back of Chester's."

"Go get 'em then," one tired guy says, producing laughter all around.

Nevertheless, two hunters went there. It was only a quarter of a mile away. There were seven deer there. They each got one.

The following year ten or twelve Tuscaroras went to the Red House area near Salamanca, New York. A certain farmer let them hunt his woods every year, so they made this two-hour vehicle trip their first stop. Tootsie wanted to go along, and they let him, even though his draggy habits put them a half-hour behind time.

When they arrived at the farm, the farmer greeted them with his arms up in the air. "Gee, fellas . . . I'm so sorry . . . I didn't think you were coming this year, so I let another group of hunters go in. . . . I'm truly sorry."

From where the group stood they could look down the road and see three Jeep-like vehicles parked along the edge of the woods in which they had so looked forward to hunting. The other hunters were emerging from those woods and making ready to drive off. The eyes of the disappointed Tuscaroras focused on Tootsie.

"There's deer in them woods," he said, tapping his finger in the air in the direction of the place that had just been hunted.

Sure, Tootsie. The hunters tiptoed around them so as not to disturb them.

Nevertheless, the disappointed group of Indians presented the farmer with a bushel of apples as they did every year, then prepared to go through the motions even though they didn't expect to find any deer.

Half went one way and half the other to form a pincer movement. This strategy would cut the time of the hunt in half. In a short time there came a volley of explosions. Soon, a gaggle of rejuvenated hunters exited the woods dragging three male deer. Tootsie was all smiles. It was as though he had perpetuated a rite of veneration. Indeed, where DID these deer come from? Irresistible apple smell? Irresistible Tootsie?

Here's another highly unusual deer incident that also took place involving hunting. For my son Tom's birthday present, I took him to Pennsylvania's Tioga Wild Boar Preserve to let him see if he could get a boar with a bow and arrow. His birthday is April 4, so the Saturday of the weekend nearest that date became the day we had reserved to hunt.

When I mentioned our plans to some of my coworkers, two carpenters who were also bow hunters expressed a desire to go with us. A phone call confirmed that this was fine with the person at Tioga who did the scheduling.

The weather on the day of the hunt was perfect. The setting is that of an old abandoned farm, maybe a large beef cattle farm covering acres and acres of rolling countryside, some of which had now become wooded. Different areas had been fenced off for the harboring of various species of exotic game.

The owner greeted us heartily. Another group of hunters had preceded us and were listening to his spiel of what you can and can't do. We joined in to listen.

As he spoke, a chromey king-cabbed pickup truck drove in and came up so close that a couple of us had to move aside. The driver wore a ten-gallon hat. With him was his eight- or ten-year-old son. It was as though the driver was saying, "I'm here, and I've come right on top of you, so you can get a good squint at these here silver-engraved rifles on this Impala-horned rack in the back window!"

Ten Gallon got out and horned right in on the owner's conversation. "Whaddaya do if one a'them boar critters charges you?"

Disregarding the impolite intrusion, the preserve owner answered, "Simple. You just stand there calmly until the boar is about three feet away coming full bore. Then you jump like you never jumped before in your life!"

Lord, did we laugh. Ten Gallon walked off to look the place over. In the meantime his son was doing just that.

Around this "staging area" were a number of cages displaying a few exotic small animals and birds. Nearby, in full view, was a good-size wire cage in which a large Chinese pheasant showed off its long black-and-white tail. The boy had been studying it. "Hey!" he yelled, taking two running steps toward us, "WHAT'S THIS?"

"Son," the owner said, "That's a robin."

"DAD! DAD!" the boy called, "COME AND LOOK AT THE ROBIN!"

Ten Gallon got the message. "Come on, Everett, let's go get a hotdog someplace." They left.

We went in as a group—the two carpenters, son Tom, a guide, and myself. I was simply a tag-along.

We had scarcely gone fifty yards when I took note of six white deer somewhat off to the right of the direction that we were walking. These deer didn't seem overly concerned with our presence, and I had this fleeting thought, "For a hunter with a high-powered rifle that has a telescope sight on it, this is HUNTING?" (The various species of game had various price tags assigned them. The rarer, the costlier.)

I assumed that we were all mainly concerned with the sighting of wild boar because no one paid any attention to the white deer. I became curious as to whether they were albinos or not. I hoped to get close enough to see their eyes better. Did they have the pink iris and red pupil, or did they have dark eyes? If we continued in the direction we were walking and if the deer did not run, the closest we would come to them would be about forty yards.

As it turned out, the deer did not run, and at this distance I could see quite clearly that they had dark eyes, the same as any other regular deer.

On we went to a full day of successful hunting, Tom making a spectacular shot on a boar. While we waited for one of the carpenters to get his boar, Tom lucked into a tom turkey and collected that, too, a feat for any bow hunter. By day's end we were a tired but happy group that left Pennsylvania for home.

In the month of August of that same year Tom and I were visiting Mad Bear. Now EVERYONE knows that if you visit Mad Bear, it is mandatory that you play chess. He just automatically gets the board out and methodically sets it up, piece by piece, and you WILL play a game. After which you WILL eat.

In the middle of the game Bear carefully lifted the game board and set it aside, saying, "I just thought of something. Just remember, it's still my turn." (Which it wasn't.) We smiled.

"Both of you get around more than I do. Both of you hunt. Some Indians in California called me; they want to do a White Deer Ceremony, but they wonder if they could ever find a white deer. Do either of you know where there might be one?"

I answered. "We both saw six white deer at Tioga in Pennsylvania in April, remember, Tom?"

Tom said, "No."

What? Well, I'm sure Tom had just forgotten. NO ONE could have not seen those deer, but I wouldn't embarrass him, so I said, "I'll just check it out and see if this place does have a white deer."

Bear replaced the game board. "OK, let me know."

The next day, Monday, I was back at work at the Eastman Kodak Company in Rochester, New York. I looked up the two carpenters who had accompanied Tom and me on the boar hunt in April.

"Remember the six white deer we saw at Tioga in April when we left the parking area to try for boar?" Both men looked at me a bit puzzled. "No," they said.

"Oh," I said, equally puzzled, "I must be thinking of a different place that I went. A different time."

I could scarcely wait to get home to call Tioga. When I did get home and made the call, I found myself hedging on asking the question that had now put me strangely in the "odd man out" category of a "who saw what" situation. Instead, I asked another question first.

"When we were there on a hunt in April, I noticed in your brochure that you had eight hundred dollars listed as the price for hunting white-tailed deer. How come so high?"

A laugh came through the phone. "That's because we don't have any. We had some, but they kept jumping the fence and running away. We raised the fence height to ten feet. Hey, that's the height of the basket in basketball. They still jumped the fence and got away. I gave up. We don't HAVE any white-tail deer. If anyone is crazy enough to pay eight hundred dollars for a white-tail deer, then they're crazy enough to let me go out and jacklight one for them." (Likely, eight hundred dollars was the fine for jacklighting.)

"Ahem. In April, when we went in for the boar, I saw you had six white deer, three bucks and three does. By any chance do you still have them?"

A silence came from the other end of the line.

Did the person I was talking to have a heart attack? A stroke? I waited. After a while the voice came back on.

"Ted," the game farm operator said, "I have exactly what you are asking about. I have six white deer. Three bucks and three does, but you never could have seen them. You see, I just got them last week."

"Great!" I exclaimed, "I know you can't reserve one of them on my say so because I'm not the one looking for a white deer, but someone special is. Some Blackfoot Elders want to do an old traditional White Deer Ceremony, but they had sort of despaired on ever finding a white deer. I'll have them call you."

"Do! You know what, Ted? I'm going to donate them the deer they want."

Before I called Bear to have him relay the good news, I reflected on seeing those white deer in April. That's right! No game farm operator would have let six white deer roam free near the parking lot. They could have just walked right on down the driveway the same way we came in. They could have run away! But if they did, one of them would have screwed up. One of them could not have been part of a great ceremony.

The place where my wife and I used to live was already not easy to find because it was about five miles up into the foothills of the Smoky Mountains plus another mile off the main road. Now we have built a place (from the White Pines that fell during the big snowstorm of 1997) another mile farther from civilization. It's ad-jacent to the Pisgah National Forest (the reason for a padlocked gate). When the real estate agent was showing Diana all his parcels of land, he showed her this one last of all because he was afraid it was too remote a place. To make things even "worse" for him, there was a light film of snow on the ground, and when they stepped out of his vehicle, what did they see but the large footprints of a pan-ther (supposedly extinct here).

Of course, Diana asked, immediately, "What are those tracks?"

Now, the agent felt trapped. What more could there be to discourage a sale? He used up all the time he dared, pretending to inspect the tracks, but actually stalling for time to think something up. It was no use. "Panther tracks."

"I'll take it!" she said.

Well, the thing about the deer that happened here can wait. Let me tell you first about what happened at the place where we previously lived.

Most all of the land around here is forested, mostly White Pine. Toward the west, however, from where our rented cottage stood, was an open area, a shallow valley, a hayfield about the size of a football field.

I play disc golf, a game much like regular golf except a frisbeelike disc is thrown instead of a golf ball hit by a golf club. I practiced throwing discs in this field, and one year an eight-point buck would graze nearby as long as I kept doing my thing. If I stopped, the white-tailed buck would lift his head and study me until I minded my own business again. Each evening anywhere from four to eight deer would mosey down from the woods and graze on into the night.

We had a large white gentle dog, Molly, a Siberian sheepdog called a Ku-vatz. She often slept on the grass in that field, but near enough to the house so that the deer no longer paid Molly any heed.

One early evening, though, six does came down from the woods with some-thing new, a newborn fawn.

So what did the fawn do? As soon as it spotted this white curly-haired thing, Molly, it trotted on spindly legs in a straight line toward the dog. The mother was frantically pawing the ground in an effort to call her baby.

I'd been watching the deer from our roofed-over back porch, and I got a sud-den strong urge to whistle and call Molly back to the house. She was getting old like I was, and maybe we were becoming testy and didn't know it. I guess I didn't whistle because the scene was too mesmerizing. What would a big dog do with a little deer? Eat it?

Just as this spotted little animal got to Molly, she woke up. She lifted her head, and the two animals smelled noses. Molly then went back to sleep. The fawn dilly-dallied back to the grown-ups and got a sharp "spank" nudge of Mom's snout on its butt.

I found myself standing up. There were some tiny beads of sweat on my forehead. I hadn't trusted the power of innocence and gentleness to come through.

The next somewhat similar deer incident may have occurred to further convince me of the power of meekness.

On past where we now live stands the old Waldroup homestead. Though no one lives there, the property is still kept up and the grass mowed around the old farmhouse. Fred Waldroup told me I could toss my discs there if I could find an area level enough to do so.

One early afternoon I drove up toward this open area. It's within walking distance but . . . carrying forty discs?

Just as I came up over the hill to where everything was easy to see, I had to stop. Here was a sight to behold.

Six grown-up wild turkeys were starting to cross the lane in front of me. This was unusual enough, but they had also formed a circle of maybe twenty feet in diameter. And what do you think was in the center of the circle? A spotted fawn.

Did they spook? Oh no. The turkeys were "riding shotgun" for the little princess of the woods, and they just smoothly continued on across the lane and into the woods, which sloped downward, and out of sight.

It was as though, in meekness, the fawn had already inherited the earth.

The Sturgeon

One day, in the *Democrat and Chronicle* newspaper of Rochester, New York, there appeared an article in the out-of-doors section that claimed that there were no longer any sturgeon in Lake Ontario. Showing the article to my children, I said, "Well, let's find out. I know a Medicine that will call a sturgeon."

By the time I finished work at Rochester and got the children, a fly-beard spear, and the Medicine root *(Arctium major)* at Tuscarora, it was near 11:00 P.M. before we were ready. We chose the old sturgeon fishing dock at the lower Niagara River, which is not far from Lake Ontario. This fishing spot was known as "the Rail" because an old bent railroad rail protruded out over the river at this place. To get to the Rail, one had to walk a treacherous little trail along the steep bank of the gorge. This trail could be reached from Art Park at Lewiston.

When we arrived at Art Park, with not another soul to be seen, we were treated to a spectacular sign—a beautiful rainbow. A light green rainbow. A huge beam of neonlike light arose from where we might have guessed. The Rail is located and curved upward and back down at about the edge of Lake Ontario.

"Look at the laser beam!" son Bob shouted. "Let's go and see the pot of gold at the end of the rainbow!"

We had to rush up the long incline at Art Park to even reach the trail and get a look down into the gorge to see what the cause of this phenomenon might be.

Serendipity. I wish now we had just stopped and looked at it. Its diameter was seven or eight feet.

I wonder now, had we had a camera, would it have let us take a picture? As we neared the point of being able to see its place and cause of origination, blink! Out it went.

Now we had to be extremely careful. Even in the daytime, a misstep in the loose shale could cause one to tumble headlong to severe injury if not death. Finally, an hour or so later, we made it to the Rail. Here we put the Medicine in the water after first tying it to a stone large enough to keep it from washing away. The children, Bob and Mike, began calling, "Ga rah!" (sturgeon), toward Lake Ontario.

We backtracked about eighty yards to a relatively flat spot, pitched a little tent, and went to sleep. Just before daylight I heard a noise. Someone walking. Two people. It was Jim Rickard and a friend of his carrying fishing rods. They were headed for the area of the Rail.

I tried to get the boys awake, fearing that if a sturgeon did appear at the Medicine, it might disappear if the fishermen frightened it, and we'd never get to see it. It was no use. The boys were too deep in sleep. Sand-manned.

I needn't have worried. In a few minutes Jim and friend came rushing back. "Bring the spear! There's a big sturgeon at the Rail!"

We managed to arouse Bob and Mike, and as a group we went to investigate. Dawn came with us and showed us the sturgeon. Its back was a few inches above the water. I didn't want to kill it, so I made a feeble stab to send it on its way. Instead it only went a few feet and stopped. This was too much for Jim. He took the spear from me, nailed the fish, and pulled it out. We took it to the Lewiston fish market and weighed it. Eighty pounds. Amazingly, one fourth of it, twenty pounds, was caviar.

I never told the sportswriter in Rochester that he was wrong. He might better go on believing that there are no more sturgeon. Or sturgeon Medicine. Or green rainbows.

This is the teaching of Medicine to one's children. It excited me to be able to do this. The children, though, jumped back into the car and went to sleep. They probably thought, "Yep. There is such a thing as sturgeon."

The following year the state of New York put sturgeon on the "protected" list. So if you want to know just when all this happened, go look up the year the sturgeon made the list.

Six Nations, One Humanity

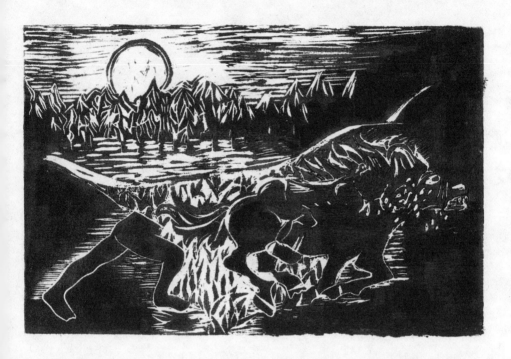

Overleaf: The Ooh du(t) cheah (Half-a-woman), which frightens men into good behavior; see "Medicines of the Universe," pp. 225–29. Woodcut by Rhiannon Miles Osborne.

The Great Law of the Great Peace

What constitutes greatness? Is it in the eyes of the beholder?

Ask a hundred different people and get a hundred different answers, ranging from different categories of priority—rareness, beauty, music, and so on, to "what degree of greatness must be present to earn that title."

For great people, we first may hear well-known names like Mother Teresa, Mohammed, Martin Luther King, Jesus Christ, Mahatma Gandhi, Abraham Lincoln, Gautama Buddha, Stephen Hawking, Charlie Parker, Keats, Einstein, A. S. Byatt, Chris Connors—until we begin hearing of lesser-known individuals and then hear names we have never heard of.

I might name Lulu Gansworth, Leon Shenandoah, Automatic Transmission, Daisy Thomas, Rashan Roland Kirk, Sadie Mann, Charley Johnson, Degonawida, Barbara Patterson, Isaiah Joseph. Dead people. Gems hidden in obscurity.

But this brings us to an important crux regarding greatness. Supposing, regarding people, one could not be called great unless one had reached enlightenment. What? And just how do we gauge that? Someone might say, "Well, let's start with Jesus Christ and go upward from there into Higher Consciousness in naming names."

Well, at the risk of naming Empty Cloud too many times in the book, I still can't think of a better example of exactly what I am getting at here.

Let us picture ourselves as having been present at this exemplary happening where, suddenly, all the bells in town start ringing, all at once, all by themselves. Then we hear someone whom we deem the wisest among us say, "Oh wow! An enlightened person approaches. Let us rush to meet them!"

So as we rush down the narrow path, at about three-quarters of a mile distance, and run into a "beggar" who is blocking our way. Bam! We knock him out of the way and rush on. The beggar, who is Empty Cloud the enlightened person, asks the last of our cascade of people what the "ado" is all about; then he, also wanting to "see" an enlightened person, joins the pack and rushes down the path, too.

How far do we "rush" before we realize that we have failed to recognize enlightenment?

The very fact that Empty Cloud was so humble that he couldn't know that he WAS a "bundle of power," an enlightened person, is a crucial part of why he was enlightened. Put THAT in your pipe and smoke it.

It must be, then, in order to get to this rarified place, we need to do something more than watch TV. So what if we all went on a huge vision quest? At the end of ten days and ten nights we would ask, "What is it we must do to reach enlightenment?"

And the answer would be, "Oh, all you need to do is love one another, all of your family, all of the Elements of this Divine and Harmonious Universe."

So great things are rare, and very great things are very rare. This, then, is why all the great Medicine plants are so rare—or actually, in many cases, just hard to see. We are just not ready yet. Many great, great Medicine plants have not even been seen yet. When that great Medicine that cures the common cold is found, it will likely be so common that we have failed to see it.

Enter the Great Law of the Great Peace. Anyone having heard a rendition of it might describe it as an epic narrative. Then, pressed, one might say, "Well, it's something like 'the Way' you know, the Tao, the Taoist 'Way' to enlightenment."

The Great Law's greatness is in its simplicity. Simple? Well, what you think you are hearing is a long bedtime story; but if you're not careful, great lessons will slide smoothly over your head.

For instance, the law of adoption.

"The adopter must love and want to adopt the adoptee. The adoptee must love and want to be adopted by the adopter. When this situation exists, the Chiefs SHALL SANCTION THE CEREMONY."

Not twenty thousand dollars, two attorneys, and a judge—no, love is the only necessary criteria.

Greatness.

Or one might be listening to the lengthy naming of the original fifty Chiefs of the confederacy as required in the Condolence Ceremony. In the process of the "raising" of new Chiefs, one might tend to daydream a bit and miss the ensuing, "And it shall be your [the inductees'] duty that your skin shall be seven spans thick, for all manner of criticism shall rain down upon you. But if you conform to your duty, which is to make this a better world for the unborn, then, if you are all confronted with an important decision to make, it will be easy for all of you Chiefs to be of one mind."

Can you imagine the Constitution of the United States being that simple? A short-cut to greatness.

Picture, then, ten days of narration, starting with the "cause" of the formation of the Iroquois Confederacy—that cause itself being the Great Law of the Great Peace.

It started with the birth of a male child in Huron country, an immaculate conception. Of course, the mother of the pregnant daughter was furious when her daughter insisted that she had not been with a man, that there WAS NO father.

This "grandmother-to-be" then plotted to kill the child of her "liar" daughter.

So after the birth of the child, one day when the opportunity arose, Grandma chopped a hole through the ice of a body of water and pushed the infant into the hole to be drowned. But this was no ordinary baby, and Grandma should have realized this when she returned home from performing her wicked deed: WHAT WAS THIS? Here, peacefully nursing in its mother's arms was the "drowned" infant. It had unexplainably beaten the grandmother back to the house.

Instead of seeing the light, the grandmother went berserk. She tried twice more to kill the child before realizing that she was part of the source of a very very special little person.

The ensuing section of the Great Law now goes on, in a sagalike presentation, to portray the growth and development of this enlightened being, the Peacemaker . One might be easily led to consider this saga as pure mythology until at some subtle point, any member of the Six Nations will realize, "Eureka! This tale has become my recognizable history!" A living thing with a consciousness of its own.

Much of the greatness of the Great Law resides within the exploits of the Peacemaker as he goes about consummating his manifest destiny of forming a "united nations," the Iroquois Confederacy.

Right from the start, as the Peacemaker drifts southward, he employs a radical concept. He needs help, a trusted aide. Does he seek the most benevolent person he can find? No. He seeks the worst. "For every degree of evil that a person or thing displays, so does he have the same capacity for good." Good is hard to see, but not evil.

Enter He a wat tut (Hiawatha), that naughty boy. Well, he is bad until he comes under the influence of the Peacemaker. His emergence into enlightenment is a powerful episode, too. At one point his wife and all of his daughters become ill and die, one by one, each death devastating He a wat tut until he all but commits suicide in grief. From this rock-bottom place, from this lengthy comatose ordeal, comes a great Medicine-like awakening. He becomes intrinsically aware that other human beings might also suffer his degree of grief, and with a vow to help them he makes the first original string of Sacred Wampum to give to suffering humanity. It would be like, "BANG! All your suffering, all your grief will go into this Wampum," and as he did, as he hung that Wampum on a rack, he became enlightened. He went on to make a series of strings of "symbols of cures" for all of our psychological illnesses. It is not easy to grasp the depth of greatness of these acts.

So when these two benevolently enlightened beings, the Peacemaker and He a wat tut, embark on their "peacemaking" journey, it is hard to imagine anything being able to stop them; and despite a host of tribulations, nothing can.

Bill Scott and I traveled from the Indian Center at Rochester, New York, to the Oneida Indian Reservation ten times, a distance of more than a hundred miles, to hear Jake Thomas, who traveled over twice that far (from the Six Nations Indian Reservation at Osweken, Ontario) to expound the Great Law. His skill at oratory engaged everyone's attention through much of his discourse, but once in a while he would use a trick or two to jar our awareness quotient.

He was telling about one of the initial confrontations between the Peacemaker and one of the potential Indian nations. The Peacemaker was being assessed with wary eyes by the senior leaders of this nation. "Who is this stranger to tell us that peace brings power and righteousness?"

When the Peacemaker had first come close to the area, he had set up a small camp. The smoke from his little fire had aroused the vigilant people's awareness of his presence, and they had thus come to investigate.

They as much as said to him, "Go back to bed! We'll discuss your dizzy notions and return tomorrow morning with our decision."

They spoke loudly, not because of any elevated temper but because they happened to be standing near the banks of a noisy, raging river.

The next morning they met again, under a large tall tree whose roots had, for years, quenched the thirst of the tree from the river. There, the Elders rendered their decision.

"We have come to a satisfactory decision. You climb to the top of this tall tree. We will then cut the tree down, and you will be dashed violently into the middle of this tumultuous river. We will then return to our homes. Tomorrow morning we will return to this meeting place. If you are here to greet us, we will commit to the acceptance of your ambitious scheme."

If these people expected the Peacemaker to depart posthaste, they were quite shocked to see him unhesitatingly climb to the top of the tree.

At this point Jake Thomas noted that, despite his narration being at a climatic posture, some of his audience was nodding off.

He said, "SO THEY TOOK A CHAINSAW AND CUT THE TREE DOWN!"

Jake brought down the house. The evoked laughter aroused the whole audience to grasp the clear meaning of ". . . and now you know the rest of the story," which was:

As dawn broke the following morning, campfire smoke was seen rising from the Peacemaker's camp.

And now you know the rest of the story.

Some time ago, around 1991 or so, Grandmother Twylah of the Cattaragus Seneca Indian Reservation initiated a series of Peace Elder conferences that were initially to span four years in east, south, west, and north locations. These conferences drew Elders from all over the world, and on their own strong momentum, they continue to find new locations. The conference even met twice in 1997.

At or maybe somewhere between the first and second one, I learned about aboriginal peoples in Australia who had among them great seers called Dream Walkers. Along with that information, it was said that these seers had put out the word that "somewhere in the world there were people called Iroquois and that these people had the secret to world peace."

Among the Six Nations, strings of Quahog clam shell Wampum have a significant usage in the accompanying of a message—similar, in general, to a notary public-stamped document. To me, though, a message with Wampum sends chills up my spine, as if I were witnessing the essence of the Creator at work.

In my first experience of Wampum-message I was a youngster sitting in the Tuscarora Baptist church. On this warm day the windows and front door were open. Off in the distance I heard a cry. Presently it became louder. The cry was "KWA UHH!" This cry came at intervals, and the loudest one, directly in front of the church, scared me. I heard otherworldliness in it. Later, my father told me that the message was informing us that a Chief of the Six Nations had died and that the runner was carrying a black Wampum.

I tell you this story because the Dream Walkers had made a Wampum-like meaningful thing to accompany their words regarding the Iroquois and world peace. It was a wreathlike object about four feet tall of sacred Medicine things. It was to accompany their message, which would be delivered at universities in various cities in the United States. I think funding for this tour ran out, and I never got to attend and hear or see a presentation. In the many semi-invisible laws of the Universe, the true meaning of this missed opportunity and the message itself may have gone over my head anyway. I say "semi-invisible" because all great Medicine things can only come to us when we are ready. We probably have stepped over many four-leaf clovers hiding among the trees.

Incidentally, Wolf Song I, the Peace Elder conference at Cattaragus Reservation, represented the direction east, the direction of dawning or spiritual awakening. Wolf Song II represented the south and came to the Thunder-Horse Ranch in Texas, hosted by Mary Thunder and her husband, Horse. Wolf Song III, it was announced, would be held at Los Angeles, representing the west. When subsequent news came that Los Angeles was out and that Australia had taken its place, I said, "Ooh la la!" recalling the Dream Walkers' message.

So I went to Australia overly excited. And just like the times when I bow hunted white-tailed deer overexcitedly and would already be planning what I would do with the deer when I got it, I wouldn't see any. The Dream Walkers did not speak English and likely did not wish to be near anyone who did. So their Medicine, just like other great Medicines that are invisible to those not ready, remained invisible.

So if one of the greater of Medicines, the secret to world peace, does reside within the Great Law of the Great Peace, it has remained hidden to the world, at least to this date.

It is not my purpose to suggest that the secret to world peace is surely hidden in a "law of right living" that is inaccessible to most people. Maybe it is. I asked Isaiah Joseph, whom I considered the wisest of Medicine people, "Why don't we get to hear the Great Law more often?"

He said, "To expose a great Medicine too often where there may be the slightest disbelief is to risk diluting that Medicine. Would you often cast pearls before swine?"

A great Medicine will be perceived as having the ability to hide. A very great Medicine, using this analysis, may then never get to be seen. So, too, by this line of thinking, will a very great concept hide; that is, it will be too deep to see, too obvious to anyone incapable of exhibiting the level of love of Soong gwi oo dee sut eh (the Creator). You have heard it said, "When you are ready, your teacher will come."

So we have the Great Law of the Great Peace, but do we have it at a level to live it?

Freeman Sowden

I was at the Six Nation Reservation in Canada, learning to do a ten-day feast for families of dead people, and the teacher was named Harry Henhawk. He had only one arm. At some point he told me a story. We were discussing how any particular cure was ever first discovered. I suggested that maybe the law that says that the more dire the illness or the situation, the faster the Medicine worked—that maybe the desperation or the urgency to do something in a person of compassion put out vibrations that called in the needed Medicine.

"Yeah! Yeah!" Harry interjected, "I think you're right. I know a man that did just that. Freeman Sowden. He's Cayuga.

"I happen to go with him to see the horse show at the Paris fair [Paris, Ontario]. While we were there, a white man came up to him and asked him if he was Freeman Sowden. The man had been to Freeman's house, and his wife had told him that he was at the fair with a one-armed man, so that's how he found us.

"The man begged Freeman to come with him and see something. He took us to his automobile, and inside was a small girl with a sack over her head. He took the sack off, and when he did, I thought I had never seen a more terrible sight. The girl's face was a mass of scabs and pus.

"The man said that he had taken his daughter to great doctors all over the world, and none had been able to cure her, not even find out what was wrong with her.

"Freeman looked the girl over for quite some time, but he didn't say anything. Then he just stood there like he was watching something way out past the parking lot. He had his eyes shut. After a while he told the man that he thought he might help the girl, but that the girl would have to live at Freeman's house for at least two weeks, maybe longer.

"The man didn't want to do this. He didn't want to tell people who would ask about his daughter that she was living with some Indians. But what could he do? So he finally said he guessed it would be alright."

Harry Henhawk shook his head. Maybe we all can call a Medicine. Did Freeman have something more than we do? More compassion?

I told him about the great shrinking of a huge tumor at Monawaki by the injection of human tears. Were they special tears? Were they from someone of great compassion? How do you gather them? If you see someone crying, do you say, "Wait, let me get a bucket and catch your tears?" Uncle Charley cried a lot while praying for people, and he certainly had compassion, or there wouldn't be any tears to gather.

But there was more to the story about Freeman Sowden curing the scabby girl. Whatever the Medicine was that came to Freeman, it worked, and the girl became completely cured in two weeks.

Harry Henhawk continued his story. "Now Freeman was a hero. The man wanted to pay Freeman a large sum of money, a hundred times more than Freeman had charged him. Freeman said no, that Medicine doesn't like that, that maybe the scabs could come back if he did. So the man, on the sly, got Freeman's address from his wife, and every year after that a package would come with new overalls and shirt with no return address.

"In those days Freeman was a big man. As he got older, he shrunk, and, after that, when the package came, he'd laugh because he knew that the clothes inside were way too big for him.

"One day I was in Toronto, and a beautiful woman came up to me and said, 'You don't know me, do you?'

"I said, 'No, I don't believe I do.'

" 'Well,' she said, 'I was the little girl with the bag over my head at the Paris fair.' "

Now, of course, I had to meet this man, Freeman Sowden. I wanted to see what such a tricky man looked like.

My chance came on a Sunday, and when I stopped at Ron Farmer's store in Osweken, called Farmer's Dell, I was told that Freeman's house was easy to find. All I had to do was go past Sixty-nine Corners and see a log cabin on the left-hand side of the road. Well, I drove up and down that road between Sixty-nine Corners and the next corner but never saw a log house.

Finally, in frustration, I drove past the next corner and came to the Medina Baptist church. I drove into the churchyard, which was quite full of cars. I sat in my car wondering what to do. I didn't have on what some Indians call Sunday-go-meeting clothes.

Just as I was deciding to leave, an old rusty pickup truck drove in. A smallish man with white hair and blue eyes came out of the passenger side.

"Sir," I said to him, "Could you tell me where Freeman Sowden lives?"

"I'm Freeman Sowden," he said.

Well, even now I don't know what got into me to say to him what I did. I think it may be like Empty Cloud being trampled by people rushing down the path to see "the enlightened one" because he looked like a tramp: I expected Freeman Sowden to look so, so special. Or maybe I tried to funny scold him as some of his peers might do. I wanted to be IN.

I said, "Why are you so late for church?"

Freeman smiled a powerful smile. He would never have to floss. His teeth did not squeeze against one another. He spoke nice and slow, saying, "Waaal . . . I walked to the end of my driveway . . . if a car came and gave me a ride one way . . . I would go to lacrosse game . . . if one gave me a ride the other way . . . I would go to church."

I knew he was big Medicine. That is the way Medicine lives. Like the great Bertha Groves would say if you asked her a question like, "Would you like a soda cracker? Or also there's pheasant under glass?"

"Whatever."

The reason I couldn't find Freeman's log house was that it was no longer a log house. He had made so much money selling a certain remedy that he had covered the log house with siding. He was even in the process of building what he called "a little hospital," after which he flashed that powerful smile.

I got to watch him put together this remedy that monetarily sided his house. His wife, who spoke so softly when she said her name that I never heard it, sat across from him at the kitchen table. Between them, on the table, were four big dishpans, each containing four different Medicines. One contained small sections of a small green vine that I recognized. One contained a buff-colored fluff not unlike that of the Oyster Plant, except a longer fluff. The other two pans contained two different kinds of bits of tree bark that I could nowhere near recognize.

Next to Freeman was a pile of bags, maybe four-by-five inches, made from unbleached muslin. He would put a certain amount from each pan into a bag and pass it to his wife, who, waiting with needle and thread, would quickly sew the bag shut. Even though Freeman was slow and deliberate, it was amazing how accurately he apportioned the right amounts into each bag with his fingers.

Each bag cost seven dollars. Each bag could cure diabetes.

No. That's too unbelievable. And that's exactly what the people who lived on the reservation and nearby towns said. So the nearby afflicted suffered and died. Of course, we know why. We know that they fell under the law that says, "An expert is a person out of town."

Who then bought these bags? Freeman and his wife could hardly supply the demand. People came in 747s from Holland, Germany, and Japan. They'd take a taxi from Toronto to Freeman's house for a seven-dollar bag of magic. But they didn't die.

On one of the occasions I came to visit Freeman, he was sitting on his screened-in porch. He could see out, but I couldn't see in. It just looked dark in there to me. Out of the darkness came his voice. "Ga jeeh. Thot n'yeah." I didn't know he could speak Tuscarora, and I laughed out loud even though he only said, "Come in. Sit down."

I told him something that my grandmother had told me—that if you chewed on a green snake, you'd have good teeth.

We used to have quite a few of these little light green snakes that ate little flies, even at night. Insect sprays killed most of them, and now they're quite rare. What happened with me when I tried my grandmother's formula was that even though I tried to be gentle in running that snake back and forth between my teeth, it still wiggled strenuously and touched my lips. As soon as it did, I threw it away. Now I knew that to tell Freeman this story would make him laugh, which it did. I just loved seeing that laugh. Then I said, "Have you ever heard of such a thing? That chewing on green snakes made good teeth?"

"Funny you should ask," he said, "I didn't think anyone knew about that anymore. But, you know, last year I got into an argument with two Cayugas about that. They were in their forties. One of them bet me ten dollars that it wasn't so.

"So I said to him, 'Well, how can I prove it to you?'

"He said, 'If the old Cayugas say it's so, I'll give you the ten dollars.'

"So we walked down to the Grande River, where the old Cayugas live. But we never even got there. Along the river were these hickory nut trees. Under the trees there were Cayugas in their eighties. They were cracking the nuts with their teeth. The guy that made the bet with me saw them. He didn't say a word. He just gave me the ten dollars, and we turned around and went home."

Freeman made me open my mouth, and he took a twig and counted my teeth and pronounced me sound. I told him that I would pay him a dentist's fee by bringing him any plant or bark that he was having trouble finding or couldn't get to because it was too far away.

He said, "Well, there is one bark I'm finding scarce now. Sycamore. Can you get me some?"

"Yes," I said, wanting to please him. On my way home, on a Sunday night near midnight, I said to myself, "Now why did I say that?" The only two trees that came to mind were at Tuscarora. One was in someone's yard and the other a half-mile from any road. I had to get to Rochester, where I now lived, to get some sleep so I wouldn't be tired on the job the next day.

The next day was a very hot day. So hot, in fact, that when I came home, my wife said, "It's too hot to eat in this house. Let's do a picnic someplace outside."

"OK," I said, "but where?"

We thought for a while, and after a while she said, "What about Ellison Park? We've never been there." So that's where we went.

We went to the lower part that looked more isolated and shady. We crossed the bridge and stopped. I couldn't believe my eyes. Here were seventy-five Sycamores with bark peeled loose by the heat, all over the grass. I filled three shopping bags.

I could safely bet anyone a thousand dollars that I would be seeing the Freeman Sowden smile again.

Tobacco Burning

First of all, everybody (different peoples from all over the world) has THE SA-
CRED TOBACCO that does big Medicine for THEM. Henry Niese, runner of
Sundance at Eagle Voice, loves to tell of being "a messenger caught in the middle." A great person of Medicine sent him to another great person of Medicine
with a gift. "Take this Tobacco to So-and-So. It is rare and precious."

Henry did. The "receiver" was blind. He took the gift of rare and precious
Tobacco and smelled it. "THIS is not the REAL thing!" So now the powerful
blind man sends Henry back with a gift of his "REAL" Tobacco. Lucky it wasn't
years ago when the king would have had the bringer of bad news beheaded.

I was telling "dowser" and "sensitive" Dr. Michael Ash from London, England, about our (us Indians of the Six Nations) use of a Sacred Tobacco, and I
was surprised when he said, "Oh yes, the *Nicotania rustica* that we planted at the
Six Nations Indian Reservation when I was there some years ago."

I thought, "Gee, this guy must be OK (pure enough)," because many Indians who may have ulterior motives regarding the growing of this plant (like the
selling of it) could NOT grow it. No matter how they tried, even procuring and
transplanting half-grown plants, it would not sprout from seeds or would die as a
transplant. So it can certainly proclaim itself as "no ordinary" Medicine.

In a Tobacco Burning that is done out-of-doors, it is customary to shout three
(some do four) distinctive yells into the sky to "herald" the coming of supplications.

At a gathering of Elders, Ru chuh'need was getting ready to do a burn, so I
yelled the three yells into the sky. Five horses in a pasture up and across the
country road from us came running up to the fence to see "what the heck are
these humans up to now!"

We "knew" it was going to rain at any moment because the sky was so black,
but Ru chuh'need went into the ceremony in his nice, slow, evenly tempered
way. When he came to the part where he was speaking of the sun, a perfectly

round hole appeared in that black sky, and a beam of light, a spotlight not unlike those used at a concert to highlight a soloist, encircled Ru chuh'need. Everyone "oohed" and "ahhed."

These were all Six Nations Elders. So now, for sure, we would be wont to say, "We have THE Tobacco!"

It never rained either.

One day I was reading one of Umberto Eco's best-sellers, I think it was the one about Joseph Stalin's badness, and someplace in the book it mentioned the poor people's use of a "rough, rugged tobacco" in prayers. Next to the word *tobacco* was this little asterisk, and at the bottom of the page was an explanation in letters that needed a magnifying glass to read. *Nicotania rustica.*

OUR TOBACCO! How did THEY get it??

So maybe what we are saying here is not so much about the Tobacco-Burning Ceremony as it is about the power of a Sacred Tobacco to "move mountains."

Oh, by the way, I got to wondering what in the world was a Dr. Ash from London doing monkeying with OUR Sacred Tobacco? Didn't you, too? So I pestered him until he said something. Well, actually he drew his answer with a pencil.

First, he drew an equilateral triangle that looked like it was standing, balanced, on one of its points. Then, as if this triangle were a flower, he put a curved "stem" on it. Then he drew what looked like the shape of an orange (fruit) cut in half with the flat side up. To the bottom of this he added a "flower stem" that curved and met up with the stem of the triangle flower. "This," he said, "is just a pretend, for simplicity's sake, of what the molecular structure of commercial Tobacco looks like."

Then he drew wavy lines coming upward out of both "flowers." These lines, he said, represented the emitting of waves of radioactivity or whatever it was that could cause cancer.

Next he drew the same symbol again, except this time, instead of waves emitting from the "flowers," he drew a "cap" on them. The triangle received another triangle to form a square or box. The "half orange" received the "other half" to form a circle or "whole orange."

He said that the halves putting out those waves were emitting them to attract a "mate," which would make it whole and would put an end to the emitting.

Then he said, "What you see in the symbol that is not putting out cancer-causing emissions is the molecular structure (in simple terms) of the Sacred To-bacco. Always already 'mated.' " Mated for life.

I dug (hip talk) hearing that. But I almost asked him why didn't he just use a couple plants for his experiments instead of, as he said, "a whole acre or more." Maybe he's just a good man, a philanthropist who gave more than an acre of *Nicotania rustica* to the person who owns that "acre or more" at the Six Nations Indian Reservation. And are the plants still there someplace?

I have hinted, every once in a while throughout this book, that many of the big wheels of the Longhouse might get after me for telling too much about the power-ful things that have happened regarding the many sacred Medicine "ways" that like to be hidden from disbelievers. (These disbelievers, having not the slightest knowledge that their own disbelief, animatingly energized by fear of the unknown, might dilute the Medicine.) I just trust that a strong disbeliever would never ever come near this book, that this book will hide like the Snakeroot flower.

Remember, not all Tobacco Burnings, or ANY ceremony, will automatically bring forth a "MOVED THE MOUNTAIN!" consummation. Soong gwi oo dee sut eh, the Highest Consciousness of the Universe, may see a better way than your supplication or perhaps reject your plea as not necessarily contributing to-ward making this a better world for the unborn.

So there's only one more Tobacco-Burning Ceremony incident to tell.

Some people don't know that many sacred and powerful masks, or False Faces, were confiscated in different ways and sold to or somehow ended up in museums. Many of these masks certainly played some part in their own "escape" and "homecoming." Many reports came through from museum curators who were frightened into resigning because of the shenanigans of the masks at night, when the museums were closed to the public. The masks would move about, change places, scream that terrifying call that they can make, or just raise cane in general, slamming things any old way, causing crashing noises, breaking plate glass display cases, and more.

So little by little over the recent years, through the Chiefs' efforts and maybe from other unknown pressures, the groundwork for the return of the masks began to manifest.

Ee'yog (gossip) had it that six masks would be released to the Oneidas. Maybe to appease the Oneidas so they might slow down their buying up (or buying back?) of so much land so fast.

An important representative from the Onondaga Longhouse went to see if this rumor were true, if the release could be expedited in any way, and if he could talk to the masks.

The rep took with him a setup whereby he might (without setting off smoke alarms) do a Tobacco-Burning Ceremony at the museum.

Everything proceeded as hoped for. The six Oneida masks were in a certain room, mounted on the wall. Almost as soon as the Tobacco-Burning Ceremony began, a very curious thing happened. A door to an adjoining room opened all by itself. All by itself?

The curator strode forward to close the door but was told, "Leave that door open, and I'll tell you why later."

One hundred or more masks were being incarcerated in that adjoining room. THEY wanted to be part of the ceremony, too, so they opened the door.

At the closing of the ceremony, the Burner received a vision. He voiced it to the masks. Of course, all of this was in his native tongue. "You'll be coming home within two years."

And they did.

The False Faces

This subject is taboo, but I want to tell you why it is. For one thing, like all Indian Medicine, masks are part of the Medicine whose power can be enhanced or angered or appeased or diluted by care (treatment), respect, or disrespect (neglect). To have a mask or masks for protection is a grave responsibility. This type of Medicine must be "fed," or it can turn against the "owner" or a caretaker's responsibility. The phrase used to describe what a mask will do if you hurt it by not paying any attention to it and, for sure, by not feeding it is, "It will eat you up."

It has to be that in the world there are masks that are harmless, but that's the catch: Which ones are the "living ones," and which are not? Under certain conditions a harmless mask can be brought to life, and the innocent "owner" can become subject to death.

Doesn't all this sound like nonsense? Well, that is THE reason you don't hear certain things talked about that belong in the powerful Medicine areas that Medicine people protect. Unawareness is no excuse.

When my family and I moved in the late 1930s from Seven Clan to Dog Street, we moved directly across the road from the Mike Jacobs family. Mike, whom we called Michael Angelo, had four brothers—Tootsie, Bought, Mooh-mooh, and Guggins. He also had a sister named Viney and a mother, Cull-line. Cull-line had a sister named Gaw-mut.

I liked Mike and his brothers Tootsie and Mooh-mooh. I didn't know Bought or Guggins very well. They were of an older crowd. I liked Mike because he was nice; Tootsie because he was always telling stories, even though they were mostly lies; and Mooh-mooh because he was quick witted and funny. One day Tootsie had a small crowd around him, listening to his stories, when Mooh-mooh came by. He went right up to Tootsie and said, "Gimme a cigarette and I'll believe you."

Certain families have more ESP-type experiences than other families, and the Jacobses were of the first category. Even another Jacobs family was like that, having produced Duke (also in this book). "They say" (ee'yog) that Cull-line's family traced a more direct line to the Tuscaroras of North Carolina, though I fail to see what that meant or matters. Just the same, one could say that this family was a bit more "Longhousey," and Cull-line herself lived in a small house apart and in the bushes some distance from Dog Street. In fact, Mike had not yet built a house on Dog Street when we first got there.

Regarding the "ghost story" nature of their lives, I remember Michael Angelo telling of coming home one night with his brave "protector" dog, Jeese-uh. It was only a medium-size dog, but not afraid to attack other larger dogs that might threaten its master. On this night, though, it barked only once, then chickened out. It began whining and hiding behind Mike's legs. Mike put his hands on it and in the dark could feel its hair bristling, standing up. Also, the dog was shivering. Mike could see nothing, no reason for this behavior.

The path to the house (Cull-line's house) was a winding one. Upon following the path around a bend, Mike saw why the dog did not want to continue on. On the side of the path was a familiar stump. On the stump, however, was a skull, a skeleton head, which exhibited a whitish glow. Mike and the dog took a big detour.

Within twenty-four hours, one of Mike's friends passed away.

There actually was a "driveway" to Cull-line's house, but it was quite inaccessible, especially after any heavy rains. This lane did not go directly from a point on Dog Street that was closest to the house, but from a point a quarter of a mile down the road. The winding path, though, was the shortest access to the house, so when Mike acquired an automobile, he would park it just off Dog Street at the top of the path.

One night something broke in the engine in his car, and he nursed it home though it protested with a clunking noise. Probably the main bearing was wanting to be history. Mike parked it at the top of the path and sat in its comfortable seat a few more minutes before facing the cooler night air.

Now he heard a "clop-clop-clop" noise like that of a horse coming from the west. A horse this late at night? No one used horses for transportation anymore.

But even so, why was the noise so oddly loud, as though the animal were hugely out of proportion in weight to an ordinary horse?

Mike waited, listening. He had backed the car in, just in case it had to be towed to a repair shop. Whatever it was on the road did not come into view before it stopped.

As in the chapter called "Duke," where Duke Jacobs conversed with a ghost, we can conclude that people like Mike and Duke do not scare easily. Just the same, these brave people use a sixth sense that can tell them, "I feel some other-worldliness here." That's what Mike felt about this noise, and a bit more, so when it came to a stop, he got the same feeling his dog got when it sensed the skull on the stump before it could be seen. Mike opened the car door, quietly stepped out, and went to the road for a look.

What he saw was a white horse standing in the middle of the road. It was only about thirty paces away. It was very nearly twice the height and breadth of an ordinary horse. Brave or not, Mike got back into his disabled vehicle and "abled" it to the "inaccessible" lane and clanked the car back to the house.

The big white horse was not a death omen like the skeleton head on the stump; no one died following this incident. I think the horse was simply telling Mike that human beings are not owls, that he should not be a night owl, that the middle of night is not the best of times, especially if you frequent the taverns.

It is the same sort of law of probability that my grandmother, Geese-a-geese, used to recite to me, "Don't go out at night."

I didn't pay much attention to Grandmother's admonitions at the time. Later, however, I could hear them again when my cousin's daughter was shot through the head with a high-powered rifle (a victim of a misplaced shot that was meant for someone else) during some of the darkest time of night, around 4:00 A.M. or so.

So, having said all this, let me tell you what happened to the families of Cull-line and her sister, Gaw-mut.

At that time a tourist could come onto the Tuscarora Indian Reservation and not find a shop where they could buy articles of Indian craftsmanship. Gaw-mut sought to remedy this problem and set up a trading post. Well, you know how tourists are; they don't know authenticity from Adam-icity, and maybe Gaw-mut was not far behind because she put up a totem pole to attract attention. Totem poles came from some other Indian heritage, as did the many-feathered war bonnets that can be seen at pow-wows.

Nevertheless, trading posts are not obligated to sell only the "real thing" of any given Indian people, but run more on the principle "let's make some money however we can."

One thing Gaw-mut did acquire that was very real to the Indians of this area was a mask. As it turned out, too real. She had gone to the New York State Fair near Syracuse, where there is a section especially set up for any of the Six Nation Indians to sell their wares. Here she had purchased this mask. She bought it from a man who had stolen this mask right out of the Onondaga Longhouse. He was an alcoholic and needed a drink, and his theft shows to what extremes an alcoholic will go to appease the uncontrollable lust of that addiction. I'm sure he wore an angelic expression on this face as he hoodwinked the unsuspecting Gaw-mut.

The mask was black and not necessarily artistic in looks as some masks are. It never sold, but maybe Gaw-mut didn't want to sell it. Maybe it was not for sale because she didn't have any other masks; but if she was using it to "dress up" her trading post authentically, this purpose may have made the mask even more angry. This mask was very very alive and very very powerful. A mask of this stature might like to be fed twice a year, but here at Gaw-Mut's place it was never fed.

Pretty soon her husband died. Then her son (the Sultan of the book *The Reservation*) died. Then she herself died. Now all of her belongings went to her sister, Cull-line.

Cull-line, though much sharper than Gaw-mut, still had no way of knowing the degree of danger she had inherited. Pretty soon both Bought and Guggins died. Then Cull-line found herself on her deathbed. A flash of intuitiveness came to her. She had Michael Angelo go and get a hold of Tootsie and bring him to her. "It's the mask!" she said, "It's the mask that's eating us up! Get rid of it." Then she, too, died.

Now the boys brought the mask to my father and told him of the dead Cull-line's wishes. Father dug a hole and buried the mask.

A drive-in garage was part of our house. Near the northeast corner of it grew a mock orange bush. Under the bush lay an old bushel basket lying on its side. The opening looked outward. Every morning my father would go outside and talk to the chicken that loved to sit in that basket and be talked to. "Gaaaa ga ga," one would say to the other. "Gaaaa ga ga," the other would say back. On the morning following the burial of the mask, however, the chicken was not in the basket. The mask was.

"Why them naughty kids next door," Father said to himself. "They watched me bury that mask. Now they want to play a trick on me, so they've dug the mask up and put it in the basket to scare me." He made a fire and put the mask into the fire and burned it.

The next morning the mask was back in the basket. Its long black hair was not even singed. (I have subsequently been told that more than one member of the False Face Society has accidentally suffered a house fire, losing everything except their False Face or Faces.)

"WHOA!" Father must have thought. "This is a live one! And powerful! How could I have been so careless?"

He carried the mask gently into the house and gave it some Sacred Tobacco, telling it, "Now, everything will be alright."

Next, Father took the mask back to Mike and told him that this was no ordinary mask, that it needed to go home, back to its rightful owner, and that although he had given it some Tobacco, all haste ought to be used in finding out where the mask came from.

How could Mike do this? He had no idea how Gaw-mut had acquired the mask. Anyway, my father had appeased it, at least for now, maybe even for good.

By this time, Michael Angelo had found himself a wife, Pat, and he had put up a live-in building directly across the road from our house. Despite having found out his obligation to the mask, Mike was so easy-going that he just assumed that life was supposed to resume helping him live happily ever after.

Not so. The time was halfway between spring and summer, and Mike now had a job on a farm someplace between Ransomville and Model City. On a Wednesday morn he was merrily cruising down Blacknose Spring Road on his way to work when "Wham!" an invisible something (like a man's fist) punched the side of his jaw and knocked his head sideways. It immediately became a struggle to continue driving because Mike's head stayed looking over his left shoulder. Somehow, though, the car was turned around, and Mike made it back home. Here, he found that he could scarcely talk. He mumbled to Pat that he had gotten a stroke, that he might not be able to work, at least for a while.

The weekend was approaching, but they did not look forward to it. Mike's neck still held his head in the "haw" position, the word people yelled at horses and mules to get them to turn left. If anyone had any notion that Mike's plight was connected to a mask that was alive, they may have told him that he was lucky, that these masks usually ate people up.

On Saturday the morning time was crowding toward noon when there was a knock on the door. Two Onondagas were standing there.

"We've come for the mask."

Pat was ecstatic. "Good show! But how did you know?"

"We've known this mask has been missing, but sometimes they have a way of coming home by themselves. This one didn't, so we decided to do Medicine and find it. We saw that you had it."

The Onondagas were in a hurry. Likely the men knew that Mike and his kin were in serious trouble. They took the mask and left. But here sat Mike with his "stroke," still with his head bent sideways, his speech blubbery.

Four or five hours passed. Suddenly Michael Angelo's head snapped front and center. "Hey!" he said clearly, "HEY! My stroke's gone. I can talk!"

At this moment in the Onondaga Longhouse a Faithkeeper was cradling the mask in one of her arms. Her other arm was busy stuffing sacred Mush into the mask's mouth.

When the Cull-line/Gaw-mut mask incident took place, I'm guessing that my father was about sixty years old. When he was younger, in his early forties, he lived with a great Indian doctor named Joo gwadee at Six Nations, Canada. This Cayuga was tutoring him about the higher Medicines. On the wall of Joo gwadee's bedroom hung a large mask. It was there to "watch-dog" and keep track of things.

One night Father was awakened by a sharp rattling noise. Along with the rattling noise was another sound that Father later described as the whinny of a puppy asking for love.

Father turned up the wick of the kerosene lamp and looked about. It was the mask. It was rocking and trembling itself against the wall and making the regular "False Face talk," which, up until this moment, Father had never heard. Beads of sweat appeared on the area above the mask's lips.

Father went to Joo gwadee's bed to wake him up, but the bed was empty.

Now Father noticed an eerie glow on the wall opposite the window. This faint light had a wiggle to it. Some unusual kind of light must be outside causing this glow. What was it?

Father went to the window and looked out. The neighbor's house was all aflame. With the fire and the incandescence of the sky around it for a background, Joo gwadee could be seen approaching. He had with him the old man whose house was burning down. Joo gwadee had saved his life. The mask had awakened Joo gwadee in time. It had kept track of things.

Being as my father had witnessed the power of this mask, it seems that he surely would have been more careful about the mask that Michael Angelo had brought to him. Maybe it was the ruggedness of the carving of the Onondaga Longhouse mask that fooled him. But that's the point. If a mask could fool my father, how much more likely could YOU be fooled? Do NOT buy a mask.

There used to be a certain hotel in London, Ontario, that, like most hotels, had a bar, a "watering" place. Also, like at most hotels for quite a few years, the old "no alcohol to be served to Indians" law had been ignored. Indians occasionally drank there.

An Oneida used to stop there from time to time and have a beer. He was a happy-go-lucky, unattached, carefree individual. He owned very little. Everything he possessed could be put into a grain bag, which he kept for this purpose. Among the things of his ownership were two small protection masks, which rode around in his bag whenever he moved. He was an itinerant farmworker.

One hot day after work he stopped in at this hotel for a beer. There he encountered a newly hired barmaid. She said, "The law says we can't sell liquor to Indians."

"But I drink here all the time," the hot, tired, thirsty Oneida exclaimed.

The barmaid became irate. "Not while I'm here. Get out before I call the police!"

Crestfallen, the Oneida departed. Thinking about it on the way home, he was thirstier and more miffed by the time he arrived. But he got an idea. He spoke to his masks and told on the barmaid. After that he felt better.

At work the next day he told his coworkers about the barmaid who had resurrected the old no-liquor-to-Indians law. After they all had a laugh, the Indian said, "I'll bet she gives me a drink tonight."

After work our happy-go-lucky friend went whistling up the sidewalk to the hotel, two of his coworkers with him.

Again, no liquor would be served. This time for a different reason. There was no hotel there. All that was to be seen in its place was a pile of smoldering ruins. Some people stood looking.

"What happened?" the Oneida asked.

"Big fire last night," someone volunteered. "But everyone got away safely. Everyone but the barmaid."

Back home that night the Oneida spoke to his masks. He told them they needn't be so rough next time.

And this is all I'm going to tell you about the False Faces. Maybe I've told you too much already. I have to mind my Ps and Qs, too, you know.

Peach Stones

I'll tell you just a little bit about the Peach Stone Game because it belongs to the Creator and is tricky to understand—sort of Heyoka-y and yin-yangy. The average bear and all WASPs would say it was gambling.

The game is played with a wooden bowl whose sides slant upward and outward. Six peach pits have been scraped flat and smoothed into "coins." One side of each is white, the other black, like heads and tails. Stones.

At the very first game there were no stones, and Creator may have been a bit worried, but six Chickadees (birds of the titmice family whose heads are black on top and white underneath) are said to have volunteered their heads to be used as stones.

This bird is special not only because of that, but because it can call to a stubborn, unconscientious person and cause that person's death. It's like a culling out of the unworthy. We call this bird the jeet daah bird. The Chickadee can change its regular call, *chik-a-dee-dee-dee-dee* to *jeet daaaa* (*a* as in "cat").

What the bird is saying is, "Meet me" or, as it sounds, "Meet meeee." If the obstinate person thinks, "Oh, that's just a stupid old wives' tale," and answers the bird by saying, "Yes, I'll meet you," that person is a goner.

My mother had a brother who did that. When he answered the bird affirmatively, everyone scolded him loudly, but it was too late. He may have had second thoughts because it took him six months to die. Six months, though, is not long in a teenager's (or anyone's) life.

Back to the Peach Stone Game. In any of the Six Nations of the Iroquois certain clans would always form one side (team) to play this game. At the Onondaga Midwinter Ceremonies where I first played the game, I found out that I was on the Longhouse side. The other was the Mudhouse side.

The scoring is maybe something like it is in tennis, where you earn so many "digits" to score a point. In the Peach Stone, ten points wins. Let's say you need ten "digits" to score one point. A "digit" can be scored in two ways. If you can "throw a field"—that is, all six stones come up either white or black—you earn a digit. Or if you can throw five of one color twice in succession, you also earn a digit. If you throw any other combination twice in a row, you lose your turn to the "thrower" of the other team. I may not have these rules exact, but I want you to see that it is not easy to win ten points. The "throwers" and "digit" points can go back and forth for a long time before a single point may be scored.

Get this straight. I am very reluctant to tell you about this game. It is one of the very sacred things that take place in the Longhouse. It is Ceremony. It is one of the very things that separate Medicine from physical consciousness. To the uninitiated, it is a test of faith. The faith aspect is where members of each side put up a thing of value that at the end of the game goes to a member of the winning side who has put up a matching article. Women may put up a beautiful quilt or beadwork or beaded dress. Men may put up a ribbon shirt or lacrosse stick or turtle rattle. So it can be difficult for the uninitiated to believe that this is not gambling. For me to tell you that you cannot lose, that upon your death you will get these things back, is risking that you will tell me, "Rubbish!" and that my Medicine will be diluted by the strength of your disbelief.

But let's say by some freak thing you did get to put up a lacrosse stick and "win" another from someone whose team in the Peace Stone Game "lost." Then, let's say this newly "won" stick becomes your favorite. One day you discover this lacrosse stick missing. You are in the process of chewing out your younger brother for taking it. The phone rings. You answer it. Someone on the other end of the phone line tells you that So-and-So, the former owner of the "missing" lacrosse stick, has just died. You apologize to your younger brother, who has been pleading his innocence.

One more thing about the game. For some reason, you are not to "put up" an article that is black. In my very first game I put up my ribbon shirt and my (genuine) wolf tail. There were some black hairs in the tail, but it was accepted. As a seven in the Enneagram, I just naturally never thought of "losing."

At the end of the day (which can be determined by the position of the sun or by clever argument), we (the Longhouse side) were losing by a score of nine to one. (Maybe some influential Elder on our side brought the game to a halt for that day.) A few years later I was the thrower and got on a lucky or power streak, and someone from the other side put a stop to the game for that day with the score nine to one in our favor. (Betty Jacobs, of our side, argued furiously, but to no avail. The next morning when the game resumed, a little girl ended my streak and went on to win the whole shebang.)

So here I was, having my first taste of the Peach Stone and finding myself on the losing end of the game being played at the Midwinter Ceremonies at Onondaga.

Noisewise, the game sounds like uproar or "disorder at the border." A big crowd surrounds the two "throwers." As soon as a thrower gets a turn or shakes the dish before "setting" it on the blanket, the opposing side members holler "SHAWWWHH!" or any zapping thing to disrupt the thrower's result. As in the song "Accentuate the Positive," "pandemonium was liable to walk upon the scene."

I said to myself, "I don't think it's fair to use Medicine here in this game . . . but that hollering . . . that's Medicine! . . . I think I'll go home and get me every power object I can find."

That night I drove back to Rochester and got all the Medicines that I could think of, including asking the Little People to help me. This came to eight Medicines in all.

The next day, ding, ding, ding . . . we began knocking off the points until we had the score reversed. Now we had nine, and they had one. I had run out of Medicines, but surely we ought to be able to come up with one point just using the law of averages.

Leon Shenandoah was the Tadadaho (Fire Keeper) of the whole Six Nations, and I've heard that he wasn't supposed to have a clan so as to not be partial to anyone. Well, then, what was he doing sitting over there with the Mudhouse gang? He was much loved, and such a position generates power. Some Mudhouser must have thought of this and in desperation got Leon to "roll the dice" for them. A tremendous roar went up when he took the bowl into his hands. And to my dismay Hizzoner began a tremendous comeback. The big Longhouse was pure din.

I closed my eyes. I couldn't see the players anyway. I was standing on tiptoes leaning over the bench in front of me, but people were standing on that bench. I was frantic. Somewhere in all the "tapes" stored in my head there had to be another Medicine.

Sometimes it seems as though it takes more than panic to force the issue.

Beyond desperation. Like begging some great dead person, a dead seven, for help. Yes. That's what it does take. Because the Medicine did come to me.

Some years before this, in the springtime, I had happened past a shop that was going out of business. The shopkeeper must have known me because she called to me by name, "Hey, Ted!" and waved me toward her.

I didn't know her, but that didn't matter; I pretended I did. What she wanted me to see was a crystal ball. You know, like a Gypsy fortune-teller looks into the future with. It was the size of a big grapefruit, and it "grabbed me." It exuded aesthetic pleasure.

Price stickers were on it. Lesser ones on top of the original one that said "$500" until now it was down to a sticker that said "$100."

"Oh, Ted," the lady said, "I want you to have this. I'll let you have it for fifty dollars."

"What would I use it for? Bowling?"

"Oh, you know what I mean. It loves you. It wants to be yours."

I bought it. I kept it in velvet with my Medicines.

One day I was thinking about the integrity of a certain person. It bothered me that integrity of that level never gets recognition. I was reminded of a Lao Tzu poem:

> A leader is best when people barely know he exists
> Not so good when they obey and proclaim him
> Worse when they despise him
> Of a good leader when his work is done
> And his work fulfilled, the people will say,
> "We did this all ourselves."

I gave the crystal to that person, and one day I got a call from them. "That crystal wants to go back into Mother Earth."

We did it in a ceremony, dressing the ball in those bluish-tinted breast feathers of a male pheasant (still on the hide). We buried it in a secret place, a Little People's place.

This is the Medicine that came to me.

The Tadadaho didn't have a chance.

As soon as I asked the crystal ball to "teach Leon a lesson," the Peach Stones came up in three consecutive fields, all white, all white, all white.

The game was over. We'd won. Noise just doesn't get any louder. I was still standing with my hands on top of the bench before me. My eyes were still shut, but I could feel something touching them.

I opened them. A little boy was standing on the bench facing me. He was wiping the tears from my face.

But guess what? Maybe it would have been good to have lost. Know why? There is no Wolf Clan in the Mudhouse. Had they won, the wolf tail may have jinxed them forever, for every ensuing year.

Songs of Power

I like to get excited about things and go hog wild over something, maybe even hardly sleeping because of it. Like about chess. But, of course, there's no end to chess—trillions of combinations—so after a while I run to something else.

In the 1970s I got excited over songs, Indian songs. I was gonna learn them all. It all ended, songwise, when I ran into Chief Pat Sandy. We were talking about ceremonies, and the Cayuga Chief said, "We borrowed one [ceremony] from the Tutelos. Forty-four songs." Forget it.

One time Randy Henry gave me a tape of himself singing as lead singer of a group. He is one tremendous singer, so I said, "Did you record this at a social or a sing?"

"Naw, it's just a bunch of us from the bush," he said, "My sister's on it, too." Hardly a spirited recommendation, so I didn't rush home and put it on.

One day I slipped it into the tape player while I was driving along, and "Judas Priest and little green apples!" why didn't I play this sooner?

There is or was a jazz school in Chicago, the Knapp School of Percussion, that had about forty would-be jazz drummer students. Only three of them "swung," and of the three only one REALLY swung. He just exuded this contagious rhythm and beat, and everyone wanted him to drum for them when they did an arrangement for ensemble group practice. Drumming on another level.

One time I went to Kleinhan's Music Hall in Buffalo, New York, to hear a jazz concert of several name jazz groups and singers. First up was the pianist Thelonius Monk. He could not stand to have a poor rhythm section. Man! He came on like ghost busters! In a few minutes he literally had the place rocking. Suddenly all the lights went out. The music stopped. A man's voice came on loud and clear on the audio system. "LADIES AND GENTLEMEN . . . WE ARE VERY SORRY TO HAVE TO INTERRUPT THIS PROGRAM . . . BUT IT IS IMPERATIVE

THAT YOU STOP MOVING AND BOUNCING TO THE MUSIC . . . THE WHOLE BUILDING, ESPECIALLY THE BALCONY, IS QUAKING AND MAY COME APART AND COME CRASHING DOWN . . . WE'LL START AGAIN, BUT PLEASE RESTRAIN YOURSELVES."

With the first drumbeat Randy Henry's tape had that same magic. But there was even a bonus. The sound was "far out." Instead of the "shum, shum, shum, shum" sound of the regular water drum and rattles, the sound was more a "shing, shing, shing, shing." It even sounded like the rattles were coming in a hair ahead of the drum.

After a while I suspected this "bunch from the bush" might be high on pot, but maybe I was just jealous. Music itself and certain "magical" songs can get this euphoria to kick in. Maybe I was just wishing I had been there. They were having SO much fun. If they made a mistake, they would all just laugh hard, maybe even scream.

At socials and sings only men do the singing—that is, originally, but now some women sing, too. In Randy's tape his sister does a masterful job of holding back, waiting for the perfect moment to give the song a lift.

This tape, to me, is pure Medicine. It might cure leprosy, but it is merely one of thousands of songs that have power. Some we will never hear because they belong to secret societies that only sing them in ceremony.

Some of the songs we sing are on the edge. That is, we might be told, "That song is not to be sung at a social," yet once in a while, maybe at a social being held at a different Indian nation, it will be sung. The Corn Dance is one such song. It is so very very beautiful. It's no wonder that the Indian corn sometimes grows to sixteen feet.

Maybe a certain song and certain persons belong to each other. One evening, standing on the back porch of my cabin and looking down into a deep wooded valley, I got the urge to sing to all the Indian spirits that ever walked along the stream below.

I brought my Medicine Drum to a steady beat and started singing a Round Dance song verse. It goes, "Hote ha'note hey'yote ha'note hey'yote hey ya ya." Not this time. I was barely able to get the first five notes to echo down into the valley before I choked up and started to cry.

Later, when I told someone about it, they said, "Oh, that's just a social song."

I said, "Maybe to you, but not to me."

Then, too, this happened to me. After I had seen the False Faces dancing to the Old Moccasin Dance Song, it became sacred to me.

Going to work one day, I began singing it. It put me in a trance. I smashed into the car ahead of me, causing a five-car pile up.

Did I learn my lesson? No. One day I took my wife's old dark green Mercedes and washed it, even washing the diesel engine. Coming home and feeling good about myself, I started singing the Old Moccasin Dance. The next thing I knew I was off the road and rolling down the side of a mountain. It is one of the best ways to "total" a car.

Did I learn my lesson *then?* Eh . . . so far.

Sometimes the REASON for a song makes power generate in the whole singing group. Every once in a while somebody on some Six Nation reservation will say, "It's time for a Sing" (to honor all the great Clan Mothers and women Elders and Faithkeepers both past and present).

Sacred song power, one might surmise, would be generated to various degrees by the aroused emotions of the singers. But what about music played by instruments?

One night I viewed a documentary on TV showing an incredible thing that happened during the ending of World War II.

German soldiers had taken over an old hotel building made of stone. A bridge over a river led to this building, but what troops were foolhardy enough to attempt to cross that wide-open bridge and risk being strafed by machine-gun bullets?

It doesn't seem possible, now, looking back on what took place, that human minds could have thought of such a solution. Allied soldiers carrying guns did not solve the problem. So what did?

A band of Scottish bagpipers came marching across, plaid skirts swaying to the eerie wail of the pipes. Machine guns did not appear at the windows of the German hotel . . . instead, white flags. Surrender.

One time in Ontario, Canada, there was a prison riot. It happened at the Kingston Women's Prison. I am calling it a "riot" because I don't know what else to call it. The guards, men, were staging a sexual attack on the women prisoners. Now it may be that hardly anyone knows about this because the account of it came through ee'yog. Why would the prison administrators tell on themselves?

If this almost happened this one time, then it could easily have happened before, if not here, then in any women's prison anywhere. It's the "criminal's" word against the authoritative figures who are ostensibly there to protect the common citizen against crime. So the inmate is at the mercy of the staff. If ANYbody knows this, it's the inmates, and, in this particular case, when one of them who lived through the attack served her time, she was able to relate what happened.

There is a strange compulsion that human beings are susceptible to. It is the same frenzy feeding or killing spree that piranhas, weasels, and the mink family display when they smell blood. It affects humans when they smell fear in a victim and when they are the perpetrators in a perpetration-victim situation. In a gang rape it arouses the sex urge, and in a prison it is like: "We are the law. We are in charge here, and we give ourselves permission to punish these breakers of the law." Whoopee. Group behavior as displayed by hyenas also contributes to a feeling of validity, and soon all involved are incapable of moral reason.

Fear made the women scream as the men advanced on them. All the more, then, did the men feel their wild oats.

The citizenry outside the prison, if they did hear the screams, mostly thought, "Well, what do you expect? It's a prison."

A few women, though, outside on the streets listened and by careful listening made out some of the words of cried-out messages. They began trying to form a group of support women, but it was not easy. And what could they actually do?

Inside the prison, among those being attacked was a woman Elder, a Mohawk. The Elder began to sing. It was as though an enchantment grasped the other inmates. They stopped screaming. They begin to sing, too. In a short time it was as though they had known the song forever.

Now a highly unusual thing happened. The men had been taking their time, arousing more fear in the "mice" in their cat-and-mouse game. They stopped moving ahead. Some invisible force was stopping them.

Outside the prison women were beginning to surround the prison grounds, and though relatively small in number, they began voicing chants of disapproval and condemnation.

The prison women continued to sing. The men backed off, slowly at first, but as more left the scene they inadvertently caused a restlessness.

Those remaining may have thought, "Maybe they [those that left] know something that we don't. Maybe someone has squealed on us. Maybe someone is coming."

Soon it was all over. Finished.

The song ended. Someone asked, "What song were we singing?"

The Elder woman smiled. "A power song. We were singing the Women's Honor Song."

All the songs on Randy's tape were women's dance songs.

After I told my wife, Diana, about the women freeing themselves from being raped by singing the Women's Honor Song, she was so taken by that great event that she wrote a poem and told me that I could share it with you. Here it is.

HONORING SONG
Here in my hours, light trickling on
Black frost,
Days of hours come mining the
Heart—true atlas of territory, this
My country.

Yeats, where are you now,
But in a suddenness of green
Forever at risk / dark phenomena
Eating at your edges, discovering
Proud fury, aging, letting go . . .
A prisoner of the sky

Something is dividing, is crucial,
Is falling . . . something you were, yes
A hero whose words are left on water—
"Do not give us peace, let us be maddened

First—let us grieve the earth, let us
Die in the square of beloved land,
Let us tear at the cross that makes

The swift knives cut / that let our
Children die . . ."

Let us grieve and be maddened first
For we are holy; we are men whose faces
Are burned and burning—ever
In your broken promises.
We are the Honoring Song
Sung from the ashes . . .

Diana Osborne Williams

Energy Places

Once when I was in Australia, one of the Aborigines took me to see the Blue Mountains. Here, he showed me three connected peaks called the Three Sisters. Legend there says that years ago three beautiful sisters of a village were turned into these three peaks to escape being taken prisoner by an attacking horde. The Medicine man who hid them thus would then turn them back to women again once it became safe to do so. Although the Medicine man hid in a cave, he was tracked down and killed, so the Three Sisters became destined to beautify the land as three mountains.

I said, "Get your didgeridoo. I'll get my Medicine drum, and let's try to hit the right magical notes to bring the Three Sisters back again."

I started a slow beat and began singing a Medicine song. When my friend cut in on didge, I got goose bumps and the willies. I had my eyes closed. After a while our music started to go dead. Soon I realized I was singing alone. I opened my eyes. Here was a group of tourists surrounding us, and more could be seen coming in the distance. They probably thought that we played there every day for coins. We left.

I used to think that I knew quite a bit about finding energy spots and energy vortexes through the tingling in the palms of my hands or by finding spots of congregation by deer or grouse or Medicine plants. But here, the whole of Australia had already been mapped by the Dream Walkers and Medicine people into grids of Song-lines and Medicine spots and holy dwelling places of their many clan people. Flies, Grubs, Birds, and so on made up this seemingly endless "people," members of their universal family. Many of these sacred spots were greatly feared as extremely powerful places because "civilization" had thoughtlessly trod upon them, unceremoniously poking at a spiritual hornet's nest.

At Tuscarora and other Indian reservations there are power spots and lines, too. It is interesting that some of the lines follow sections of paved roads, suggesting that early walking paths, which later became roads, were first "felt" spiritually, then followed.

One of the larger power places is the woods at Tuscarora called the Commons. Adjacent to it, or even a part of it, was the area west of it called Old Saw Mill. Here, when some pasture land was plowed up and two fruit orchards planted, pottery, flint arrowheads, and human bones surfaced. A long ridge of limestone that is part of the upper section of Niagara Falls extends eastward to include the Commons Woods. The soil atop the limestone is not very deep, so this bone-strewn area at Old Saw Mill is not likely to have been a gravesite. Brass buttons found there also suggest that a skirmish between some Indian settlement and certain troops took place here. This is not a place that can be reached by a paved road.

Andrew and Blanche Davis and their family lived in a house that was the nearest dwelling to Old Saw Mill. Their long driveway from Upper Mountain Road put them less than a mile away. They reported hearing, many times, as they sat out on their lawn on a summer evening, singing and drumming and Indian-sounding whooping coming from Old Saw Mill. Someone asked Andrew if he ever went down there to see who was dancing.

"Not me," he said, "Them were ghosts. They weren't singing in any language that we know of around here!"

This property, owned by my father, is said to have had a sawmill on it at one time, hence its name. Two great Medicines grew in this area, and when I was about four years old, Father took me on a Medicine-gathering walk to this place. The distance from Seven Clan was about a mile, but I thought we were never going to get there.

When we got there, Father said, "You stay here while I get the Medicine; maybe you'll find some arrowheads."

Probably all my questions and my skeptical nature had him decide not to let me see the Medicine. I might question it. Presently he came back ready to go back home.

The first thing he said was, "I forgot to tell you something; these are human bones you see here, bones of people that used to live here. Don't pick any of them up. Don't take them with you. If you do, what will happen is, you'll get sleepy. You'll get so sleepy you won't be able to stay awake. You'll fall asleep, and I won't be able to wake you up."

To myself I said, "Well, what do you know! Here I have my back pockets full of choice bones. Fingers, toes maybe, teeth. I was going to see if someday I might get enough to make a whole skeleton. Now he says this! I bet it's just an old folks tale."

We started for home. I was trailing Father two or three steps. We probably got about 150 yards when BLAM! my eyelids came down shut like heavy castle gates. No warning. NO getting sleepy first. I wish everybody in the world could have this happen to them just once so they'd know what it's like, so they'd know I wasn't telling lies. Buddy, you ought to have seen them bones fly out of my pockets. I flipped them out frantically. I couldn't see where I was stepping. Maybe I'd fall far behind. Maybe I'd run smack into my father if I hurried too much, and now I did begin to get very sleepy. Them bones came out like machine-gun bullets. When the last bone came out, my eyes popped open like springs because I'd been trying so hard to open them. WHEW! There was Father walking about three steps ahead of me. The whole thing must have lasted no more than seven or eight seconds, but I thought I was doomed. I was shaking.

I never told Father about this, but I wish now that I had. I'm quite sure that he knew about them bones in my pockets, although he never said anything about it either.

Many years later, maybe 1970, I told Isaiah Joseph of Six Nations Reservation, Canada, about my bout with the bones. He laughed.

"Wa thaw skit-naw-ree(t)" (You were skeletally entranced), he said in Tuscarora. This, then, was a well-known phenomenon and had likely happened many times.

The Commons Woods—now here was a surely tricky thing, sort of a sleeping giant trickster, a Heyoka, that left you alone 90 percent of the time. At least, that's the way it was with me; maybe it pounced upon other people more often, maybe never.

I'm just guessing, but I'd say that the "living trickster" section of it is roughly 100-by-250 yards, a sort of rectangle that starts at Blacknose Spring Road and extends westward. By age twelve I'd been in it many times without incident. That is, until this one day.

Seven Clan lay only a half-mile south of the Commons Woods. On this one day three of my school companions, around the same age, decided to go looking for arrowheads with me. They were Webster Cusick, Leroy Ferguson, and Ducky (Duane) Anderson. We would walk from Seven Clan.

Through the length of the Commons Woods, from Blacknose Spring Road to Old Saw Mill, was a drainage ditch. We would enter the center of the woods and walk north until we reached the ditch; there we would turn left and follow it to Old Saw Mill. Simple. We did this. We got to the ditch, which was now dry, turned left (west), and continued on to our destination.

The first clue that something could have been amiss was the appearance of a "new" bridge or culvert between the two fruit orchards. "Look!" I said as we approached, "They've taken out the old bridge and put in a culvert."

When we got to the culvert, we were not at Old Saw Mill. We were standing on Blacknose Spring Road. We looked at each other. I'm sure all of the others had chills running up and down their spines as I did. Someone started running. For home. We all started running. Fast. To heck with arrowheads.

Maybe this bothered me the most because I had been in that woods many more times than the others. The feeling was that we'd been transported the space of a mile in the blink of an eye.

Lots of people have been embarrassed and tricked by this great woods, even seasoned woodsmen and hunters. One late fall day five Indian hunters spaced themselves evenly apart and lined up on Blacknose Spring Road. They would walk and stay abreast through the Commons and drive any deer to waiting hunters at the other end.

It was many years later that Gary Patterson told me this story because he didn't want anyone to know how the woods tricked him. We grew up as neighbors in close proximity to the Commons, and he had been in these woods many times, so he considered himself very knowledgeable about them. This hunt, this "driving" of the woods, was done in the fall time and maybe even more than once.

Of the five hunters lined up on Blacknose Spring Road, Gary was "center man" because of his experience. He would coordinate the drive. At his signal the five drivers entered the woods.

Shortly thereafter, Gary looked up to see one of them "dream" bucks that all hunters hope to someday see. He drew up his trusty .308 and aimed carefully. Just as he began squeezing the trigger, the deer disappeared. In Gary's words, "It didn't run. It never moved. It was just instantly not there anymore. I couldn't stop myself, I pulled the trigger."

At this point I got an urge to interject, "Oh yes, Gary, the woods got you! Charmed you with that deer. Now you were under its spell where time and space were no longer perceptible," but I said nothing.

The loud discharge of the gun brought Tommy Greene over from his position to see what Gary had gotten. Gary told him his gun had gone off accidentally.

At the time of the incident Gary was unaware of having been thrust into a different conscious state, but what he said next was very interesting, incriminating of that fact.

He said that when Tommy Greene left to go back to his (Tommy's) position, "He went the wrong way."

When Gary resumed his own place, "down the middle," he came out instead into a field on the south side of the woods. So Tommy did not go the wrong way, Gary did. Even retelling the incident, Gary seemed to slip back into "how it felt" back then.

Gary hurried back into the woods to the place where he knew he ought to be. Not that easy. Not while under the spell. He soon found himself back out in the field again.

This was too much. Gary knew his situation was beyond repair. He took his stock and home did trot as fast as he could scamper. But I don't know if he went to bed or covered his head with vinegar and brown paper.

Eli Rickard was plowing the fields on the north side of the Commons. His wife, Lena, and his sister would bring him his lunch. But why walk all the way around the woods to do so? The women would take a shortcut—go right through the Commons.

Yeah.

Now this is hard to believe. In the relatively small distance through that woods they were held, circling in it, for six hours.

They began to cry; and they ate Eli's lunch up.

Maybe that's the key. If you're going into the Commons Woods, take a lunch with you.

◆ ◆ ◆

We could say Duke Jacobs was a bit "ghost crazy" . . . yeah, but let's see how he makes out with the Commons Woods.

We already had an inkling that Duke was not an ordinary, everyday person— or every night person, either, because he wasn't afraid of the dark. There is a favorite fisherman's fishing spot at Lake Ontario near Wilson, New York, called Ban geh (Ben's Place) by the Indians. I don't know what Duke and Rose and their son, Edwin, were fishing for, but because it is eight or ten miles to that place, it was about three in the morning when the trio started past the Commons Woods having walked from Ban geh. They were sleepy and tired. They were on Blacknose Spring Road with about three more miles to go before they got home.

As they proceeded to a point where they were abreast with approximately the center of the Commons, they saw in the woods a light. It was a lit-up window. It looked exactly as though someone had built a cabin in the Commons Woods and had not yet retired for the night because their light was still on.

"Look at that!" Duke says, "Somebody's living here now. Let's go and see who it is."

"Not me," Rose responds, "I ain't going in there."

It could never occur to Duke that he might be passing a spooky place, and what with his addiction to such things anyway, he plunged into the woods, saying, "OK, just wait here, I'll find out who's there. Maybe they'll let us rest there for the night."

Now the great thing about the Commons Woods is that it just doesn't do one thing, one way. It zapped Gary Patterson with a giant deer, and now it zapped Duke with a lit-up window with innuendos of a place to snuggle down and get some sleep. For just a moment or two, let's think about what goes on here. To be "charmed" by the Little People or the Commons Woods and the like is to enter a world of no time, no space. The women who spent six hours circling in the Commons may have perceived this time as being about thirty minutes, but the onset of darkness is what scared them.

Now here went Duke, toward the light with his perception of time gone— also his perception of space, because as he went toward the light, it receded into the woods at a very subtle rate, just enough to give Duke the impression that he was gaining on it. It is very hard to believe that the "no space" perception can be SO intoxicating to awareness.

How long was Duke gone from Rose and Edwin?

The eastern sky was hinting strongly of dawn before Duke gave a yell to Rose. NO answer. Again, louder. Still no answer. Finally, the third time, she heard him and answered. But as far away from each other that they were at this moment, the light must have sucked Duke into at least one large circle because if Duke had never seen the light, he would have walked far enough to have gotten home.

Duke ended his telling of this little traipse through the woods by saying, "I don't know how I could have ever made such a boo boo, but I was right about one thing. I knew Rose would be mad when I got back. I was right. Boy, was she ever pissed!"

Before we leave the Commons Woods, I'll tell you about one more small happening. I've always wanted my children to get a taste of the Heyoka (powerful clown) of this woods, but it doesn't work this way. You don't will a power spot to do something.

One day my oldest son, Tom, and I went into the Commons to get some Medicine. Tom has a green thumb for Medicine, and whereas I might need a purification to find a certain plant, he can just go into a woods and say, "Is this what you're looking for?"

We drove our vehicle through the fields on the north side of the Commons as far as we could go, parked, and went into the woods. Almost immediately we found what we came for, and after the proper gathering procedure we took what we needed. With plenty of time on our hands we went farther into the woods, crossing the drainage ditch and continuing in a southerly direction. Presently we came out on the south side of the woods.

Being in no hurry, we just ambled back to the car. When we got to the field where we had parked the car, there was no car. That was because we were back where we had started on the south side of the woods.

The Commons had not needed a deer or a light to charm us, and finally it had shown one of my children what it could do. Fine, and according to my watch, we hadn't lost any more time than if we were now at our car. But we really had to be leaving soon.

OK then. This time we would sight a south-to-north line using whatever of these old virgin trees that fell in that line as sign markers. This we did, and it seemed so simple. Why didn't others who had gotten lost in this woods do this?

Well, we found out why. We came out of the woods exactly where we had started—again. We laughed, but Tom pointed to the southwest. Rain clouds. We might get wet. Very wet. Should we chance circling round and round while we did? No. We took off running to Old Saw Mill. The rain never materialized. Maybe the dark clouds and the Commons were in cahoots.

So the Commons Woods doesn't have to charm you to trick you. Or if it does, the charm is so subtle it may not deprive you of time and space. It only takes away the compass in your head.

Wait now. Just one more thing. Just one more tricky little incident with which to close off this chapter. Chief Tracy Johnson was the Subchief of the Tuscarora Turtle Clan, of which my father was the Sachem Chief. A clan is like a big family, so Tracy and I sat and told stories and enjoyed this family feeling whenever we got the chance. As far as being experienced concerning "ghosty" things, Tracy was what you might say just a more sophisticated version of Duke.

Tracy and I were having one of these visits when mention was made of the Commons Woods. Right away it reminded me of a Medicine called Dut eehn yuks that I had been wanting to show to Tracy. I suggested that we go right on down there, and I would formally introduce him to this Rx. Off we went.

We parked on the Commons Woods side of the road because there was a wider shoulder on that side. Such lushness of shrubbery grew along this sun-accessed side of the woods that it appeared impenetrable, but none of it was thorny, and we made our way through it.

But yipes! It was quite wet in there. It was springtime, and, indeed, we ourselves had to spring from dry spot to dry spot or get wet feet. But this was nothing compared to the cloud of mosquitoes that greeted us. This visit was going to have to be fast or not at all.

I was leading the way. We had hardly gotten into these woods, ambling only eight or ten paces, when I turned left and went parallel to the road for about twenty paces. Here we came to the Medicine. I introduced them to each other, Tracy and the Medicine, telling it that "Tracy was a good man who possessed humor, would not take too much of you if he needed you," and so on, ending with, "But we are being eaten alive by these mosquitoes, and with your kind permission we would like to take our leave."

Now we hurried on back out to the road. Simple. So let's all of us go through it again together. We walk ten paces west, we walk twenty paces south, and we walk ten paces east.

The places where we started, where our vehicle was, should then have been to our left, north, twenty paces away. Well that's where it should have been, right? Well, it wasn't.

Just like anyone would automatically do, as we stepped out of the bushes, we looked to our left to see our car. I glanced at Tracy. He had a little smirk on his face.

Sure enough, when we looked to the right, there was our vehicle, twenty paces the wrong way. We both let out a good laugh. Neither of us said anything; it would have spoiled it. We just walked to the car and got in.

I'm sure the Chief noticed, as I did, our tracks leading from the car into the woods. What a nice feeling to know that the Commons Woods was alive and well and just as naughty as ever.

The Vision Quest

Regarding my vision quest, I said to myself, "I'll write about it, then decide later if I give myself permission to put it in the book." It is not a thing to tell everyone about, yet people on the path to enlightenment need the reinforcement and encouragement that the experiences of others can give them.

One day Carmen Ramos asked me if I wanted to do a vision quest. Most people would be leery of, as it is often called, being "put on the hill" unless the person in charge of their being there was super in every way. Visions of bears coming to eat them and all kinds of catastrophic expectations like lightening striking them can suddenly come creeping into their minds.

I don't want to make a big list of all Carmen's great attributes, his doing sweats and shamanistic drum meditations for twenty-five years or so, and all the degrees of black belt of different martial arts he has, and so on, because it might go to his head. So I'll just tell of an incident about him and let that suffice.

One day Carmen was doing his own quest or whatever secret stuff he does on his own up in the Adirondack Mountains. He was probably in the Lotus position, next to his sacred little fire, meditating. I don't know if I'm even supposed to tell you about this, but if it does get into the book, maybe he won't read it.

Sometimes a meditation drifts into a depth or level that leaves the practitioner physically immobile. Carmen had attained this state but didn't know it at first.

There had been little rain, so the woods were dangerously dry, and the governor had warned all campers to be extremely careful about fires. Once a fire got away, thousands of acres of inaccessible timber could go up in smoke before firefighters could arrive and bring the forest fire to bay.

So here was Carmen next to his little fire and under the spell of his meditative state, which had rendered him immobile. How he came to realize that he could not move was that he noticed his little fire had decided to sneak off on its own, but when he attempted to curb it, he discovered that he couldn't. He was not in the physical consciousness. He was frozen, but he could see. He could see his fire getting away.

Now here is something good to know. In this other conscious state that Carmen was in, one has power, but Carmen didn't preknow this until the moment arrived when the need to have this power came.

Carmen said later, "Though the fire was getting away, in the state that I was in, I just KNEW that I could direct that fire."

I had to laugh when he told me about this part because I pictured Carmen as treating the fire as though it were a naughty child. With his mind he said to the fire, "WHERE DO YOU THINK YOU'RE GOING?!! GET BACK HERE!!!" The little fire "obeyed mama," turned 180 degrees, and went back home to the main fire. Carmen went on meditating unperturbed. This is the kind of ceremonial leader you want watching over you when you're on a quest and that bear comes. ("WHERE DO YOU THINK YOU'RE GOING? GET BACK INTO THE FOREST AND GRUB FOR TRUFFLES!")

Actually, I had thought several times of doing a vision quest on my own, but just plain laziness kept saying, "Oh, one of these days." After all, my friend Ta wi da qui had done twenty-one days all by his little self, a commendable accomplishment. But we Indians don't give much praise, our attitude being, "Oh, I could do that if I wanted to."

Just the same, some tricky things came to Ta wi da qui, and he has given talks about it. Two talks, because he can't (or won't) tell it all in one session. Maybe he thinks, "If it takes ten days to expound the Great Law, then I'm entitling myself to more than one day."

Maybe one day he'll write a book and include this quest experience as part of it, so I will only tell you about one of these tricky things that happened to him.

Vince Johnson took Ta wi da qui (at Onondaga) and put him "on the hill" for a quest. Well, you can go any direction from Onondaga, and you'll end up going upwards, so this special place could be any of a jillion places.

Upon seeing Vince for the first time, you might think you are seeing a sumo wrestler rather than a man with more than a sixth sense.

About seven days and nights pass, and Ta wi da qui was cold and wet, but also determined because he had said, "I'm not coming down until I see Creator." Nevertheless, he realized that he had misjudged what the quest would be like, so he took the time to compile, in his head, a list of what he would bring next time if he ever did this again. He carefully came up with six things.

The next day he heard a noise. A deer? No, too heavy. A person? Ta wi da qui lay very still. Maybe the hiker or hunter would not see him. But the footsteps only got louder, indicating that the maker of the footsteps was coming straight at him. The quester took a peek down the hill; maybe the person was a good tracker and was tracking him. There was no one there.

Ta wi da qui arched his back and looked up the hill. Here came an Onondaga Elder of the False Face Society. It was Vince. He was carrying all six things that "the man on the hill" had wished he had brought and who was sure that no one knew of his whereabouts. Coming from the top of the hill no less.

All the bringer of good tidings said was, "I thought you might want these things," threw them on the ground, turned around, and went back the way he came.

Would I participate in Carmen's vision quest? Yes, but I would bring my own little compiled list of allowables and not wait for Divine assistance.

Carmen's rules were quite simple. The total length that one could be on the hill was from Wednesday morning until Sunday. A Sweat Lodge Ceremony started it on Wednesday morning. Of the forty members of his shamanistic drum group, maybe a dozen would be doing a quest, and they could come in on Thursday or Friday or even just do an overnight of Saturday to Sunday. Every eight hours Carmen would do a Drum Ceremony whose sound would reassure everybody. All this took place on Bare Hill, which I thought people were calling "Bear Hill." In a way, then, just to be there was already to "be on the hill."

A large acreage that surrounded the Sweat Lodge was wooded with hardwoods. One needn't go far from the lodge in the quest, and for first-timers this option might be the deciding factor: they could be alone in the woods at night, yet not really alone if the "leader of the band" was only as far away as the lodge and site of ceremony.

So on the first day five of us or so did the Sweat Ceremony and set off in different directions. Some or maybe all of the questers except me already knew where they were going. This shamanistic drum group had been sweating here for some time already and likely had taken walks in and about the area. Also, any of us could stop and come out anytime, or plan to do only one or two days at the start rather than at the end of the five days. I chose a southwesterly direction, into the wind, like a bear smelling for honey. Also, this was the direction of higher elevation, and I thought that the top of the hill would get me closest to Higher Consciousness.

As I walked, I was quite unaware that the quest had already started, but I found myself walking as though I were hunting. I just assumed that I was feeling my way along to the top of the hill. Soon I was lost in seeing all the things I had never seen before. Every tree, every rock, every blade of grass was a member of my universal family that I had never met before. I had no idea how large Bare Hill was. I had gradually left the constituent called Time somewhere in the dwindling physical consciousness behind me. I was now, distancewise, at the edge of hearing Carmen's every-eight-hour Drum Ceremony.

Now I came to a dense thicket that somewhat resembled a wall. After two feeble attempts to skirt it, left and right, I picked my way into it. It wasn't very thick, more like an overgrown bush line, and I came out onto a huge, flat, open area. If I had known that I was on Bare Hill and not Bear Hill, I might have said, "This must be the 'bare' of the name of the hill." To this day, I still don't know if this was the top of the hill because the far western edge continued to taper upward.

The first clue that I might be in a special place, in the "right" place, was a grove of Medicine shrubs ahead of me. I walked into them. They were the Nu hee(t) uh Medicine that made multivision of things, a sort of vision cloner. This miniversion of the regular Nu hee(t) did not grow everywhere. It is rare.

This was the Medicine that, along with another ingredient, could cause, say, the opponents in a lacrosse game to have double vision of the ball, so that their chances of catching the right ball was only 50 percent.

It could also, if you kept urging it, "cooking it," make more multiples until one visualized hundreds of the same thing. Twelve Indians drove a company of British troops over the cliffs at the Devil's Hole massacre, but the official report said, "Twelve hundred Indians."

The other ingredient needed for this Medicine was the scrapings of a tooth from the skull of a dead person. Now isn't that just ducky? Here I am telling of a Medicine shrub that is partner to being able to make a person see multiple images of anything. That statement alone might stretch your belief system, to where I probably lost half of my readers. And then I may have lost most of the rest by saying that now we need the scrapings of a tooth from the skull of a dead person.

And to make this explanation even thinner, I was told that the reason the scrapings had to come from the skull of a dead person is that the owner of the tooth had to give permission for this particular use of this tooth because the Medicine could not believe the word of a living person to always be true. It's no wonder there is such a separation between an Indian doctor and a "regular" doctor. And it shows how even among Indian doctors, some are greater than others.

All this aside, here I was simply continuing to walk on by impetus as though part of a flock of sheep. This mindset also happened to me as a paratrooper in a plane over the drop zone when we all stood up, hooked up, and blindly followed the guy ahead of us on out the door. I do remember the good feeling of seeing the Nu hee(t) uh, and after pushing through the wall of dense thicket, it was like, "Oh, hey, I've broken out into a whole new world. Let me explore it."

Halfway through the copse of Medicine, I came to a circle of nothing. No stones, no plant life. Being able to think back to it now, I wonder why I didn't wonder about it. Was it some sort of arena of the Little People? I have not much ever been into UFOs, but if someone who was a believer was with me, they may have said, "It looks like a flying saucer landed here."

What stopped me was a small tree, the only one around. At first I thought it was two trees, twins, but then I saw that, at about four inches above the ground, they were joined. A nice cradle, a nice U shape separated the two trunks. It was a White Pine tree. I stopped to rest. But I never got to go any farther. As soon as I lay down and put my head into that White Pine cradle, I knew there wasn't anything beyond this. My pineal gland was resting on the symbol of the Great Peace of the Six Nations.

The circle was about eighteen or twenty feet across, and I made a Medicine Wheel about half that size inside of it. The tree became one of the Four Direction markers, and I sprinkled some Sacred Tobacco to mark off the circle.

I'd fasted a day previous to this, but in such situations it always seemed that I couldn't stop expecting that I might need to urinate or defecate—here or at Sundance or at the Ten-Day Fast at Ta wi da qui's. Now I was enclosed in this circle. It was my "home," and I lived in it until Sunday. It's like metabolism took a vacation.

At night the deer would come to eat nearby. Some would walk right up to the Tobacco at the edge of the wheel and stop. They'd peer at me, and I would purse my lips as to play trumpet and let out a squeak like maybe a mouse would.

The deer would spring back a half a step, then slowly creep forward again, and be squeaked at again. Then maybe this deer would go back and tell another deer. "Hey. There's something strange in our dance circle. Go look, see what you think it is. It can't talk good." Then here would come another deer to go through the same little ritual of curiosity.

It's no wonder, then, if I was fooling around like this, that by Saturday I was still wondering why some "great vision" hadn't appeared to me. One day a vulture came floating along, and I pretended to be dying. I lay still but did a "dying tremor" with my legs. The female vulture did one circle, then said, "Oh for heaven's sake, just another man trap, and a very poor imitation at that," and it soared on out of sight.

Then at another time, a Great Blue Heron came daydreaming along, and slightly misjudged the elevation, and suddenly here was the ground, with me on it, coming up to meet it. With a squawk and some frantic wing strokes, it shot upward to safety. So strong was the "lift" that those long trailing legs fell downward, and had I been mischievous enough and alert enough, I could have grabbed that bird.

When Saturday came, I began thinking about all of what I was doing, and I said, "Why, no wonder nothing of a spiritual nature is visually manifesting. You didn't ask for anything. You haven't been awaiting a specific answer." And it was true. It was as though I were questing just because Carmen gave me the chance.

What do I need? Nothing. Well, then, what do I want? How about the knowledge of Medicine? How about what is the Medicine for AIDS? I closed my eyes and began sending out the question (and I'm not sure how one is to do that): "The Medicine for AIDS . . . the Medicine for AIDS . . . the Medicine for AIDS." On and on.

Now I don't know if I nodded off and had a dream or if I just began daydreaming. What I saw was a picture of musk oxen eating lichen. "Well," I thought (still seeing them), "If these animals can peacefully go about their daily functions in forty and fifty degrees below zero temperatures, then they must be getting some disease-countering strength from that lichen." But then I wondered if I might not just be trying to force the issue.

Late afternoon came, and I began getting antsy. Tomorrow was "go home" day. But what did I expect? For sure, to get antsy was the opposite way to go. I couldn't help it; I wanted something to happen.

Some years earlier I had made a Medicine rattle out of Slippery Elm bark. For no reason, I put some Freeman Sowden Sycamore bark salve on the handle, and even now it still smells like a cross between Lilac and Hepatica blossoms. In mock desperation I picked up that rattle and said, "If nothing's going to happen, I'll MAKE it happen. I'll throw a party!"

I then smacked the rattle against the palm of my hand, and "ZAP!" all the lights of physical consciousness went out. All fifty Chiefs of the original Five Nations were standing before me in the big circle. I don't know how I knew who they were; and even if I did know, I would have expected them to be stern and serious looking, but here they were more like children, giggly. Talk about a freak-out. I imagine my mouth was hanging wide open.

But they were Medicine. It was like they put a "charm" on me, and the next thing I knew, I was like them, giggly. I even felt a bit cocky. I said, "We're having a party, and I'm putting you guys at the head table, and I'm closing the head table."

They shook their heads, "No."

"Well, who else do you want?"

They named the Peacemaker.

"Oh, of course, how could I forget?"

(At the time of this conversation, it never occurred to me that it had to be done by telepathy. All communication was absolutely clear, though how could they know the English language?)

All this was taking place in broad daylight, but now, at the back of the group, an aura appeared. I assumed (or maybe knew by special communication) that the Peacemaker had arrived, so I said, "OK, we're closing the head table now," and to be funny I continued, "And we're going to have a second head table for the scrubs like Crazy Horse and Geronimo and. . ."

BAM! Geronimo and Crazy Horse were standing there grinning, and the rest of the bunch were in stitches. (Again, how could I even know that this was Crazy Horse? It is said that there are no pictures of him, yet I just KNEW.)

This was too much. Though I was grinning with joy, I was reduced to a blubbering mess, but here was yet another proof that some "Higher" Communication was taking place. I thought to myself, "This just doesn't get any better."

To which either Geronimo or Horse or both said, "Oh no?" and PRESTO, there stood my mother and father (both deceased).

Now here was too much on top of too much. I could only motion and send the message, "Have the party any way you like. Invite whomever you wish." And they did.

Beeman Logan came with his wife, Arlene. The party was well under way before I suddenly realized, "Wait a minute! Arlene is still alive!" as though only dead people could come. But then, she and I WERE the only living ones at the party, and I never moved from my spot; in fact, I acted the most dead.

Heeengs was there, and because she was noted for chasing rain clouds helter-skelter, I said to her, "Don't let it rain on me."

"Just stay there a minute," she said, as though I might make a run for it. "I want you to meet someone."

In a little while she came back with this tall, bony-faced (like hers) Indian, and by his dress he came from west of the Mississippi. "Meet Split-the-sky," she said. His name hints that he may have been her teacher.

The singing and dancing were tremendous. It may well be that these songs and dances were meant for my education, but I can only remember one called the Medicine's Medicine Dance.

Most of the social dance songs do not have words to them. The exception may be in songs that have been borrowed, with or without permission, from other nations because of their "universal" popularity.

For a long time I wondered about this because I sang quite a number of social dance songs, not knowing if I was making a statement or not. Unlike any other group of songs, all the women's dance songs contained a codalike phrase, "Nowiyo(t) hay'yu(t)."

I thought, "Surely so much repetition of that phrase was saying something." I went to Chief Pat Sandy (Cayuga) and asked him what "Nowiyo(t) hay'yu(t)" meant.

He put his hand to the side of his lips as though he were going to divulge to me some important secret information, as though he might even have to whisper it. Instead, he said quite loudly, "Nothing."

Alright, back to my attempting to reconstruct the "vision quest party."

The Medicine's Medicine Dance was surprisingly fast. There were only five or six dancers, but they were very very good. The song had recognizable words in it (Tuscarora), and that's why I think this dance may have been a ceremonial tribute to Medicine, maybe an old forgotten Tuscarora one.

The dance started with the dancers walking very slowly in a circle. A single singer struck a drumbeat (water drum) every once in a while. Suddenly the singer began singing and drumming at a very fast pace, equal to Smoke Dance or faster.

"Oo(t)ju(t), Oo(t)ju(t), Oo(t)ju(t)," for thirty seconds or so, then "N'yow weh, n'yow weh" (thank you, thank you), "n'yow weh, n'yow weh" (for another thirty seconds or so, in a tone a fourth lower), then a loud yell, "Jawwwww Hoo(t)!" And the dancers went into a very slow walk again. When the dancers were dancing, they danced in place and exhibited a near "show-off" exuberance.

About eight or ten Medicines were named and sung to, and I don't know if there was a deliberate pecking order to the names. I doubt it because that would be anti-Longhouse thought. Also, many great Medicine names would necessarily have to be left out because they are too long. At any rate I did manage to recall the first two names, Oo(t)' ju(t) and Wa'rodge (Pepper Root and St. John's Wort).

Other things may have taken place, but it's not clear to me because the whole thing was very much like a hazy dream that wanted to fade out when I came back into camp the next day. If I did sleep at all that night, I bet it was with sugarplums dancing through my head because I was superhappy. As I became aware of the faintest approaching aura of daylight, I could also feel an acute awareness of gratitude toward the things of life that we simply take for granted, that we might even arrogantly claim as our "given." My five senses, my heartbeat, my breath.

I didn't want to leave my sacred circle. I was, by far, the last to come into the Closing Ceremony. The walk back was a subtle transition walk, back into the world of the ordinary. The first thing I noticed was that everything was wet. People were drying their clothes by the fire, but Heeengs and her boyfriend, Split-the-sky, had not let it rain on me. The next cute little rarity came when someone said to me, "Boy! You were sure singing up a storm last night. I never heard those songs before."

"Maybe it wasn't me singing."

"Oh, it was you all right, you was the only one that far up on the hill."

I haven't told many people (if any) about this quest, and for sure not in length or detail, but it hasn't been for lack of trying. For months, if I started to tell it, I would burst into tears, and my throat would swell up. After a while, when I thought about it, I said to myself, "Why tell it? It's not believable anyways." Now, though, I realize that the story might be reinforcing to the "Red Road pilgrim" or to the Indian with one foot in the ship and the other in the canoe.

As a kind of mini-epilogue to this chapter, let me tell you what became of that Slippery Elm Medicine rattle with the Freeman Sowden Sycamore salve odor. One night Carmen Ramos had all of his sacred Medicine paraphernalia stolen from him, so I gave him my feather and that rattle. I haven't heard much from him, but it may be because he may have struck that rattle against his palm and been struck spellbound, too.

Medicines of the Universe

If everything in this Universe has a purpose, it sometimes seems that some purposes are very well hidden. Maybe there's no such thing as purpose. Maybe there's only the yin-yang. Maybe it's more accurate to say that there is Medicine in all things, but that the part that is Medicine can be very well hidden. In Medicine it is as though there are different degrees of accessibility. The greater and more powerful the Medicine, the more elusive it is.

Take the Fire Lion, the Ga hus stee'nis. It is not thought of as a Medicine. Hardly does anyone know of its existence. I could scarcely find anyone who had seen it. So the average bear would say, "It's just a mythological figure, a figment of the imagination."

Tuscarora has no word for mythology, and I don't know of any Indian nation that does.

In a story that traces its roots to North Carolina Tuscarora story-telling we hear of a Tuscarora that called to the Fire Lion for help. He was extremely fearful of the Fire Lion, so what induced him to beseech a thing that he feared the most? Desperation. For him, that was the key to tapping into a power that solved a problem—imploring this previously unthought of source as a Medicine to come to his rescue. He was being chased by another fearful thing, and in desperation his own Higher Consciousness said, "If I fear the Fire Lion more than I fear this monster, then it obviously has more power. My only hope is to find out. I'll call on it for help."

Not only, then, is this a story of a man in dire need of help who received that help from the least expected place, but it is also a story that offers more than Aesop's moral lessons; it tells us that the objects of our greatest fears are also potential friends, potential Medicine.

Both Peter Joseph and Bob Mt. Pleasant, both Tuscaroras at Six Nations, Canada, had seen the Ga hus stee'nis. Both had been scared out of their wits.

Automatic Transmission, another Tuscarora from the same place, told of how his grandfather, as a boy, saw the Fire Lion come in for a landing. This fearsome thing lives in bodies of water. It was described as "like an Osprey dive-bombing a fish under water into the Grand River." An overwhelming curiosity compelled the boy to summon the courage to steal carefully to the spot where this flying animal had plunged out of sight. After all, so unbelievable was such a sight that he needed corroboration. Just the same, he didn't just rush to the edge of the water. He had to wait until his jitters subsided.

The water was fairly deep there at this drop-off section of the bank, and the boy was able to crawl through the grass and lay on his stomach to peek over the edge. One of the most astonishing features of the Fire Lion was its eyes. They emitted sparks like a Fourth of July sparkler. What about under water? Did sparks keep on coming out even under water? Were the sparks hot? If so, did they make the water sizzle? The surface of the water was calm.

The movement of the flowing water did not allow the boy a clear image, but he did see the lion. Between wanting a good look at it and wanting to run once he saw that it wasn't an illusion, the boy made out that the eyes of the beast were closed. He had taken too long to dare approach it. It had gone to sleep. Still, what luck! He could observe it undetected unless it awoke.

One thing that the boy noticed was the lion's mane. The hairs of the mane were very coarse. Each strand of it waved around in the movement of the water like a baby snake. Oooh! And what if it woke up?

The boy backed away carefully, then dashed home. He told everyone who would listen of what he had seen. Some of the Elders said, "Oh my! You had one of the greatest opportunities to own one of the greatest power objects known. All you had to do was yank out just one of them hairs from that mane."

Because of sparse sources of knowledge of Medicine, I have touched lightly here on only one of thousands of unknown sources and their possible multiple uses. Has anyone even seen the Ga hus stee'nis in the past fifty or sixty years?

And what about our other family members, other powerful member Elements of the Universe? A note to ourselves is in order here: that we have "pull" . . . that we can call on our sisters and brothers for help. Also, that the farther "out there" we go for that help (the Four Directions, the Four Protectors, and so on), the more ethereal and powerful the help.

♦   ♦   ♦

What about the Ooh du(t) cheah? Now here is something much more people related. Naughty people related. It is an entity or being that is truly meant to scare a
person deserving to be frightened badly as a form of punishment. It can be called
a universal Medicine because no human "sics" the Ooh du(t) cheah on the
human culprit. The Universe does.

What does this frightening thing look like? A half of a woman. The bottom
half. It is reported to be black in color, but, then, it only operates at night.

Who does it chase and why? It chases men who continually have not taken
care of their wives and children, but instead spend their time and money on another woman.

The theme of this "Medicine" is somewhat like the case of the woman who
continually beat her child over her own frustrations. In such an instance, it is the
Little People, who are like "children of the Universe," who step in when a child
has suffered too much. The mother is frightened when she sees a little plate that
the Little People have provided in the feast (the feast being a powerful ceremonial form of Medicine) for her child. The plate symbolically says, "One more
time! You strike this little girl just one more time, and we'll be calling her again!
But this next time she won't be coming back. You'll never see her again because
you don't deserve to have her." This is the "fright" Medicine that zaps the mother
to the reality of her own inappropriate behavior.

A hundred years ago all the Indians of the Six Nations and maybe more
knew of the Ooh du(t) cheah. This word in Tuscarora means "hips," though the
entity is much more than hips. The Mohawk word for this entity is *Oo no(t) sa*,
and the Seneca word is quite similar.

So let's imagine a typical scene in which the Ooh du(t) cheah attacks her
victim.

A man, maybe even a dapper fellow riding horseback on an equally dapper
steed or even in a sporty carriage, is on his way home from spending half the
night with a secret girlfriend-woman. His children are at home shoeless and have
had little or nothing to eat.

Suddenly the horse whinnies and shivers nervously. The driver halts the
horse, thinking that it may have sensed danger up ahead, maybe a robber lurking
in the bushes. It is unusually difficult to stop the horse, but the driver is able to
do it.

The horse stops for only one or two seconds then bolts into a full gallop, nearly sending the rider from the saddle or the driver from the carriage seat. In that wee intermission the "bad" man knows what's happening. He hears the Ooh du(t) cheah coming behind them and closing fast.

"Ju(t)-ju(t)-ju(t)-ju(t)-ju(t)-ju(t)-ju(t). . ." His hair stands up by itself, as does the hair on the horse's back. It is not long before the horse is oozing a bubbly white sweat and is frothing at the mouth. It cannot run any faster. Its eyes are bulging whitely. The man has wet his pants and maybe more, but doesn't even know it. The Ooh du(t) cheah is running easily and gracefully alongside the man. It is on "cruise control" and doesn't run out of gas.

My father told me that when he and a group of ice-skaters at a night skating party at a remote pond saw the Ooh du(t) cheah chase a man, the noise its feet made sounded like it was running in slush. "Ju(t)-ju(t)-ju(t)-ju(t). . ."

When I told Jonesy this story, he lambasted me. "OH, FOR CHRIST SAKES, TEDDY! GET WITH IT! Them wasn't the Ooh du(t) cheah's feet making that noise, and you know it. That was her snapper snapping away. That was what was puttin' the fear of God into the poor sucker. She was saying, 'You want strange sex, Jocko, I'll give you strange sex.' "

And what if the "victim" is a man on foot or even with his dog? Without the clippity-clop noise of the horse's hooves, he will hear the Ooh du(t) cheah coming much sooner. The dog hears it first and will stop and bark a whining scared bark, with its hackles rising. Then it will implore its master (with its eyes and short runs), "Run!" By this time the master, too, hears the Ooh du(t) cheah and runs for the safety of his home with all the physical capacity that he can muster. His dog will not stay to defend him, displaying a never seen before "it's every man for himself" behavior and willingly leaves the master to his fate.

Dooh gwog had this happen to him, and he didn't even have a dog to do a protective double-cross. (Dooh gwog, whose name means "guinea hen," was the man who got caught using a guinea hen egg, which is stronger than a chicken egg, in the annual Easter egg fights and got hung with that name for the rest of his life.)

Dooh gwog, at the time, lived in Elton Green's house across from the Mission Church. The Ooh du(t) cheah likes to play a little game of sort of holding back, as though it might be getting tired, so that the pursuee keeps going beyond any normal capacity. It doesn't care who dies of a heart attack or of fright.

Dooh gwog made it to the house with the Ooh du(t) cheah right behind in a fake lag. He ran across the room and flopped into the big cushy armchair, exhausted, "Almost dead," as he put it. In this position he lay petrified and transfixed in fear, unable to move except to gasp for breath.

The Ooh du(t) cheah, as though to produce more drama, if possible, paused for effect, to make a grand entrance so to speak; then with a short run like people use to help launch themselves across a creek, it jumped up and landed squarely on Dooh gwog's face.

The smell was of woman's smell to the tenth power. Dooh gwog passed out.

This happened on a Friday night in the middle of the night. When Dooh gwog woke up and came to his senses, he assumed it was Saturday evening. No. It was Sunday evening. He had lost a whole day. He had spent it learning a lesson somewhere deep in the heart of womanland.

After this episode of drama produced by one of the Medicines of the Divine and Harmonious Universe, Dooh gwog became the most conscientious family man you would ever want to meet. Even at night, all you women.

Quantum Physics

Somewhere around the mid-1980s Mary Thunder and Horse got me Sundancing, and I have been, from time to time, dancing ever since. Sundancing and vision questing and much of the spiritual mechanics that take place among members of the secret societies within the Longhouse are things that take place strictly between the individual and the Higher Consciousness and are deemed too sacred to be shared at random. This is because sharing can be construed as bragging and therefore subject to the law that says, "Bragging dilutes one's Medicine." A second part to the same law says, "The energy of sacred experience is diluted even if the sharer of that experience is not bragging, but when the uninitiated listener believes that the innocent sharer is lying." Again, I hear my father telling others, "Don't let anyone see you gathering this certain sacred plant. Don't let anyone see you taking it [imbibing it]."

Apart from those personally kept secrets, other sharing among friends and Medicine people has the opposite effect. It reinforces the strength of the believer in Medicine. These special and scintillating sharing times never get out of hand; humor is a form of Medicine, and Indians are never without it.

At one of the Sundances I attend, there is a separate sacred fire we all gather around at night to hear announcements: who will be waking everyone in the tenting area at 5:00 A.M. with a song, anything special about the next day's schedule, any violations of Sundance protocol, and so on. If the atmosphere of the meeting may begin to feel unnecessarily demanding or strict, an Elder may interject a dose of humor to diffuse that atmosphere.

One can imagine the difficult task it is to organize and administrate a large Sundance — making sure that no drugs or alcohol get past the checkpoint gate and doing all those other things that years of trial and error have revealed are necessary but may otherwise never been thought of. So, about halfway through a

230

dance (after a week of preparation, including covering the whole hundred foot diameter arbor roof and dancers' rest area with pine branches for shade; fasting for four days; piercing and breaking four days; doing a healing round; gathering wood for the Fire Keepers for sweats at 5:00 A.M. and approximately 5:00 P.M.; and so on), the head honcho is starting to feel wrung out. So this nightly gathering around the sacred fire is a nice respite.

One night at this particular dance, after we all had started taking it for granted and more and more instances of little broken rules began popping up, the "CEO" of it went into a spiel to remind everyone of the enormity of his job. He went on to add that "some things did not simply appear from out of the blue, for instance the Johnny-on-the-spots (rented portable toilets) cost about three hundred dollars."

"SO DON'T BE USING THEM!" yelled an Elder, who sensed that this was the appropriate time to diffuse the atmosphere with the Medicine called humor.

Toward the ending of the dance, as in all Sundances, a joyfulness began creeping in like an anticipated crescendo, and a night of poetry reading and story-telling took place around the sacred fire (these activities are not done at all Sundances, though). The stories are about actual incredible and magical experiences from all of "Indiandom." Right after the head honcho's spiel was humorously aborted, he announced the special story-telling time by saying, "And now it's time for the Elders to tell examples of our concept of quantum physics."

I cried. I cried because upon hearing story-telling equated with quantum physics, I was instantly transported backward twenty years or more when I sat listening to the great Isaiah Joseph at Six Nations, Canada, saying something that gripped my attention: "Someday science will explain how the phenomena produced by our Indian Medicine people comes from their ability to tap into and direct the energy of the Universe to do their spiritually mental bidding."

I was crying because there was something more beautiful in Isaiah's words, like I could see him nodding his head "yes" to the whole concept. Here was the uncertainty principle of quantum physics. Here was the concept of certain energy particles drifting freely, as though "looking for action," free to be directed or attracted or repelled by magnetism or by gravity or by the overpowering energy of Uncle Charley's need for food or by "whatever," a favorite expression of the great Ute Red Earth Woman.

This chapter then is simply a collage of the same type of examples of "quantum physics" that have taken place among the Indians of the Six Nation Iroquois of Canada and of the United States.

These experiences are best portrayed in this chapter because each incident is not long enough to be a whole chapter in itself. Just the same, one single incident can parallel the psychological impact of Greek mythological figures, though likely the impact of the former is more subtle because such incidents deal with unknown spiritual laws of the Universe and not just with human behavior.

Long, long ago, before white people came about, the Tuscaroras used to put on an annual talent show. If it were done today, church people might call it a contest of witchcraft or voodoo power. Then, it was just a day of entertainment, a display of magic tricks, and no different than a day at the circus.

If we of today witnessed one of these shows, we would be raving about the unbelievable display of power we had witnessed. In the past, however, such displays were expected, but once in a while something unexpected might happen, like the occurrence I'm going to tell you about. Such an incident would be told and retold from generation to generation to the present, and so now you can pretend you were there.

At this particular "talent" show the "stage" chosen was an open beach on the shores of a placid little lake (said to have been near what is now Roanoke, North Carolina). The slate of participants, the "magicians," was open to anyone, though of course one had to be quite adept to go up against the great tricksters of that time.

Among the performers was a new and unknown Medicine practitioner who some say was a visiting Tutelo. So let us use the name with apologies to the Tutelo. At any rate he considered himself very powerful and could scarcely wait to show himself to be the star of the show and to out-do the local Tuscarora talent.

What the newcomer didn't know was that these displays of "power" always started gently, with the beginning "acts" being those of apprentices. Now, an apprentice could be of any age, not necessarily a youngster, and on this particular annual affair the first man up was about fifty years old. The assembled Tuscaroras thought it quite cute that this man, at his age, was the opening act. He was just, as some white people might say, "one of the good ol' boys." He had never been a participant in this magic show before, ever. Secretly, though, he had been sneaking in some lessons from one of the great ones. His tutor now stood among the crowd, watching with interest and hoping to be proud of his pupil.

The pupil went to the edge of the placid water of the lake. There he stood for a moment, a bit shy, then he held up his index finger for everyone to see. He pointed it at the water and slowly began to wave it back and forth. Wherever he pointed, a ripple was produced, and soon he was swishing a little frothy path back and forth as he increased the speed of his motion. The crowd cheered.

"HAH!" thought the Tutelo, and his mind said something like, "Oh for Pete's sake! Is this all the Tuscarora Elders can do? Here, let me show them some REAL POWER!"

It was OK for this newcomer to go up and do a trick because much of the show was ad lib (like if one could insert something funny or add a complementing little twist to the previous act, then by all means one should do it before the timing of it was lost).

So it was OK for the Tutelo to step up now, but not to do what he did when he got there. He pushed aside the apprentice, who had just endeared himself to the crowd. He then pointed to the water.

From the depths could first be seen a bulge of water. What was in the bulge? A white buffalo, which as soon as the water fell off and subsided, became an impressive sight standing there on the surface of the lake.

What happened next happened quickly. It also put an end to the whole show right then and there, and that's why the reporting of this event has passed on through generation after generation and on to now. Never before and never since was the talent show ever stopped, abruptly, as this one was.

As soon as the Tutelo pushed the apprentice aside, the secret tutor stepped forward. If anyone had known exactly what was taking place, they may have expected to witness the "buffalo maker" being thrown into the lake with the buffalo. Instead, hardly had the water spilled off the buffalo before the tutor stepped between the Tutelo and the lake.

The white buffalo's time in the limelight was short-lived. At the snap of the tutor's fingers another creature, the much-feared Fire Lion, emerged from the lake and immediately began devouring the buffalo. Not in one gulp. It was as though the Fire Lion's face took on the look of the blower mask of the False Face Society, and, instead of blowing, it sucked the white buffalo through its puckered lips like spaghetti.

This took just long enough for the tutor to collect his apprentice and flee.

Flee? Yes, flee, because of what happened next. The Ga hus stee'nis (Fire Lion), having caused the buffalo to do a disappearing act, now turned its attention on the crowd. It sprayed forth a stream of fire. Go!

The intense heat produced panic, and soon nothing—no people, nothing—was left beside the lake or on it. The party was over. The only injury to anyone was to the pride of the audacious newcomer trickster whose hair was all burned from his head. He was seen leaving, but never seen returning.

There are wanna-bes and there are wanna-see-bes. Wanna-see-bes are just people who go to pow-wows and Indian reservations and wherever there are gatherings of Indians, especially if they are Elders, with hopes of seeing some kind of miracle performed. It's as if they are thinking, "I wanna see one of them gosh darn real Medicine men or Medicine women that I keep hearing about, and, dammit, it's getting so I'm losing faith that such people exist. It's getting so's I'm wondering if they're nothing but the same as Santa Claus."

Elders at gatherings have often not seen one another for years and so look forward to the joy of such an occasion. When they do get together, one or the other or both are usually scheduled to appear on a panel or talk in fifteen minutes or so. No sooner do they meet to greet each other and gab, but here comes a wanna-see-be to butt in.

This happened one time to Beeman Logan and Rolling Thunder. They had already "run away" from the crowd and had strolled out into the countryside.

Not good enough. Here comes this poor sap of a guy trotting up behind them. "Hey. Hi!" Beeman rolls his eyes up into the sky. Rolling Thunder laughs.

They are "onto" the wanna-see-be because both have been around a long time, been all over, and have seen all kinds of buttinskies, and they can tell that this one looks desperate: "I'm giving Indians just one more chance, then to hell with all Indians; they're all fakes." I have called the guy a "poor sap" because of Beeman and RT's take-no-guffness.

Sure enough, the guy was desperate. So desperate that after walking only a few steps in group formation, he says, "I can turn a tree into a cow."

(When Beeman was telling me about this incident, repeating what he had just heard, saying, "Those were his first words, 'I can turn a tree into a cow.' I don't know how we kept from bursting out laughing, but we did.")

The "cow maker" got no answer. After a bit, he thinks, "Maybe these two codgers are deaf," so he says again, louder, "I CAN TURN A TREE INTO A COW."

In the meantime RT is thinking, "Hail Mary Poppins full of Grace! This man's GONE! How can Beeman keep a straight face? How can I for that matter? There is only one way to get rid of this guy. Let's do it."

RT stops walking and winks at Beeman. Then he says to the wanna-see-be, "Let's see you."

Exactly as they both knew he would say, he said, "I will if you show me what you can do."

On the ground nearby was a thin stick, a dead tree branch. "Look at that stick," RT says, pointing at it. About five seconds goes by, and the stick moves and crawls away as a snake.

Beeman thinks, "Well, I guess it's my turn," and he tells Wanna, "Look at that pond."

Below them is a small pond, which they all look at. Above the pond, on a hill, is a gnarled old wind-blown pine. "Now look at that tree," Beeman commands. They do.

In just about the amount of time it took to appreciate the classic beauty of the tree, Beeman says, "Now look back at the pond."

There was no water in the pond. Fish were flopping about in mud. "Better hurry up and look back at the tree, or you'll kill all the fish!" Beeman barks, feigning alarm.

They look quickly back to the lone pine.

"OK," Beeman says, "All done."

The water was back in the pond. Beeman and RT looked at the cow maker, who stood there in some kind of heavenly daze. He would be making no cows. His eyes glistened.

Just before he walked away, he broke into the silliest grin ever seen on earth. He had a new name. Have Seen.

Little Wesley was big, bigger than his father, who was called Big Wesley. At one time, though, Big Wesley was bigger, and that's when Junior was little.

Little Wesley spent some time in the U.S. Navy with another Tuscarora named Johnny Pem. Johnny told Wesley, "Whatever you do, don't do what I did.

I asked Eleazer Williams to make me some love Medicine. He said, 'No.' I said, 'Yes.' He said, 'No.' I said, 'Yes.' He said, 'OK. YOU ASKED FOR IT!' "

Johnny then went on to say that he was besieged by women who fought over him right in front of kin and that he was juked out so bad that he joined the navy to escape.

Of course, Little Wesley didn't believe him. It just sounded like any other lovesick sailor's macho wet-dream ramblings. But Johnny persisted. He persisted to the point that Wesley was forced to use all his powers of selective hearing, which led Wes to a state of tuned-out boredom. He had an attack of wanting to act outrageous, anything that could distract Johnny Pem and his lying. It was like Wesley couldn't stop himself. He pulled a black navy sock over his head and "looked" at Johnny.

"No!" Johnny screamed. 'DON'T DO THAT, WESLEY! DON'T EVER DO THAT! That's bad luck to do that. Very bad."

Well, thought Wesley, my ruse worked.

Wesley had been raised to discount and deny the existence of ESP, so although he pulled the sock off, he just "knew" that there wasn't any such thing as bad luck or luck of any kind.

Which may indeed be true, but the next day Little Wesley had occasion to wonder. He was informed that a message had arrived for him. The wire informed him that his youngest sister had died instantly the day before in an auto accident. Wes kept his black socks on his feet after that.

The years went by. One day after both Wesley and Johnny had returned to civilian life, Wesley went to visit Johnny. When Johnny opened the door at the sound of the knock and saw that it was Little Wesley, he grinned and motioned with his head, "Come on in."

Little Wesley went in. He couldn't believe what he saw. There were three voluptuous women in there. They were arguing over Johnny Pem.

When Wesley left, he was scratching his head.

We can't just leave Johnny Pem there, fighting off women, because he really was a living alarm clock—a "warner" or harbinger of future boo-boos. He didn't "see" everybody's accident before it happened, but when he did, if he warned you and you ignored the warning, it WOULD happen. Many people were afraid of him.

They couldn't seem to see that he wasn't the CAUSE of accidents, but rather more like the preventer. Maybe these people had ego problems. Maybe they thought they were kings—the kind that cut the heads off of messengers who brought bad news.

Johnny Pem had different ways of seeing. He didn't have any control of when. He told me that one of his most prevalent ways of seeing was through dreams. In a dream he would see the person who had an appointment with an accident riding on a machine. The larger the machine, the larger the accident.

Chief Tracy Johnson, who, in another part of this book, received the "miracle kill" deer from Pennsylvania, told me what happened to him and one of Johnny's premonitions .

Johnny Pem took his time giving Tracy a phone call because it was Saturday morning, and Johnny thought that everyone slept in on Saturday just because he did. Well, when he did call, Tracy was already up and gone. But Johnny just thought that the Chief wanted to sleep and wouldn't get up to answer the phone.

Finally, about 1:00 P.M., Tracy answered the phone. "Watch it, today," the seer said, "I dreamed I saw you riding a power mower. Better watch your driving today, or you'll have a minor accident."

Too late. The Chief had already slid across the icy entrance of his driveway and into a tree. He thought of Johnny Pem as a lifesaver of people, and this time, because all he suffered was a fender bender and a sore knee instead of death, he could afford to joke about it.

After Tracy reported the accident and remarked that alarm clocks should wake people up sooner, all he said to Johnny was, "Better luck next time."

Let's just for a moment wonder, Where the Dickens does the knowledge that something is scheduled to happen come from? Also, if this knowledge comes as a message from Johnny Pem, or anybody else, and we act on it and prevent the event from happening, could it have been that it wasn't going to happen? If this knowledge comes from, say, Johnny Pem's own Higher Consciousness, then why can't we all get those messages? Is Johnny Pem a nine in the Enneagram (the center of the intuitiveness of the compulsions eight, nine, and one)? If so, because a nine is also compelled to smooth any rippling of any waters, then he must be quite suited to arbitrate between the women fighting over him.

What about the Four Protectors (sometimes called the Four Messengers), our universal kin as stated in the Thanksgiving Address? Might they be an intuitive person's connection to the knowledge of future events? If so, are they our only connection? Nobody (that we know of) has seen the Four Protectors, so what would they look like? (Somebody said, "Daisy Thomas," and we all laughed.) And what about Daisy Thomas and all the great seers and readers who use different things (playing cards, tea leaves, Sacred Tobacco, and so on) to tap into this Higher Consciousness of knowledge: Do they need these things? Daisy said, "No, not once I get started."

Questions, questions, questions—beautiful and highly interesting questions, but Indians don't seem to need to ask these questions. It only matters that it is possible to see the future and change it. Sometimes, to make that change is simple. Johnny Pem calls you up and says, "When you go to your dentist appointment on Thursday, don't go by way of Hyde Park Boulevard, or you'll have an accident." So you just go a different way. But what do you do if you are Vernon Jack in this next incident?

A group of six or seven Indians were drinking beer one weekend night at the Marlboro Inn in Sanborn, New York. They were seated around a round table, and one of them was Johnny Pem. For "no reason," as we sometimes say, he lit a cigarette and placed it in an ashtray in the middle of the table and announced, "Whoever smokes this cigarette will die!"

Gasps could be heard. Then several voices.

"WHAT did you say!!?"

Johnny Pem was slow to answer. "I don't know what made me say that."

Everyone was thinking the same thing. Preposterous! Johnny Pem just doesn't SAY things like that—"Whoever smokes this cigarette will die"—but I heard it clearly, and from HIM! WOW! THAT'S ALARMING, bone chilling even.

It was as though time and sense came to a halt momentarily. In the brief interim that it did, while everyone at the table sat stunned and aghast, in through the entrance door to the inn strode Vernon Jack, unnoticed. Right up to the table of consternated Indians. Right to the "no-no" cigarette, which he blithely and flippantly put to his lips.

The horrified group sounded cries of "no" and every kind of verbal warning. Well, you know that if everyone talks at once, nothing makes sense; it's just garble. And normally, this taking of a cigarette is just a cute little trick, a naughty little ice-breaking introduction, a mini "crash the party" trick, a drum roll. Vernon took a drag.

But gradually he got the chilling message. "GOT 'NEH OOT' GIT! [Really demonic.] Can I get out of this quandary?" (The way out had already passed, though. It was to NOT smoke that cigarette.)

However, Vernon Jack did get safely home, with or without help, and went to bed. Nothing had been said about WHEN he was to die. Maybe it was all just a big joke—bizarre, yes—but that was not Johnny Pem's way. Vernon slept past noon.

When Vernon woke, he lay there thinking. He was hungry. Jonesy, across Dog Street (which is just a local nickname; on a road map one would see Mt. Hope Road), had chickens. Maybe Vern could scrounge a couple of eggs from him. Vernon got up, got dressed, then looking both ways started across Dog Street.

On the other side of the road stood Dan Bones and Vivian. They had just been kicked out of the house by Jonesy. They had gotten drunk and pissed on the couch too many times. Jonesy had finished his "GET OUT" speech by saying, ". . . and take the fuckin' couch with you!"

So Dan said, "Hey, Vernon. Help me get this couch on the flatbed."

So they got one end of the couch leaning up against the back end of the flatbed truck. Vernon climbed up on the truck, and—with him lifting and pulling, and with Dan Bones pushing upward from the ground—they got the couch on the back of the truck. Then Vernon dragged the couch toward the front of the flatbed.

Vernon Jack was a great talent on the Tuscarora Indian Reservation. Some of his oil paintings are probably in museums somewhere today. There are only so many of his paintings anywhere because after the day he helped load Dan Bones's couch on the flatbed, he never painted another picture.

Already up on the flatbed, leaning upward against the cab, was a big old heavy wooden storm door. It had a nice big window in it. As Vernon came chugging backward, dragging the couch, a gust of wind came along and blew the door over, smashing the window on his head. The jagged shards of glass severed his jugular vein. Vernon Jack died from loss of blood before he could be gotten to the hospital.

Plant Medicines

Medicine is in so many things that the category of plant Medicines can start to fall through the cracks.

I have a book called *American Eclectic Dispensatory*. It has 1,391 pages. I mean, just how many illnesses and remedies can anyone expect to have in one lifetime?

In the times of my grandmother, Geese-a-geese, every family had a sensible knowledge of remedies that took care of all the common afflictions of that time. Unless anyone planned to be what my father was called, an Indian doctor, why would you study and accumulate a large collection of herbal Medicines, especially if you hardly ever got sick?

Also, after you absorb the overall meaning of this book, you will know that you can influence everything in the Universe, including the degree of healing by remedies and more (i.e., "The amount of cure that you get from any Medicine is directly related to the amount of reverence you have for it"). You will see that we don't need to hoard anything. There are many good plant remedy books in bookstores that can be a good start to giving you a feeling about which plants you might start talking to. "Oooooh! I like Yooooou! I know you can heal me goooood!"

But because I probably ought not to leave out the names of ANY plants and should play "nice guy," I'll rattle off some of the names from the top of my fingertips.

First, there are a few what we might call "emergency" plant remedies. And then there are some rare or "more sophisticated" Medicine plants that like to play hard to get, such as Pennyroyal *(Hedeoma pulegiodes)*, whose name in Tuscarora is Wa chee'ha ruh, or "You-chase-it." You might see Pennyroyal until the day you need it. Better take some Sacred Indian Tobacco or silver with you in looking for the plant, or you won't see it.

Obviously, if you have been bitten by a rattlesnake or even by a rabid dog, you don't have time to be doing any lengthy ceremonies to any Medicines. That's why plantain *(Plantago major)* is so plentiful (at least here where I live and also in New York State). Its Indian name means "Along-the-road-species." Just grab a leaf, chew it into a good spitball, then press the juice into the snake- or dog-bite hole (or the hole made by stepping on a rusty nail).

Another "don't need big ceremony" herb is Sweetflag (root), with the botanical name *Acorus calamus.* Keep some half-inch pieces of the dried root handy to be used to offset the beginning of a cold or to break up phlegm in a scary tight chest cold. Or to offset heartburn.

In this same category is Wild Ginger *(Asarum canadense).* In this one the snakelike rhizome can be used cough-drop fashion, like the Sweetflag, when you are suffering from a cold. It's for when you start coughing and can't stop (so can't sleep). Pop one of these one-third-inch cough drops into your mouth. It has an anodyne effect (suggestive of Novocain because, like the Wild Ginger flower, it can be hallucinogenic).

In all of these "don't need big ceremony" remedies, though, it wouldn't hurt to say "Thank you" now, would it?

Another "good buddy" plant is Mallows *(Malva parviflora),* which, as a tea of any part of the whole plant, stops convulsions. Dip a clean cloth into the hot tea and wave it through the air (to cool it) then, with the "convulsee" in an upright position, put the "Medicined" cloth into their mouth and hope they don't choke.

How about Catnip *(Nepeta cataria)?* A great nerve Medicine. We used to put the tea of the leaves in a crying baby's bottle and soon could ask, "Where did the crying go?" But we grown-ups don't need to tell anybody that we use "baby Medicine" to get to sleep. Or for therapy.

Touch-me-not *(Impatiens capensis* and *Impatiens pallida)* is the poison ivy remedy. Just say "Thank you" to this plant, crush the juicy stalks, and rub this pulp on the afflicted area.

Goldthread *(Coptis groenlandica,* also called *Coptis trifolia)* is for mouth problems. Just pretend you're a snuff user and put a small wad of these golden threadlike roots in your mouth and live happily ever after. Some Indians say it's also good for anything wrong in your head. If you feel goofy, try it!

Basswood *(Tilia americana)* is a tree Medicine, the tree False Faces are

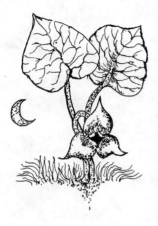

*Wild Ginger (*Asarum canadense*).*
Drawing by Diana Osborne Williams.

made from, so I would say "THANK YOU!!" very fervently first. The inner bark is used as a poultice to draw out unseen slivers or toxic substances.

Creeping Bellflower *(Campanula rapunceloides)* is a "man's" Medicine, and in your family the use of it could be controversial. Someone always has to ask, "Is this an emergency?" As a clue to what it was used for, gigglers called it "stifferene" (for erection purposes). (The leaves and stalk must be DRIED OUT first.)

One more plant Medicine.

The Tuscarora name for Spicebush *(Benzoin aestivale)* is Daw ehn yuks. It, too, might be thought of as a "man's" Medicine by women.

Let's say Mr. Goodbar is getting ready to "go and buy some lumber." But his wife suspects that he might be coming home a bit later because one doesn't need to shower and shave or overdose on aftershave lotion to buy lumber. So at that evening meal, before he leaves, she serves Spicebush tea. (The opposite of "stifferene.")

Now let's go on to a "next" level of plant Medicine. These Medicines can be a little trickier. You might, for instance, already use Goldenseal *(Hydrastis canadensis)* root powder for the flu, and four times in a row, ZIP, it has knocked the flu for a loop. So you take it for granted. On the fifth time, though, it gives you a lesson. You feel like you're going to DIE from the flu this time (perhaps you forgot to say "Thanks").

Also tricky about this category is that something in it might not even BE a plant.

The use of a green snake *(Opheodrys vernalis)* is a situation where, nowadays, you first have to FIND a green snake. This exact species. And WHEN you do find it, would you do what you need to do to use this Medicine (what the Indian doctor told you to do)? You want to have good teeth? Then you have to chew lightly on the snake's body as though you were playing a mouth organ. The snake will emit a Medicine substance that will enable you to crack hickory nuts in your old age.

Another "unplant" (more a shrub) is Prickly Ash *(Zanthroxlum americanum)*. This shrub (dark bark with roselike thorns) will have small reddish berrylike seeds. If you keep some on hand and get a toothache (especially in a cavity) and the dentist's office is closed, you can put a seed in the cavity (or near the tooth) and find relief from the pain. "Goodnight Irene."

If you say that a Medicine is for certain parts of the body, then Boneset *(Epatorium perfoliatum)* fixes up the chest area. It is also used for chills and fever and as a tonic (tea). What makes this Medicine belong to the "tricky" category is that it has been used in certain charms.

Cobwebs and Puffball dust *(Calvatia craniiformis)* are blood clotters (use either one). Put either Medicine on a bandage (liberally) and cover a cut, or put it on cotton batting and poke the batting up a nose hole to stop a nosebleed.

Heal-all *(Prunella vulgaris)* is the Medicine with a smallish squared stem and purple flowering wheatlike beards that the great Dug dih HANa'ree used so successfully that we Tuscaroras gave that Medicine his name. The name Heal-all says why (although there may be ten other plants with that nickname). Women use it for all their female troubles, and everybody uses it like catnip for nerves and sound sleeping.

The powdered root of Goldenseal is also a great antibiotic. It's strong, so if you have the flu or have stomach problems or need a tonic to strengthen yourself, go easy; trust its infallibility. I put a pinch of the root powder into one-fourth cup of boiling water and stir it. I sometimes use the end of the handle of the spoon as a miniscooper. It's not easy to get it to go into suspension. Then add apple or orange juice to it so it won't be so hot and to get past the root's bitter taste. I have also used this powder on the fresh torn-flesh holes at Sundance so the scars will be hardly noticeable.

Bittersweet *(Celastrus scandens)* is for the healing of broken bones. The

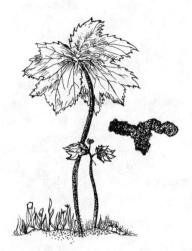

Goldenseal (Hydrastis canadensis).
Drawing by Diana Osborne Williams.

Medicine part is the red paper-thin root bark. It is taken as a tea, but it is very very strong, so use just a pinch of it for each cup (and only once a day).

Wild Grapevine *(Vitis vulpina)*) are the long vines you see in the woods, hanging from high limbs. When red squirrels were plentiful, you could always see their nests at the top of the vines. They used the stringy bark to line those nests.

Maybe this Medicine, the sap of the vine, ought to be placed in a higher category because sometimes it discriminates as to just whom it will help. If it likes you and you are growing bald, it will grow new hair. The trick is to get that sap without making the vine angry. Talk to it. Look for a vine that has a pencil-thin shoot that you can clip the end off of and poke downwards into a bottle (in the springtime). Good luck!

Blacksnake *(Coluber contrictor)* is the snake on which you will see a black-and-white checkerboard pattern (little rectangles) if you tip it over. The oil of the fat of this snake is what you want. It is good for rheumatism. So if you see a dead snake on the road that has been run over, look at its underside. If it's early in the year, they won't have much fat yet. Heat the fat to render it into oil, and keep the oil in a bottle for when you get old and decrepit.

In the meantime, if you weigh less than one hundred pounds and you see a big blacksnake, chase it, and if it climbs a tree, grab it quick.

It will pull you up the tree. I don't know how much I weighed when I was about eight or nine years old, but one pulled me up a Black Walnut tree, and that snake was only about six feet long. Uncle Charley and my father saw one that was twenty feet long.

(But is being pulled up a tree a form of Medicine?)

This next group of Medicines has a strong "mind of their own," and some of them ought not to be fooled with if you don't know what you're doing. For sure, don't ever make fun of them unless you want to be reincarnated.

Sacred Ceremonial Tobacco (*Nicotiana rustica*) can take a supplication to wherever miracles come from and entice that Highest Benevolent Consciousness to "move mountains." Or the Tobacco can completely disappear. Some great Medicines won't appear unless you come carrying some of this Tobacco (or silver) to give to them. Or, you might bring some of the Little People's Tobacco, the wild *Lobelia inflata*.

Then there's the "Redwhip" that western Indians use (and smoke) that I don't know the botanical name of, but in Tuscarora we say, "Ga jee(t) roo rud gwa ri yi(t)."

If you don't have any of these Tobaccos for the exchange in gathering plant Medicines that are "big time," then use a good grade of silver. Sometimes a Tobacco that is extremely rare and hard to obtain will also work, as though rareness is part of being "ready" or not.

Indians who do a powerful Tobacco-Burning Ceremony do not use firewood that is older than one year (wood cut from a living tree that has been spoken to).

I also put the tree root bark of Sassafras (*Sassafras albidum*) in this category because its great potential has not even been reached yet. It hides under the supposition that it is just an ordinary remedy. It might be able to heal ANYTHING, though. What you do is make fresh root bark into a tea using the purest water available. Of course, it is understood that a Ceremony of Thanksgiving accompanied the gathering of this Medicine.

Then let's say a quart of this Medicine is put in a CLEAN quart jar. Now you put your hands around that jar and "love it to death," and maybe have great good people touch it next and sing to it and tell it that it can do ANYTHING.

Now, don't you think that ANYone can be cured of ANYthing if they drink this? It is a blood Medicine and will travel to all parts of the body.

Northern White Cedar (*Thuja accidentalis*) is a Medicine that is in this category because of what it can do. It doesn't seem to try to hide or anything; it just

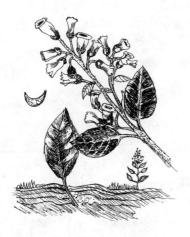

Sacred Tobacco (Nicotiana rustica).
Drawing by Diana Osborne Williams.

IS. What it can do is change people's minds, and not only just change a mind. It makes it GET THE FLIP SIDE!

Supposing a young lady has gone to Daisy Thomas and is told, "Someone has hired a killer to come and kill you next Thursday night at ten o'clock. Just smudge the house with White Cedar around 9:45. Then on Friday give me a call and tell me what happened."

On Friday Daisy gets the call. "At 10:00 P.M. this stranger rings the door bell, and I let him in. He gets a whiff of the White Cedar and pulls his hand out of his coat pocket. Then he pulls out his wallet and hands me a thousand dollars and walks back out. AMAZING! I could see the bulge of his coat pocket where his gun was."

(Or something like that.) You can't believe the power of this Medicine until you see it work.

American Spikenard *(Aralia racemosa)* is the alcoholics' Medicine, the drastic one. (Remember it hid on me for twenty years, then appeared when Chief Beeman Logan did a Purification Ceremony on me with an eagle feather?)

It is also called "The old man's tonic Medicine." Some Indian doctors used it as a blood purifier, so that's likely what helped clear up the alcoholic's "alcoholic thinking."

I've already mentioned how Pennyroyal likes to hide. It is mostly thought of as a "woman's" Medicine, though if a man were dying from pneumonia, it wouldn't hesitate to pull him through.

Pussytoes *(Antennaria neodioca)* might also be called "Dwarf Pearly Ever-

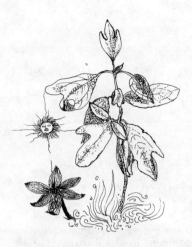

Sassafras (Sassafras albidum).
Drawing by Diana Osborne Williams.

lasting." The leaves of each of these plants look a lot like each other, but the "dwarf" of a plant species is often where the "power" lies. It is even so with the Little People; they are much more powerful than we bigger ones.

The name of this Medicine in Tuscarora tells of what it does. The name is Oo(t) naa wog wo(t) noo ree(t) (Ghosts-it-ushers-away). If you have a haunted house, all you need to do is gather two or three of these small leaves, telling the plant why you are doing so and leaving some Tobacco or silver. Then hang these leaves on a wall of that house.

Some people so badly want NOT to believe that their house is haunted that their denial lets them sleep at night. But maybe the baby is continually fretful. A leaf above the crib will take care of that.

Eastern White Pine *(Pinus strobus)* is the symbol of the Six Nation Iroquois Confederacy. This great tree may have languished in anonymity if it hadn't served as this great logo. And would it otherwise still have the tremendous power to heal that it does have? What it can do is lift a person from the depths of deep depression if the afflicted one can but lean against it. It is more likely that now every time some person looks upon that symbol (as in a photo of that pine or when Chief Jake Swamp is planting one in a strong ceremony), all the White Pines become more powerful.

So if you know anyone talking suicide, show them what a White Pine Tree looks like.

One last "Medicine" is one that, if we could "crank it up" to a high enough degree, would be all we would ever need: our own selves.

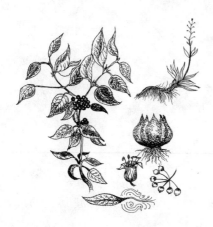

American Spikenard (Aralia racemosa).
Drawing by Diana Osborne Williams.

A good example of "high degree" would be the one in which children hugging frozen puppies cranked up enough Medicine to bring them back to life.

As soon as a problem strikes us, our first reaction is to feel bad about it. We may not feel strong or positive enough to do anything about it. But if we are such a high percentage of water, why not use this family member Element to help us?

Why not get a glass of the purest water we can find and put our hands around it (hug it) and pour forth our love and our feelings into the water, telling it what the problem is and telling the water to "fix it."

The degree of intensity of the problem affecting us would dictate how much we need to "zap" the water. A dire emergency situation could cause an "instant cure" to be made. This "love hugging" can also be done with any tea we have made from plant Medicines.

If the problem is a person's illness or something affecting one's own self, then one need only drink the Medicine water. If the problem is affecting another person living nearby, then that person could drink the sacred water. If the person lives far away, then the glass of water can be set on a picture of that person or even set on a piece of paper on which you have written the person's name.

If the problem involves something like the foreclosing on a piece of property or, say, the clear-cutting of a virgin woods or mountain, then the water can be thrown on that land area or the glass of water placed on top of a map of the land with the problem. Maybe many people taking turns "hugging" the water would create a very potent Medicine.

If the problem is VERY unusual, you might have to use your own creative head.

. . .

So . . . even plant Medicines extend past merely healing sick people (including mental illnesses). They have been used as oracles to take a peek into the future or to "see" (name) who is the criminal in a crime.

They have been used to "trick" the opposition "visionwise" in games of sport or even in wartime. Some Medicines have been a "never-to-become-tired" elixir for individuals in a sporting event or for long-distance runners bearing an urgent message.

They have been used for protection. Sacred Tobacco is often scattered across the doorways of a house that has been cleansed (smudged) so that no negativity can reenter. Or it can stop anybody or anything with bad intentions from entering the premises.

Plant Medicines have been used to ward off or scare witches, ghosts, or skeletons (even when these entities meant no harm) just to "make sure."

Most people have never seen some of the most powerful Medicine plants that "hide." Just the sight of any one of these plants can convince anyone that some kind of "power" is being emitted from that plant. One such plant is a fungus called "witch catcher." It is in the shape of a small brown barrel, easily overlooked. But to look into the barrel and see a white hand in there, ready to "grab," tells you, "WHOA! THIS IS NO ORDINARY PLANT!"

Another use of plant Medicine is to purify and induce the sought-for vision in a vision quest. If these Medicines are shown in a plant book, they will often have the picture of a skull and crossbones beside them as a warning: POISONOUS!

All in all, it is as if with unlimited faith our use of plant Medicines is limitless.

Snow Man

Let us borrow an incident that took place near the Six Nation area, or close enough.

David Wahyahneethah was driving in the wintertime toward Sault Sainte Marie from Michigan. At the time he was staying at Manitoulin Island. He was going to see his foster daughter, whom he had raised since she was eleven years old.

A bad snowstorm came up, but he was too far along to turn back. As he kept chugging along, it became harder to see; the roads were narrow, with not much of a shoulder. It required extra careful driving because other cars and trucks were slipping and sliding here and there.

Presently he came to a more open area, and he could see in the distance ahead of him the dark figure of a person walking in the snow.

David stopped, and this old Indian man got in. When David asked where he was going, the man just indicated "that way" with a thrust of his chin.

The old man had that slow old-fashioned way of speaking English when he did talk. As he spoke of "the way it used to be," David thought, "This guy goes way, way back."

At the slow speed that they had to drive, it was a good five hours that David had this passenger for company. It was only later that it came to David that the old man had been very much like a good luck charm. That is, while car after car and even trucks "spun out" and were abandoned, David's car never slid on that slippery road.

Finally, they came to a place where the old Indian indicated that he lived. David's passenger got out and with a good-bye wave of his hand went on into his house.

David realized that he was now only about eight or ten miles from the place where Sheila, his foster daughter, lived, and he was able to continue on and get there with no problem.

Years later David found out where Sheila had grown as a child. On a summer day he went to see that place. It was somewhat near where he had visited his foster daughter on that cold wintry trip.

When he got to this "early-Sheila home," it was vaguely familiar, but the elderly lady there was a stranger. Stranger or not, David was a bit taken back when she said, "What took you so long?" She then cooked up a smashing breakfast.

In the ensuing conversation David discovered that this woman was Sheila's foster mother. On top of an old radio or TV was a picture. Oh—no wonder this place seemed familiar—here was a picture of the old Indian in the storm and of the house to which David had brought him.

When David asked about the picture, he was told, "Oh, that's Sheila's grandfather. He died in 1912" (some seventy years earlier).

The road passing the house was named John Paul Road. The grandfather's name had been Wahsahnasik, but missionaries had changed it to John Paul.

When David told the lady that he had given the man in the picture "a ride to this house," he expected her to marvel at such a thing. Instead, she just nodded, as though to say, "Oh yeah, his spirit comes to visit once in a while."

David subsequently found out from local Ojibways that the old man who had ridden with him through the terrible storm was known to have powers to move large objects at will and that the name of the house where he had lived (where his picture sat) was called Dream's Rock.

So it must be that Chief Seattle knew what he was talking about in his famous speech when he said, "There is no death, only a change of worlds."

New Age and Ancient Wisdom

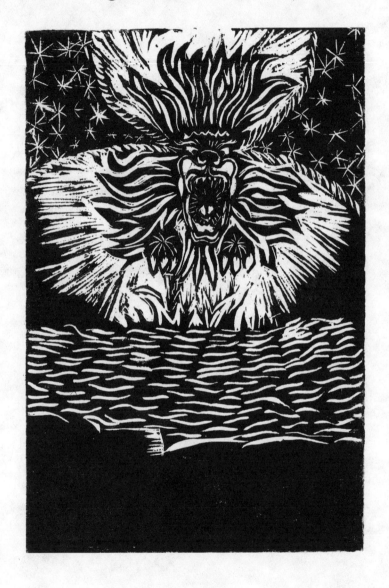

Overleaf: The Fire Lion; see "Medicines of the Universe," pp. 225–29, and "Quantum Physics," pp. 230–39. Woodcut by Rhiannon Miles Osborne.

The Odds

Many babies have died at birth, and there has never been a guarantee that any of us will live beyond that first day. Or any other day.

My aunt Minnie lived for 23,741 days, plus part of another day. When she was born, what were the odds that the day she would die would not only be her birthday, but the birthday that multitudes of people wait for, her sixty-fifth, when she would retire and draw Social Security. She was not even sickly. A complete stranger stabbed her to death. He needed money to sustain a drug habit.

Elsewhere I tell of winning three jackpots on the one-armed bandit machines at Las Vegas. What are the odds of anyone using only three quarters and CONSEC-UTIVELY hitting a jackpot with each coin? Most people have the courtesy of putting in another coin after a win and pulling the lever to erase the winning symbols on display. I didn't know any better. I was in love. Not erasing upped the odds. Even being in love has its odds.

Now let me tell a story on (like telling on) my dead (former) mother-in-law and father-in-law.

George and Dorothy went on a vacation in a Volkswagon Bug. This was not unusual, but they seemed to have to make it unusual by taking along George's sister-in-law, Elda.

They went through parts of Mexico. Now, three in a Volkswagon Bug HAD to be crowded, what with all the luggage three people think they need on a long vacation. It was dangerous to open the front-hood trunk because, like a killer jack-in-the box, it would fly open from being under pressure. Still, Dorothy managed to squeeze two bottles of Mexican champagne into that death trap because the rest of the Bug was jam-packed, too. Dorothy bought them because they only cost two dollars apiece. George lambasted her for buying such "crap." (When they got home and George tasted the "crap," he lambasted Dorothy for not buying more.)

Next, they blew into Las Vegas. George fell in love with Vegas. He wished he could clone himself. Have Georges running around taking over the place. Playing the big spender from the East, he blew a wad.

Dorothy and Elda, though, did very little but gawk at the lights. They didn't know "broccoli from George Bush" about the games being played noisily all around them.

After quite a long time they began to fear that George was lost amid the hubbub and set out to find him. It wouldn't take too long to do ten miles in Las Vegas without knowing it, so they eventually stopped. Their feet hurt. The only chairs available were gaming chairs, so they chose places where the game of keno provided a few open seats. Let George come to them.

Discovering that the game could be played for as little as one dollar, Dorothy nevertheless asked Elda, "Do you want to go halves with me?"

Elda said, "Yes," but being what we at Tuscarora call "Yeh g'we(t) rooks" ("She's stingy," though the phrase actually implies "Her excrement is bound up"), she did not open her purse.

Dorothy had to have the game explained to her until the explainer was rolling his eyes upward almost out of sight.

Dorothy won. She was handed twelve crisp one-hundred-dollar bills. She put them in her purse.

Elda said, "Where's my half?"

Dorothy said, "I didn't see any fifty cents come out of your purse."

Now what are the odds of these two women loving each other up in a crowded Bug as it wended its way from Las Vegas, Nevada, to Niagara Falls, New York?

Enough silliness.

The odds that somebody would see something only once in their whole life could be more than a thousand to one. If nobody has ever heard of that something, then the odds could be doubled. The Patterson boys, Titus, Short, and Manny, saw such a thing. That is, the whole experience is part of what they saw.

At the time they lived at the old Patterson homestead. The house was large and had a roofed-over porch facing south. Across the road and a little to the east was the home of Tommy Farnham. He was just a young man, but he had some-thing wrong with his neck or maybe his whole spine as it was connected to his head. That whole section was stiff, as though he were part mannequin.

Tommy had somehow picked up the nickname Jug Head, but he acquired it before his neck fused, so nobody thought anything of it. Still, how would you like that name if your head froze to your body? Later, though, the nickname was passed on down to his younger brother, William, as though it were an heirloom or an outgrown piece of clothing.

One Sunday afternoon Short, Titus, and Manny were sitting out on the porch talking about any old thing. In the yard and in-line with Tommy's house was a large Honeysuckle bush.

A large light-colored dog came meandering across the lawn and disappeared behind the Honeysuckle bush. Even though the dog had a red ribbon tied around its neck, none of the teenage boys said anything about it. After all, Mt. Hope Road was, by a mile or so stretch, a dogleg shoot-off of Dog Street.

Still, why didn't the alert Patterson watchdog, Rover, see the foreigner and bark?

Ten minutes or so passed by when Manny says, "Hey, you guys . . . did you notice that dog with a ribbon on its neck walk past a while ago?"

"Yeah. I don't think I've ever seen that dog before."

"Me neither. It went behind the Honeysuckle bush and never came out."

"I know. I've been waiting for it, too."

"Let's go see if it's still back there."

It wasn't. There was nothing. The boys went into the house and told the rest of the family what had transpired.

The Patterson family were early risers. They had a large farm. There were cows to milk. The next morning they were all at the breakfast table when a soft knock came on the door.

It was Mrs. Farnham. Her eyes were all red. "Tommy . . . (sniff) . . . died last night."

There was silence. What was there to say? When Manny did speak, though, everyone looked at him because of the sound of his voice. Like a judge at a mur-der trial identifying the name of the killer, he said, "The dog with the ribbon."

There was a quorum of knowing nods.

·   ·   ·

We all know when the voice of someone we are speaking with rings true. We meet many people who say, "How are you?" and keep walking right on past, like it would be an effrontery for us to answer them.

At the Wolf Song Peace Elders gathering some years ago at Mary Thunder's place in Texas, I met a man named Bob Powell. He was a small black man, and we hit if off immediately. Just from snatches of conversations here and there, I came to love him very much. He is a physicist, but I didn't know that then.

On the day before the ending of the gathering, I was walking westerly, and here came Bob walking in an easterly direction. If we both kept on the same lines each of us was on, the closest distance we would come to each other was about twenty-five paces. I thought to myself that in the melee of everyone packing up and leaving on the following morning, Bob and I might not see each other. Maybe never again. I called to him, "Hey, Bob! We better hug now because to-morrow we might not see each other."

"Taad," he called back, "I kin hug you AAAny time I want to."

We both laughed loudly. Tears came to my eyes. I had been given an acco-lade of such great proportions. He knew that I knew that there was no such thing as time or space. We never saw each other again.

Ten years went by. I received a letter from a man named Harvey Grady. I'm not sure where he lives, maybe Sedona, Arizona. I'd met him at a place called Council Grove in Kansas. Harvey is not the average bear. I don't know what all Harvey does, but one of the things is highly unusual.

Probably you have heard of Seth. Seth is an entity that came, first, I think, through the Ouija board that was being "operated" by a woman named Jane Roberts and her husband, Robert Butts. They lived in Elmira, New York. How many people in the world would smile (or laugh) if they were told, "Some highly intelligent messages are coming through the Ouija board in Elmira. You better get over there and see. Maybe these words will solve all your problems."

Of course, this is carrying things too far, but you get the point. Seth subse-quently used Jane as a "channel" and came through verbally. Robert grabbed a tape recorder, and these recordings became the well-known *Seth Speaks* series of ten or twelve or more books.

I have read most of them, and maybe it's going too far afield to continue any-thing much more regarding Seth and Jane and the channeling, but I just want to insert something that I found quite interesting.

Jane and Robert formed a class or study group that met at their home on Thursday nights. Questions could be asked of Seth, but one Thursday night Seth said (or words to these effects), "Tonight you're in for a treat. I'm going to try to put you in touch with another entity much higher up the ladder of consciousness."

After a couple of aborted attempts, a different voice did come through. This voice was later reported to have sounded "reedy." Members of the group looked at one another. Was this a man's voice or a woman's, they asked.

The answer was, "Neither. At this stage we don't need male and female. I am both." Anyways, all this about Seth is just to say that channeling of entities, the same as a radio channel's radio waves, does take place.

Harvey Grady goes a step or two farther than Jane Roberts. However he does it, he tunes into about fifteen entities. Out of that many, if they all are "experts," one out of fifteen certainly could give supersage advice on any matter. But I don't mean to advertise Harvey here. In fact, people like the Peacemaker or Empty Cloud or Christ or Automatic Transmission know that the more humble one is, the stronger the Medicine. That may be why you may never have heard of Harvey.

One day Harvey wrote to me. He had composed a poem about me. It made me cry. It was equal to Bob Powell's salute to me. I wrote to Harvey. I told him that this was the second time in my life that I had received such a great thing. I then told him about the first one, about Bob Powell and what he had said to me ten years ago.

I was sealing the letter to Harvey. The phone rang. It was Bob Powell.

Coincidence? What are the odds that it was a coincidence?

Isolated Phenomena

What attracts phenomena? Sometimes when you are thinking of someone, the phone rings, and it's that person. Surely, the bulk of unusual occurrences take place when we are at ease, daydreaming. We even "expect" such things in a meditation and more so in a vision quest.

I have seen the aura of a person but once. I was at a Sunday morning service at a church called Christ Unity. This was in the early or mid-1970s, when I tried several churches to see if I might find a great "WOW! this is it!" church, a sure-fire guarantee-to-heaven church. The minister of Christ Unity Church was a woman. Partway through her sermon, she sprouted a nice big light yellow aura about her whole head. There was a slight greenish tinge to it. Behind her, on her left, were three big wooden thronelike chairs, the center one having an ovalish aura, as though an invisible person with a whole body aura around them sat in it. Following her sermon, the minister went and sat right in this chair and covered the chair aura, but she retained her head aura.

When the service was over, the congregation formed a big circle, held hands, and sang the peace song. Then the minister walked down from the pulpit, broke through the circle, and went across to the other side, breaking through again and standing by the exit door. The circle then became the line that shook the minister's hand and told her what a fine sermon she gave.

When the lady minister came down and broke into the circle, the aura was still around her head. But when she got to the center of the circle, the aura went out as though she turned her "on" button off.

As I shook her hand, I told her that she had this aura around her head during the sermon, describing it. Then I told her that it continued until she reached the center of the church, and there the light went out.

"That's very interesting," she said, "that's very interesting indeed." And then she leaned closer to me and said in a low voice, "When I got to the center of the circle, I thought of my daughter who is in Kansas, pregnant without a husband."

Later, the thought came to me, "Yes, we can be in a strong healing mode, but if someone or something strikes us negatively and pushes that button in us, BINGO! we lose it. We might even go all the way to a place where we, ourselves, might need a healing." On my quest for spiritual knowledge, I had come to, or been led to, an experience I have not forgotten.

About this time, the mid-1970s, I became addicted to visiting different people, trying to dig out of them any experiences they had had that were of "ghost story" nature. I was writing the book *The Reservation*, and I thought there ought to be a chapter of anecdotes that, though we would say, "Let's tell ghost stories," were really just about any oddball happening experienced by the teller or by someone the teller knew. Soon, I had much more than a chapter of these stories, and, in fact, I could see that the total of them was much greater than the sum of the parts.

There was no end to them, and no end to the addiction except that the dying of the old great story-tellers tapered off the finding of gems. I was also then learning to play chess, and there was no end to the learning of that game either. Before I realized that I ought to be prioritizing my hunt and visiting the oldest people before they passed into oblivion, I sometimes would badger those people who swore, "I NEVER have experiences like that."

One such person was Kenny Rickard Sr. I must have sat with him four or five hours as both of us told hunting or fishing or naughty stories, and I'd interject ghostly or witchy stories, trying to bait him into recalling one of his own. Finally, the witching hour of midnight came, and I gave up. I was going home. It was then that Kenny told of an experience that I like very much. It had an abstractness to it that took it deeper into the connectedness of all things.

"I did quite a bit of tunnel work in my time," he said, "and a lot of tunnel men have also worked in coal mines. There is a big 'no-no' among tunnelers; you just never never whistle in a tunnel. Something about the vibration of a whistle, maybe the echo, makes it strong enough to cause the ceiling or walls to cave in. Men have been trapped and died from such a thing—from a whistle.

"Well, I've never had to worry about that—I just don't whistle. I mean, I can, but I don't. So one day we were working at Stauffer Chemical in Niagara Falls, and I was sawing away on a board when I heard myself whistling. Man! That was so rare I remember I stopped sawing. Did I whistle? Yep, I swore I heard myself whistling. So I started sawing again. Whoa! Here I was, whistling again. Even though on any job there's lots of noise, trucks, a bulldozer, guys hammering, I knew for sure that I'd caught myself whistling.

"Just about that time I saw movement, I looked up and here came a bunch of factory workers running. One was coming nearby, and I asked, 'What's happening?'

"He was motioning with his arm to come on, get out of here, and he yelled, 'THE TUNNEL! THE TUNNEL BLEW UP!'

"I followed him. In a chemical plant one explosion can set off the whole shootin' match. Luckily, it didn't. What they called 'the tunnel' there was a covered walkway across the top of the roof of one of the buildings. I don't know why it blew up. Maybe a gas leak and a cigarette. They hush things like that up, try to keep it out of the newspapers. So I don't really know what happened. I don't even know why I whistled."

I went home. I had to drive about seventy miles, and I never got sleepy. I didn't whistle either.

Kenny's experience about whistling brought another incident to mind. My mother told me about something similar that had happened to her. One day she heard herself whistling. Well, we all might absentmindedly whistle, and my mother knew that. It wasn't just the fact that she was whistling that shocked her; it was the song that she was whistling. It was the funeral hymn.

The phone rang. She picked it up. It was the news that her sister Barbara had just died.

When we accept that we are intimate kin to all of the Elements of this Divine and Harmonious Universe we can begin to see that some of our kin can see future events better than we can. Our ancestors were much more alert to this than we are today. If they saw sturgeon jumping in the river or chickens roosting any small distance from the ground in the daytime, they would hurry on home and take the dry clothes off the line before it rained. They also paid closer attention to more subtle Elements.

Grandmother Geese-a-geese showed me the northern lights one night. They were bright red. She said, "A big war is coming, lots of blood spilled." The aurora borealis indeed predicted the coming of World War II.

Two Senecas at Cattaragus were sharp enough to listen to a tree. The incident started with a trip into the forest to cut wood for the stove. Before they left, they loaded up the stove in anticipation of being gone for most of the day. One of the men normally walked with a cane, but since he wouldn't be walking much, he left it at home.

After they had been cutting for a while, they began sawing, with a two-man crosscut saw, some splittable-size blocks of wood from a fallen tree. Back and forth the sawblade sang, "Zing zing, zing zing."

Now, if a tree were to start talking, in any manner, we would probably at least say that the tree would have to be a living tree. This tree was a dead one. A dead dry tree. But it started to talk.

From "zing, zing" it went to Seneca words. "Stop, stop . . . stop, stop . . . stop, stop."

Neither man said anything. It was just kind of cute to imagine the tree telling them to stop. But then the words changed.

"Go home . . . go home . . . go home."

Still the men said nothing to each other. Neither was tired yet, and each one was thinking, "I'm probably the only one of us who thinks I hear the tree talking." Two blocks had been cut off. Now the third. The voice changed again.

"Fire, fire . . . fire, fire . . . fire, fire."

The men looked at each other. "Do you hear what I hear?"

"Yeah. Let's make one more cut and listen."

The tree said, "Now! now! now! now!"

The men wasted no time. They hurried back to the house. The house was full of smoke. They had left the damper wide open. The stove was red hot. The cane that "Hop-a-long" had left at home had fallen against the stove and was now half burned up. The fire it was creating would have soon set the woodpile and the house afire.

The four blocks of wood that spoke were never burned. They were stood in the yard so people could sit on them and tell stories. And I thank Fred Kennedy for recalling this incident.

The Little Lights

When I was in Puerto Rico for one of the Wolf Song Elders gatherings, I slept in the basement floor of an old stone building. The window near my bed was just a window-size hole in the wall, but since it was so warm there, any night breezes were welcome.

During the night I woke up and said a little prayer of thankfulness. As I was going back to sleep, I noticed a tiny light outside the window. My sleepy mind said, "Neat! . . . Hello there. . . . Oh do come in!"

In came this little speck of a light. It was greenish in color and moved slowly and steadily through the night air. One might say that it acted as if it weren't too sure if it ought to be in "here" or not. Then, as though it survived best in only very pristine places and as though the rest of this area and I weren't quite up to par, it slowed to a "crawl," made a four-foot or so circle, and went back out the window.

In the morning I meant to ask the local people about the tiny light, assuming that they would know all about it, or them. But you know how day and night are so different that "night things" sort of belong in the night, so the incident drifted away like a dream. As time went by, I forgot all about it until years later. Hey, maybe I was dreaming.

Years later my wife, Diana, and I adopted, as a son, a man we call "Mc-Naughty" (Clyde Hollifield). He is Diana's age, but he is so magical that we couldn't let him get away without putting some kind of semilegal "gotcha" leash on him.

Of McNaughty's many magical "delving intos," he is obsessed with "night lights" . . . ANY night lights. He also putters with puppets, scaring people when the puppets "come alive." He is also good at doctoring animals and birds that have accidents.

But his fascination with "night light" things fascinates me, too. He loves to do things with foxfire (damp rotted wood that glows at night).

One night he showed us this other form of night lights that "grew" in the lateral cracks of boulders along a small freshwater stream. One reason why foxfire and this "rock-crack" cousin are so fascinating is that when you shine a flashlight beam onto the lights, you see nothing special at the very spot of the lights. In the cracks of the boulders you'll see some moss or maybe nothing.

Now I'm sure lots of people have seen most of the various types of foxfire and other things like glow worms, and find even fireflies fascinating.

Now we can stop here and, like most people, say, "All these things are quite well known and scientifically explainable." But here's more. It's like there's a line here that crosses into unexplainable areas. Or, at least, unexplainable by the average Joe or Josephine.

Native American Medicine people all were into playing with and respecting "night lights." One of the rules of plant Medicine gathering was, "No gathering of Medicines when the lightning bugs appear, and until they are gone."

Years ago, before the advent of automobiles for travel from place to place or even the use of horses (not a mode of travel among Indians of the eastern United States), many Indians did shape-shifting. That is, they would turn themselves into birds or animals, usually dogs, to travel more quickly and easily from place to place. Then, of course, upon arriving or near arrival, they shape-shifted back to a person again.

Even as a sport, some Indians would chase and try to capture the glowing balls called "Jack-o-lanterns" that cavorted about at night. The "word" was that one could attain a certain "power" if a ball of light could be captured. Perhaps some succeeded in shape-shifting into a Jack-o-lantern and therefore were able also to "see" at night, by their own light.

What brought on the "No gathering of Medicine plants at night" rule was that it became known that some "witches" (Medicine people who often came to be called witches by nervous Indians) shape-shifted into lightning bugs. And sometimes even just nosy Indians learned the trick of shape-shifting and could look into people's windows at night, posing as an insect. Remember, two of the rules of Medicine as told to me by my father, Eleazer, regarding certain great, powerful Medicine plants are, "Don't let anyone see you gathering this Medicine" and "Don't let anyone see you imbibing (taking) this Medicine." Thought waves can penetrate, mingle with, and dilute (or enhance) things, including Medicine. Certain Medicines are so precious that all caution must be used to keep them at their highest potency.

So now I want to tell you about some little lights that are here in the area where Diana and I live that act like that little light I saw in Puerto Rico. It seems most likely that they are insects, given that lightning bugs also dot the night landscape with little lights.

Enter McNaughty. The phone rings, and McNaughty says, "I want to show you these other little night lights. They can be mistaken for lightning bugs, but they are quite different. For starters, you can't see them in daylight or artificial light. They're smaller, and they don't blink on and off like lightning bugs. If you go near them, the lights go out or move off. They seem to favor the areas of freshwater streams, but they only stick around about a week, then they will next be seen at a thousand-foot elevation higher. A week later they move up again. They don't seem to like evergreens."

We went to see them. Sure enough, they were everything McNaughty said they were. Tiny lights with a consciousness all their own. We respected them and left them alone.

Each year, though, we would think of them again and try to "feel" just when they might be about so we could see them again. Usually, McNaughty would have "tracked" them and let us know. I think he even had a yearly date. Maybe in the month of May was when he would expect them.

Some of the things of this great Universe of ours that fascinate me the most are the many things just such as lightning bugs. Or electric eels. Or those fish in the deep depths of the Arctic Ocean that are like glass and you can see through them. No blood. Do they eat? So many things that have more magical ability than a human being.

What is extremely intriguing is some creatures' ability to have instant communication, such as flocks of birds or schools of fish that can move as one. And more so, this thing about honeybees that was discovered at Princeton University. Testing was being done to see just how fast honeybees can find a food source. Now in the chapter about my uncle Charley, I wondered if his ability to "charm" a rabbit or pheasant came about because his feeling of NEED possessed him to that extreme a degree. He feared that his mother might starve to death. In the case of honeybees, they all (the whole hive) might starve to death if no food were found.

So here's what happened with the bees. In the first test a source of food (maybe sugar) was put out and was rapidly found. When that food source was moved to a new location for test number two, a bunch of bees came swarming in very rapidly.

But now get this! When the food source was moved again, lo and behold, the bees were already there waiting for them. Little "mind readers," no less.

Maybe hornets are not slouches at mind reading either. I can remember, as a boy, looking for a stone, picking it up, and making ready to throw it at one of those big gray paper hornet's nests up in a tree. Before I could throw, out of the nest came a hornet on a beeline (pardon the pun) to my forehead and stung me.

So what about the communication abilities of the little night lights? They might be insects, but I am not too sure. It got so we began forgetting about them. Once we'd seen them, it was not a yearly springtime "Stop the presses! The queen has arrived!" situation anymore. Certain things—great Medicines, for instance—will disappear if their use is discontinued. Even in use, they follow the law that says, "The amount of cure that you get from any Medicine is directly related to the amount of reverence you have for it." And what about the False Faces? What if you do not feed them? Diana says, "The Druids say, 'He who likes the fire must tend it.'"

So maybe those delicate little lights exist at the cut-off point of physical consciousness and can disappear into Higher Consciousness. At the Findhorn Gardens in Scotland the god Pan was surprised to find human beings able to see him because he had never before encountered people who had risen above the physical conscious state. So if the little lights prefer to stay aloof in a more pristine existence, then they might also hover just out of reach of everyday thoughts, like a fading dream does upon our awakening. So what might jar our memory of them?

Enter homeopathy. Even though all the Elements of our Universe are related in seemingly such unknown ways, ANY Element might come to our aid when we least expect it.

Diana is a homeopathic doctor and has practiced homeopathy for nearly thirty years. Homeopathy is a system of medical practice that treats a disease by the administration of minute doses of a remedy that would in healthy persons produce symptoms similar to those of the disease. Does this seem "too far out"?

Well, so were the first thoughts that the world is round, not flat. I think the amazing results that homeopathy produces are quite magical.

Diana says, "The remedies we use come from all the different kingdoms, and by the time the remedy is finished being prepared, its physical presence has all but disappeared."

I don't meddle into her practice. What if her father told her, "Don't let anyone see you preparing this Medicine"?

Well, one time, I didn't mean to, but I saw her preparing something anyways. Maybe she was diluting a drop of silverlike hummingbird defecation into one one-thousandths. Whatever, but she had this vial of dilution, and she struck it against her forearm exactly a hundred times.

I said to myself, "Cool! I like that! That one hundred thing. I'm gonna do that, too. I'm going to some way use that one hundred formula one of these days."

But, of course, like a kid, I think stuff like that all the time, and if somebody challenges me and wants to know "when" I am going to use it, I'm liable to say, "In my next lifetime."

Another instance of my "Oh cool! I like that" way of thinking occurred one day in a drug store when I saw a cute container of something called BLUE-EMU. Well, I HAD to have that, even though the cost, twenty dollars, almost stopped me from having it. In fact, I was already out of the store in my car before I succumbed to the "Oh, why fight the feeling?" inner impulse and went back in and bought it. Even THAT little fight with sensibility made me all the more sure that I should have such a rare thing.

Some time later, when I was sitting on the "throne" of our bathroom, looking at two dark ugly spots of varicose veins on my legs, I thought, "I wonder if that emu stuff might get after them spots. Emus don't have varicose veins." The jar of that blue pastelike stuff was within reach. I began rubbing it on, but now here's where that formula of "one hundred times" came to my rescue. Every ten rubs I'd say, "Emus don't have varicose veins," then would continue with the count until I reached one hundred. One hundred rubs for each spot. And, I'll bet by now that you have guessed that the dark varicose vein spots have disappeared (after eight or ten rubbing sessions).

OK, I'm sorry we had to go through all that, but, hey, it's part of all things being related. So, back to homeopathy.

Diana had studied homeopathy in England, from the Druids in Wales. The same place that spawned the word *bonkers* is also the source of a wild array of homeopathic remedies. Diana had one labeled "Eagle Remedy." Where might one ever use that?

Lest we forget that all things are related, here's what happened next.

For years, Diana had organized, with the help of volunteers and solicited funds, one and sometimes two Native American Elders gatherings per year. It became a taxing thing on her, and as she tried to wind down her role, she would say, "This is the LAST one I'm going to do."

At the most recent "last one" a surprise-party type of honoring was bestowed upon her. As part of it, Lloyd Elm (Onondaga), whom I think of as a Sundancer holy man, did an Adoption Ceremony and adopted her as his sister. As part of it, Diana was presented with an eagle feather. Eagle feathers can be big, big Medicine when treated with reverence. This gathering took place on Mother's Day weekend.

Diana meditates daily and takes a daily walk. These practices have put her in touch with trees and plants. Among the messages that she got at this time was to "listen to the eagle feather."

The messages from the feather are a private thing between the feather and Diana (some likely regarding the homeopathic treatment of some of her patients), but she disclosed to me that the feather had said, "It's time to take that eagle Medicine."

We both took it. What happened to me, as a result, was that whatever was sacred to me became even more sacred (in my awareness).

What happened to Diana was that she began seeing and hearing the messages (from the trees and other Medicine plant life) more clearly. Among the messages came a reminder of the little lights, that we should not forget them.

Up until now if we went to see the lights, it would be from an invitation and reminder from McNaughty. In our minds we knew he would have been keeping track of them "for" us, so maybe we had become somewhat spoiled. So this time we said, "Let's do this on our own. Let's find them by ourselves."

Knowing that these lights hung around freshwater, we drove first to a place where we could swim later at Spring Creek. It was maybe at a thousand-feet elevation, a good starting point. Nothing. So up we went to a higher point of elevation. We sat around the stream of water there in the dark until we became disappointed enough to leave. Maybe, we thought, we were too late. It seemed as though it was nearly time for the lightning bugs to appear, which would signal "too late." But we didn't see ANYthing. Home we went.

Our house is up near three-thousand-feet elevation. Past our house is an old abandoned farmhouse. It is higher yet in elevation and sits surrounded by a rolling meadow. There is no water, no freshwater stream, near either of these two places. Both of us, Diana and I, were feeling bad that we hadn't found any lights, so we said, "Let's go up to the old farmhouse and sit and watch the moon come up."

So we went and sat on the mowed lawn of the farmhouse. (The owners, friends of ours, still took care of the place.) It was a serene atmosphere, but we yearned to see the little lights. Both of us are stubborn about such precious things and couldn't give up. We stared into the dark until the moon came up. What did end our hopes was that we began seeing a few lightning bugs. Reluctantly we went home.

Our house is on a knoll within the vast white pine woods. Remember, Mc-Naughty said, "They don't like pine woods." No water anywhere. But when we got to the house, what do you think was there waiting for us?

Just like the bees waiting for the food source to arrive, the little lights were there waiting for us. We cried.

Diana stayed at a spot just below our house where we first saw them in our approach. As these lights are wont to do, they had drifted a bit. I went up to the house to see if any were there. No, not by the house. (They stayed on the north side, like Ginseng does.)

Presently I heard Diana singing. Slowly the lights came to her. Not to be outdone I began whistling the Old Moccasin Dance song. Up the hill came five or six lights. These lights always move at a height of about three feet above the ground (average).

One of the lights that came to the house zoomed up to our upstairs window and peeked in. Then it came back down.

We were half out of our minds with elation. I'm sure these feelings of elation permeated the area around us. The lights were "drawn" to this feeling, and they came and mingled right with us.

Diana said, "You know, Ted, this possibility of people communicating with all things goes on all the time. We've just been looking at the little lights phenomena as a separate thing. It's really all one continuous possibility. Like 'He who likes the fire must tend it.' "

So it doesn't matter to Diana or me if these little lights are bugs, bugaboos, or tiny entities like the Little People who can be seen by some people and not by others.

If the Little People like to be given marbles to play with, then maybe the Little Lights would like something smaller.

Maybe granulated sugar.

Seeing Things

The phrase "Oh, you're just seeing things" has often been spoken to children. It means, "You're lying. Such things don't exist." Some parents might even be thinking, "Oh God! Maybe my child is insane!"

I have been fortunate to have had my children with me when certain things have appeared, and we saw them together. One of the most beautiful and unexplained things we saw was the light green rainbow at night as told in the episode of the sturgeon. It looked like a huge neon tube, and we wonder, now, had we carried a camera, would it have shown up on film? The producing of the sturgeon by Medicine was good for my children to see.

One afternoon my children and I walked out of the western door of my mother's house on Upper Mountain Road. The sun was three fists high yet from setting, and the sky was cloudless. Starting from someplace over our heads and streaking westward to set before the sun was a nice white round meteorite or "falling star." It never burned up or disappeared like those seen at night, which often last only long enough to make short streaks.

As though I had to say something, like quickly wishing aloud on a falling star before it burned out, I heard myself say, "Look! There goes Nixon to San Clemente!" We all laughed.

I must have somewhere picked up on the words *San Clemente* because after I said it, I thought, "What a foreign thing to say."

The next day the newspaper headline read, "NIXON TO SAN CLEMENTE."

I saw another unusual thing twice. I was driving from the Six Nation Reservation in Canada to Rochester, New York. As I drove, a small round cloud with bursts of lightening behind it preceded me. That is, it stayed in view in the upper right-hand corner of my windshield until I reached the tourist-attracting lights of

Clifton Hill at the bridge at Niagara Falls, Ontario. One hour and fifteen minutes or so.

Though that was a phenomenal thing to see, it could be thought of as a very
rare thing of the wind to carry a cloud at the same speed as I was driving, for such
a distance. So, for that reason, I didn't think too much more about it, even
though another thing made it rarer still. Clouds don't usually keep their shape
for more than ten minutes and may even dissipate.

Enter Duke Jacobs. Maybe certain people "draw" things to themselves from
out of other conscious states. People like Duke, who saw so many things. Two
weeks after seeing that little round cloud, I went to the Six Nation Reservation in
Canada again, this time with Duke, his wife, and his child. The little cloud did it
again on our way home at night. This time I had corroboration. All three other
people could keep watch for the lightning flashes without having to keep their
eyes on the road as they would if they had been driving. I may have been "lucky"
to have this happen once, but I think Duke influenced the cloud to come back.
It took us to the bright lights again before disappearing among them.

Even some great people are phenomena, and to have my children meet them
and adore them is like having them see the pot of gold at the end of the green
rainbow. Automatic Transmission was one of these great people. I introduced
him to them as "Hardy or Artie Johnson" (I, being partially deaf, never knowing
which name I was even hearing, and he, being also partially deaf, not correcting
me).

He immediately told my children of once hearing a small bird on a harrow,
hollering *jig a jig a jig a jig a jig*. When he went to see what was wrong with it, he
saw that a snake had hypnotized it and was slowly easing up to it.

Mike asked, "Did you rescue the bird?"

"Oh no. The snake was probably starving. Maybe that's how it got the power
to charm the bird. I let it have the bird also because it put on a free show for me."

Speaking of the influence of parents on children (especially regarding the development or retardation of their Higher Consciousness or intuitiveness), there was
an example of it next door to where I was born.

Joan Patterson (born on a Christmas Day of the same year as I was, 1930)
slept as a child in the attic bedroom of their house with her older sister, Leah

May. One night she woke up and saw a ghost. It was an old woman walking about in the room with a long thin walking stick. She was making tapping-the-floor motions with the stick, though no sound came from it. (Maybe one of Joan's grandmothers.) It scared little Joanie, and in the morning she told her mother, Alta, about it.

"Oh no," her mother said, "You were just dreaming."

Joan believed her and never saw another thing outside of physical conscious-ness for the rest of her life.

Joan is dead now, but before she died, she attended a family reunion of her brothers and sister. Her mother had long passed on. Her older brother, Wesley Huh, told everyone that as a small boy he had seen a ghost in the attic, an old woman tapping the floor with a long thin walking stick.

"Yeah! Yeah!" Joan exclaimed, "I saw her too . . . but Mom told me I was just dreaming."

"That's what she told me, too," Wesley said.

My parents did not tell me I was dreaming when at three I heard the ghost snare drum corps announcing that "Uncle Sam's boy," Bill Uh, was dying. They probably thought, "Hmmm, that boy's a handy watchdog. We better keep him that way."

Every once in a while throughout my life, despite my being so skeptical, I'd be shown something unbelievable by the Universe. Remember the aura around the head of the lady minister, Harriett Baumeister, which went "out like a light" when a negative thought came into her head? One time this "aura thing" hap-pened in reverse.

I was writing to a Tuscarora man who was living with his wife and child in New York State. His wife, Mary Ann, was Algonquin and came from the Man-awaki Indian Reservation some ninety miles north of Ottawa in Quebec. Their child of four years or so, a boy, was affected with Down syndrome. Albert had been a schoolmate of mine and a neighbor. Not having seen each other in a good number of years, we had a lot of verbal catching up to do.

Albert and Mary Ann were, of course, used to their son's Down behavior, but I was not. It was as though I secretly and compulsively wanted to cry for the sake of the boy who slobbered and waddled about, buzzing like a big bumblebee with his tongue hanging out.

To myself I said, "I'm going to try to give this boy some healing with my hands without Albert or Mary Ann knowing it." As casually as I could, with my cupped hands I "aimed" beams of healing at the boy as he cruised back and forth in perpetual motion.

Within a minute or so the boy came directly to me and tried to crawl up onto my lap. I picked him up and hugged him, placing his head looking over my left shoulder. He promptly stopped "humming" and fell asleep.

I had been keeping a strong eye-to-eye contact with Albert so he wouldn't notice what my hands were doing. If you ever do Medicine of any kind, including ceremony, you will find that the LEAST amount of anyone's influence is MOST desirable to success.

After a while I happened to look at Mary Ann who was sitting in her third of a triangular seating. Her eyes, big as the proverbial saucers, were on me as though awestruck. I asked her what was the matter.

"There's . . . a big blue light all around you," she sputtered.

Neither Albert nor I could see it, but this must be the way that it can be. In a church full of people I was the only one who saw Reverend Harriett Baumeister's aura.

I don't know if any lasting healing help came consequently to the boy, but I do know this. From then on Mary Ann thought I could do anything. She might call me in the middle of the night and say, "My sister up in Manawaki has a headache. Fix it."

I have had a couple more experiences connected with Mary Ann's reservation, Manawaki.

Around 1981 or 1982 I heard that there was to be a gathering of alcoholic Indians at Manawaki. Its purpose was to reinforce the spiritual strength needed by anyone who wished to stop or continue to refrain from drinking alcohol. The event was to be held at Bitabee Lake. A group of us decided to go, and we rode up in one of those camperlike motor homes.

The man in charge there was named Peter Commanda. He may have been a Chief, but before long I found out that he was big Medicine.

The first Medicine thing he did was already done before we got there. When we pulled in, I took a walk to see what herbs grew there that I might recognize. Before long I could see a very dark swatch of clouds coming from the southwest.

I hurried back to the gathering. As I walked past Peter Commanda, I pointed to the ominous clouds, now very visible. "Look at THEM babies!"

He smiled. "Oh, I've already taken care of them."

I kept walking . . . toward the safety of our vehicle. Before I could get to it, someone, maybe Peter, began calling, "ATTENTION EVERYBODY! ATTEN-TION EVERYBODY! COME TO THE LAKEFRONT! COME TO THE LAKEFRONT! OUR FIRST SPEAKER IS THERE NOW. HE IS WAITING FOR US!"

People began reluctantly straggling toward the gathering place. It was less than a hundred yards to the lakefront, but the clouds were almost upon us. I was actually closer to the gathering place than to our vehicle. I looked to see if, by chance, the Algonquins had erected an overhead rain tarp-umbrella or tent. No, but there was Peter Commanda standing there looking like a gentle Genghis Khan and giving me a "come on" movement with his head. I came.

As soon as I saw Peter's likeness to Genghis Khan, I also thought of Tito Puente, the Latin drummer. He had composed a song to the late great drummer Tiny Khan. He had entitled the song "Tiny, Not Genghis."

When I approached Peter, he said, "You're staying until Sunday afternoon, aren't you? We're having a moose barbecue. Mmmm good."

"I'm at the mercy of the mixed crew I came with. If they stay, I stay."

"Well, you better stay because you never tasted anything like this before. It is rare to see a moose here anymore. You gotta go a hundred miles north to hunt. I mean the hunters do. But me and Drum, we do Medicine. We did Medicine two days ago. The next day we heard a grunt. We took a rifle and went back of the house. Here was a big bull looking at us. He will be the barbecue."

The sun shone on Peter's beaming smile. The black clouds had split. It was raining so hard on each side of the gathering that, to the east, we could scarcely see across the small Bitabee Lake.

I looked up and said, "I think you did more Medicine than just the moose Medicine."

Peter winked at me.

I don't know whatever possessed me, but I said, "What about beaver tail?" I had heard that it was one of the greatest of delicacies.

"Oh . . . yeah . . . I never thought of that." He started an immediate fast walk toward the fire of the open-air kitchen.

"I was just kidding," I called, but it was no use. The miracle of the split sky had summoned more scaredy-cats, and the program schedule waited for them. I could hear "Hi, hi," "Hi, hi," "Hi, hi" as Peter hurriedly met them on his way to the fire.

I watched as Peter took a bag of Sacred Tobacco from his pocket. He spoke to the fire and tossed the Tobacco into it, then came back.

The speaker had not finished his talk before a beat-up old truck came huffing and puffing up to the kitchen. A big man got out and went to the back of the truck. He walked a few steps toward the cook. From each of his hands hung a large beaver. In one motion he plopped both beavers on the ground and turned and drove away.

After the talk I went up to the cook and asked him if the guy that brought the beavers had said anything.

"Yeah. 'Here.' " The farther north you go, the less words are needed. Some Eskimos won't even talk to you.

We couldn't stay for the Sunday barbecue, but I was spiritually on top of the great White Pine (Tree of Peace) as we started for home.

A few miles under way we came to a curve to the right in the road. I was up front talking to the driver, John, and I had just finished saying, "Man! I feel like I could heal anyone of anything right now." Just then a motorcyclist came roaring past us, but misjudging the sharpness of the curve, he lost control and sailed into the ditch on our side of the road. Cyclist and cycle went airborne, both doing somersaults before landing and bouncing to a stop. He wore no helmet.

John pulled over and began calling for an ambulance on the CB radio. I got out and put my hands about six inches from the man's head. I was full of what I had seen, so I zapped some of that Peter Commanda Medicine into the healing. Blood was oozing out of the unconscious man's ear. In a minute or two we had a small crowd of rubberneckers.

The cyclist abruptly opened his eyes and, seeing such a motley bunch staring at him, may have thought he was in hell because he instantly struggled to get to his feet. The motorist who was next behind us and who had witnessed the magnitude of the accident began yelling, "No. No. Don't try to stand. Your back may be broken!"

To no avail. The man got to his feet, uttered a few French expletives and limped over to his motorcycle. He stood it up, "spanked it," and it started. We all watched him ride off, the handlebars aimed wrongly.

Back on the road we'd gone but a short distance before we met the ambulance rushing to the scene. It was busily sirening people out of its way. It was on a wild goose chase. Maybe it was caught up in the yang of the yin that Bitabee Lake had given us.

Now I'm going to tell you about something that I wasn't going to tell you about. The reason I wasn't going to tell you is that maybe I didn't have anything to do with it. Maybe I didn't have any affect on the motorcyclist, either, but at least it was part of the Manawaki trip.

This other thing has to do with splitting a rain cloud. The first time I ever heard of such a thing was when Mocks Johnson ran into Heeengs in the woods and was having a nice conversation when the sky threatened rain.

Mocks was ready to take off for home even though he would never have beaten the rain. Heeengs said, "Oh, don't pay any attention to them clouds; I'll take care of that."

She thumped the bottom of her walking stick into the ground and thrust the other end toward the rain clouds. "No!" she said, "You can't come here. Go around us." The clouds split and only a few wind-driven raindrops hit them.

The next time I "met" Heeengs was after she was dead. During my vision quest I asked her (as she appeared to me in spirit form) not to let any rain fall on me. All other vision questers, except Carmen and me, got soaked (Carmen, because he was running the quest and could get in his car or tent, if he had pitched one).

The part I wasn't going to tell you about was when the split sky happened again, here in North Carolina.

I belong to the Professional Disc Golf Association (PDGA), and I go to the world championships. There are age groups or divisions. For instance, the Senior Grand Master Division starts at age sixty. My division is called the Legends. You qualify for it by reaching seventy years of age. In order to make a decent showing scorewise I try to practice all I can.

By the year 2000 I still hadn't found an eighteen- or even a nine-hole disc course anywhere near my home. I was living with my wife, Diana, way up in a hard-to-find place near Bluff Mountain, building a house in an even harder-to-find place. Out in our shallow-valley backyard (140 yards long) I put a disc golf basket. This "backyard" is a hayfield. By the end of April the hay is already trying to hide any errantly thrown disc. Two or three of a dozen discs that I would take to the world championships are real favorites of mine that would be irreplaceable if lost.

By the Fourth of July some of the hay was up to my shoulders in height. Our landlord had given this hay to a neighbor living some miles away, and I was listening every day to hear Lionel Brooks's tractor come put-putting up the mountain. Lionel also grew Tobacco. He was tied up in whatever Tobacco farmers get tied up in to preserve their cash cops. In three weeks I was supposed to be at the world championships.

Finally, one day, around noon, I came home to find Lionel sitting next to his hay-cutter eating a sandwich. I rushed over to him and gently praised him for coming. I say "gently" because I didn't want to overexcite him in any way. He was older than I was, and I didn't want him to die before he cut that hay. So with the barest number of good words, I left him alone.

About halfway to the house I happened to look back toward Lionel. Words even fail me now to try to describe my feelings about what I saw. The whole western sky behind him was black. At first I just wanted to cry. If we got this storm and maybe more days of rain, there'd be no telling if the hay would ever get cut. It had to be dry to be cut, or it would mildew.

Then I got mad. The angry kind of mad, although some insanity may have crept in, too, because I pointed my finger (like Uncle Charley charming a pheasant) at the center of the clouds and said, "YOU CAN'T DO THIS. YOU CAN'T RAIN ON THE HAYFIELD!"

I went into the house in devastation. I threw myself on the bed and stared up at the ceiling. I heard the tractor start up. A half dozen or so big raindrops hit the roof of the house. Then silence.

Through the open window I heard a sound like wind in the distance. Or was it rain? I could hear the tractor again. I guessed Lionel was high-tailing it for home. But what was this distant noise? I went outside to look.

This time I did cry. The whole hayfield was swathed in golden sunlight. Lionel was nonchalantly chugging along cutting hay like a good little farmer should. I could imagine him whistling, "Maresy doates and dosey doates and little lambsy divey." The woods on both sides of the hayfield were being drenched with rain, causing a sound "like wind."

Here's another unusual thing that happened. One day I was visiting my grown and married son Bob in a town named Hilliard, northern Florida. I took a walk. In those times I had taken to smoking cigarettes, but, knowing that a number of forest fires had been started carelessly, I left my cigarettes "home" because the woods were all superdry tinder. Maybe even a cold lightning bug could have started a fire.

I was just walking along nicely, minding my own business, when, oops, here was a snake in my path. Not knowing every snake around these parts, I gave it a good inspection. It was very light blue, maybe even slightly toward the color called aqua. I said to myself, "That snake is not poisonous. I'm going to catch it and show it to Bob. Maybe he'll know what it is."

I approached it slowly, smoothly, and gracefully. Maybe I could be so graceful as to charm it. Well, it had grace, too. It let me get about eighteen inches from it, then it gracefully began to move away from me at the exact speed (low low gear) that I was moving toward it. I increased my speed. It increased its speed.

I sprang forward and lunged my hand toward its head, intending to grab it at the exact spot where it could wear a bow tie if it wore a bow tie. All I was able to grab was its tail, which promptly broke off as though the snake were made out of blue cheese and could discard some of itself whenever it wanted to.

Now I had to run to catch up to the rest of it. Same thing. A lunge, a grab at the head, a piece of tail. The part that I didn't get went zipping down into a hole. All I had was a three-inch piece of snake. Well, this would have to do. I started back to Bob's place with my little prize in my hand. It had a good feel to it.

Looking at plant life I hadn't seen before in my life, I sort of forgot about the "thing" in my hand. Now I've told you enough times that I'm a seven in the Enneagram, but I didn't say much about what else I can be.

In the Enneagram, a seven, under stress, goes to the number one, the "nitpicker." When the seven is emotionally in a strong opposite place owing to stress, they go to the number five, the "observer." Well, I was enjoying the peacefulness of my walk so much that I had become a five. Everything I saw was exceptionally interesting. That's where my mind was, not on the thing in my hand.

While I was in this pleasant daze, the urge to smoke came sneaking in. Without another thought I just automatically put that "snake cigarette" in my mouth and took a drag on it. YIPES! When that cold thing touched my lips and woke me up, I flung it into the blue. Of the sky. It took me a while to find it again.

Bob said, "Oh, that's a glass snake. You can't smoke 'em."

I'm telling you about things I've seen. I don't know what suddenly has reminded me of something that happened when I was five, in 1935.

The house we lived in at Seven Clan had an enclosed stairway between upstairs and downstairs. One day I came down those stairs to go outside and play. I wonder now, Is one born already with a certain compulsion per the Enneagram (nine different-numbered compulsions) or what? I'm a seven now, and I was a seven then because all I wanted to do then is play, as I still do.

So here I was on my way to play when I reached the bottom of the stairs.

Oops. There, in the living room in his favorite rocking chair, sat my father reading the *Niagara Falls Gazette*. I backed out of sight. Father could come up with the most unthought-of chores, even surpassing creativity. ("Here . . . take this bucket and this stick. Go up to all the stems of the potato plants and put the bucket under them and tap the leaves with the stick. You will be surprised at how many potato bugs that you don't see will fall out into the bucket. When any bugs try to climb out, hit the bucket with the stick. Ring it like a bell. The vibration of the bell toll will send the bugs back to the bottom. After a while they will get tired of climbing and will stay at the bottom. Then bring me the bugs," and so on.)

I couldn't stay hidden forever. I might die of starvation. The seven's need for play overcomes his abomination of work. I walked devil-may-carily past my father, who continued to read as though I didn't exist.

Out the door I went, skipping to my Lou, my darling. One of my favorite places to hang out was the woods' northern escarpment, where I could dare myself to climb up and down the tricky embankments. A path led to this place, and I headed toward it. At the chicken house I took one step toward going around it and stopped. There, up ahead, coming out of the woods on the same path I was meaning to use came my father with a burlap bag of Medicine over his shoulder.

What is this?! I ran back into the house and looked at the rocking chair where I had seen this same father reading only a minute or two before. The chair was empty. I ran back and met my father. "You know what?" I said confrontingly, "I saw you reading the paper in the house just now!"

Father often laughed a lot when he was talking with someone, after every paragraph and sometimes even after just one sentence. I guess you could call it more of a chuckle. He looked at me, and this time he laughed even before he talked. "Anybody can do that," he said, and then he kept right on walking past me on into the house.

When I worked in construction, I came to crane work of different kinds. At the start of it, I worked with a great crane operator named Bill Farmer. As an apprentice, I drove a mobile crane for him. He was from the Six Nation Reservation, and I think he was Mohawk. We worked out of the Niagara Falls local operating Engineers Union.

One of the jobs we got was roofing a series of new substation buildings for Niagara Mohawk Electric Company. These new buildings were in various towns and cities south of Niagara Falls and Buffalo and on down into Bradford, Pennsylvania. The roofs consisted of long prestressed concrete slabs brought in on the long flatbed trailers you see smoking up our air on any superhighway. Our thirty-five-ton PEH crane did its share of smoking, especially on long uphills. On downhills, I had to be careful not to get rolling too fast, or the speed of such weight would overcome the stopping power of the brakes, and we might tip over on a curve or come to a "T" in the road where we had to go either left or right.

Between jobs, we tried to be ready for the next job and be set up before the trucks got there. So on this one day, we were barreling along on this gradual downhill, and I was tempted to "let it sail" past the safety speed because I could see that the highway went back uphill and would slow us of its own accord. Still, there were some curves.

Before I could really make a decision, I found myself putting on the brakes. We were "right on the bubble"; I mean, the brakes almost didn't hold, but gradually they grabbed, and, as though "being told," I brought the crane to a stop and put the "stop" blinkers on.

Bill said, "What'd you stop for?"

I said, "I don't know."

He said, "Maybe something's wrong, let's look." Most operators would have wanted to keep going. In fact, I never would have expected Bill to say what he did. He was very gung ho about getting things done.

As I was climbing down from the cab, something shiny caught my eye behind the front tire. There was only about a two-inch or less gap of viewing opportunity behind the tire at all. Something shiny?

I started the truck motor back up and turned the wheel for a better look: the steering rod on the left side had only one more thread to go before it would disconnect from the wheel. The shiny part was all the other threads from which it had vibrated loose. I'll let you conjure up what could have taken place had the steering come apart just as we reached a speed of sixty miles per hour.

Some years later, at the Eastman Kodak job in Rochester, New York, I was told to take over the Linden crane at a certain building under construction because the coworker who normally ran the crane had just called in sick.

You have seen similar such cranes atop high buildings. We would be pouring concrete unless the wind velocity was too high. This day was looking to be calm and peaceful.

I started to go to the roof through the building stairway, as anyone would do. In fact, it was the only way up unless you did what I did.

The boom and counterweight of these cranes sit on a "stem," a T-shaped affair with a square mast or tower of sections of steel construction that go all the way down through the building to a concrete base at the bottom. A ladder can be climbed up through the center of this mast. Maybe I thought I needed some exercise (heaven forbid), but I went up that ladder instead of being normal and using the stairway.

As I climbed, I casually checked the nuts and bolts of the mast, and the higher I got, the more careful I became. As I came up through the plywood flooring (part of the ceiling concrete forms), I was sort of giving myself a pat on the back for being a good "prepared" boy scout.

From my position halfway through, I got a good look at the electric swing motor. It looked a bit out of kilter, or maybe that was just the angle from which I was looking. I went and got a better look.

Of the four large bolts that normally held it in place, only one remained. Once the mechanic arrived with four new bolts, it did not take long to secure the swing motor. In the meantime I went over to the job "super" to tell him what the problem was. He was on the phone, and before I could say anything, he put the phone down and said to me, "The concrete plant just called and said the first load will be a little late. Some bolt came loose someplace."

"OK," I said, turning away.

Some days we just "live right."

I'll end this chapter with a small but fitting anecdote. It has to do with the sense of hearing. A sense of the ear.

Some people have perfect pitch. That is, you can have them blindfolded while you go to a piano (or any in-tune instrument) and strike the B-flat note. They will say right away, "That was B-flat." You can't fool them.

I don't have that ability, but I have a fine sense of the beauty of a song or even of a phrase or riff. Having played jazz trumpet with a jazz group, I am very familiar with the phenomenon that any one of us could have a "grooving" solo, where an otherworldly beauty comes out in the tone quality, the emotional and spiritual feeling, the ideas, everything. It pulls the whole band up and inspiration simply takes over. Then, just when you think it can't get any better, someone will send chills up everybody's spine, and we will scream and carry on like idiots just for that one "overthrill." Maybe you know what I'm talking about, but even if you don't, when it happens, you'll KNOW it.

I mentioned already that Diana and I were living in "far-out land," a place where days could pass before we would see another human. But I found out that we still weren't far out enough where ceremony is concerned—it is strongest if no other person, no other soul, is anywhere near by. So we built a place farther up the mountain, with a locked gate a half-mile or more from the house. The gate, having been there for a long time, was kind of rusty.

One day I was so excited with the way things were going in the building of the house that I hated to quit, but I did. I went back down the mountain in the old four-by-four Nissan pickup, unlocked and swung the gate open, drove through, and stopped to relock it.

Hating to stop when things were going to smoothly, I held the gate still for a long moment before I gave it a nice soft push, and it closed by itself.

I don't think I can tell you about this incident correctly. You would just need to have been there with me and hear what I heard: it was that bone-chilling beauty of a soloist gone "beyond." The rusty gate played "Taps" like I've never heard "Taps" before. "Taaaaa . . . ta . . . taaaaaaa. . ."

It was even a bit scary, but I got the message. "You were right in stopping work when you did. It's time to rest. Day is done and the katydids are waiting in the wings."

Elemental Communication

It is one thing for us to say that we are family to all the Elements of this Divine and Harmonious Universe, but do we attempt much communication with these Elements? And do these Elements attempt to communicate with us? Most Indians know that the Elements do try to communicate, and that it is up to us as an Element called People to at least voice thankfulness. Most people, though, don't go much further than voicing some variation of, for instance, "Nice doggie" when a pet dog wags its tail. Some people do talk to their flowers and maybe to the veggies in their garden.

My mother raised her voice one year at her Christmas cactus. She'd been taking care of it for four years, and for the past three Christmases it hadn't bloomed, or even ever.

"I'VE BEEN TAKING CARE OF YOU FOR FOUR YEARS, AND YOU WON'T BLOOM," she said. "I'VE GOT A GOOD NOTION TO THROW YOU OUT!" This was two weeks before Christmas. At Christmas time and every year after that the cactus was teeming with blooms.

At the church on the Tuscarora Reservation that we referred to as the Presbyterian church (though the Indians who went there likely didn't know one denomination from another and might go there because it was closer to their house or because they were just plain nosy or any such relevant reasons), there occurred an event of phenomena.

A funeral took place at this church five weeks before Easter. After the funeral the family of the dead person gave the flower arrangements to the church and hoped they would look no worse for wear at the following Sunday service. At the midweek Wednesday night prayer meeting the flowers looked as beautiful as ever, so quite a few prayers were for them and to them to stay beautiful. On Sunday, sure enough, they looked as though they had just been picked, so even more fervent urgings and praising of their beauty took place. Uncle Heal-by-Prayer Charley was there praying and crying with joy.

Someone, maybe over-elated or half jokingly, said, "Let's make them last 'til Easter." Well, that's all it took for the joy-filled members to take up the challenge. And each Sunday as the flowers remained unwilted, the "oh yes you can make it" urgings rose to a fever pitch. Of course, with communication of that high an order the flowers had no choice.

On Easter Sunday those flowers communicated more than just beauty. They were saying, in essence, "Your faith and your belief can bring miracles."

On Monday came another communication. June Johnson lived across the road from the church, and he acted as janitor. That day he walked into the church and couldn't believe his eyes. Every flower was wilted and blackened as though it had been dead for a month. The message was, "You get what you ask for."

As a teenager I used to get a chance to talk with an Elder woman whom some people referred to as a witch. Her name was Heeengs. She was some slight relation to me, though I don't know if she really ever married Dan Williams or not.

What Heeengs told me was that her mother used to take her to the Green Corn Ceremony. When the ceremony was concluded, most everyone went home except those few, including her mother, who had to stay and clean up the place. Little Heeengs wandered out to the cornfield, where the corn was about half grown. She saw there a fascinating sight. Every corn plant sported a bright halo about two inches above it. Heeengs sat down transfixed as the whole field of corn gave off a tremendous amount of light. She said the whole field was alive because each halo jiggled as it tried to follow the movement of the plant beneath it playing in the breezes. When her mother came to get her, she fought back a little because she wanted to stay longer and look at that sight. She said, "I remember my mother taking me by the wrist and pulling me away."

I said, "Could your mother see the halos, too?"

Heeengs thought a moment. "I don't know. Maybe she had seen this so many times and was so tired she could just walk away from it."

On October 13, 1999, my daughter Donna, whose Indian name was Wot naad gi(t)'th (the Aura of Dawn, which is also the name of the direction east), died from cancer. In around 1970 I had been told by the great seer and reader Daisy Thomas of Six Nations, Canada, "I see you are doing Medicine. You are undertaking a tremendous thing. If you continue, you may lose your youngest daughter. That is a traditional condition that can happen if you dedicate yourself."

"Well," I thought to myself, "My father did Medicine, and now he's dead, and my sister is still alive." I'd forgotten that our father, Eleazer, had already lost a child (years before we were born) in an earlier marriage. Also, I thought that if I was worth my salt and that if my youngest daughter, Lisa, was to take sick, then I'd cure her, wouldn't I? And then, bam! Lisa was struck by a panel truck as she rode her bicycle on Williams Road.

When I told Daisy, "You were right," she cautioned me. She knew, without my ever telling her of my family, that I had another daughter, Donna. "I told you that because you were doing Medicine, you needed two protection masks and that you must join the False Face Society of Healing; when you did that, you dedicated yourself. You are protected. But I see that you have an insatiable thirst for Medicine knowledge. You have gone to see Isaiah Joseph, haven't you? You have another daughter, you know."

In the ensuing years I came to find a special deep kinship with other members of the False Face Society. Leon Shenandoah (the Tadadaho, or Fire Keeper, of the Six Nations), Lloyd Elm, Eulale Moses, Da ya wan dut (Wally Green, who did my Induction Ceremony), and especially the two Tuscarora brothers, Ta wi da qui and Ru chuh'need.

One day toward the ending of a certain year, Ta wi da qui called me and invited me to a Ten-Day Fast. It began on Christmas Day. Sixteen people came into his house, and he took the phone off the hook and locked the door. No food, no water, but he allowed us one capful of aloe vera from a bottle per day. One night in about the middle of the ten days a Yoo snek kreet (Great Horned Owl) came to the window and in that low low voice that they have told us that Daisy Thomas had died.

That was about ten years before Donna's death. I don't know if there is any connection between my pursuance of Medicine and what Daisy said and Donna's death, but birds came again.

Each morning my wife, Diana, gets up in the dark and meditates into first light. On three successive mornings two sparrows came to the window before Donna died and one, in particular, would beat against the glass in front of Diana.

Donna in Florida, Diana in North Carolina. Then at 2:30 A.M. of October 13 the phone rang with the message of Donna's death.

At the funeral service I mentioned our connection as a family to all the other Elements of this Divine and Harmonious Universe, asking them all to join us in the funeral service and to pour forth their love and comfort and healing and balance and grace and purification into our minds and bodies and spirits. I also placed a soft leather beaded pouch of Sacred Indian Tobacco in Donna's casket for her to share with my father because he might be getting low in supply, having died in 1966.

Two friends of ours, Dennis and Christine, were there, too. Dennis is a pipe carrier and after the burial did a Pipe Ceremony. Two Bald Eagles came and flew over the spot of the ceremony.

Ten days later I did the Ten-Day Feast for Donna. The purpose of this feast is to acknowledge that it is time to release the spirit of the one who has just died into the caretaking of the dead who have gone on before them and who are here waiting to do that; that we now celebrate the freeing of this person to enter Higher Consciousness.

In this feast certain traditional foods are prepared, including the Sacred Sisters corn, beans, and squash, and a special place is set for the departing one.

A day or so before this feast for Donna I was thinking that I would like to include in the menu a dish that Donna especially liked. Half jokingly, I thought of caviar. No. Too salty. Lobster. Well, I don't know; if a dozen people come, I might not be able to afford that. But still being a bit silly, I considered pheasant under glass.

Well, back to reality, the last pheasant I'd eaten was in 1953 in Chicago, but what happened next was tricky indeed. The door opened, and in walked Diana carrying a pheasant. On her way home the car in front of her had struck the pheasant and broke it's neck. So we all had pheasant, not under glass, but baked in creamy gravy in crockery, Donna having the largest portion.

The ceremony concludes with the words, "We have done all we can now for Donna, and we turn her over to the dead here waiting, and they know what to do, for they know more than we do."

The ceremony was over, but I wanted to show our guests what a great artist Donna was. I unrolled a canvas that she had painted in oils of herself sitting in a forest of huge trees and sunlight coming through in sheets. One of her hands is reaching upward, and a Baltimore Oriole is about to land in it. But something was in her lap that we hadn't really noticed before. Two long pheasant feathers. One last elemental communication. "Meat is a requirement of the feast, and providence supplied it. Bird."

Of all creatures, birds are the best "seers." Here then are two more incidences that tell us to pay more attention to them. The first occurrence happened to Horatio Jones's daughter. And of all the names of women that there are, the name of the woman who had this experience had to be Birdie. Maybe that is also why she knew, immediately, the message in the communication.

Quite a few Indians used to like to make extra money in the summertime picking fruit. Birdie was one of them.

Oh, one amendment. There was one woman, Bernice, who, though she did like to make extra money, didn't really make extra. Maybe she didn't pick fast enough because the pay was by piecework. At any rate, she had to pay the babysitter more than she made.

Birdie, though, as did many pickers with small children not yet in school, had relatives who loved seeing their small kin and would gladly baby-sit for free. On this particular occasion Birdie and her neighbor Vivian left their children, three in all, with an Elder woman named Pearl. Pearl was nearly blind, but she had sat with many children many times.

At about 10:00 A.M. while Birdie was atop a ladder filling her picking bucket with sour cherries, two sparrows suddenly fluttered in her face.

"Something's wrong!" she shouted, "Something bad is happening at home." She rushed down the ladder and told Vivian that she was leaving, that something wasn't right and she must get home and see what it was.

At that moment the three children at Pearl's were trapped in a burning barn. They had been playing with matches and making small fires along Chew Road until some state road repairmen came by and scolded them. They then ran and hid in the barn, making a small fire of hay, which got away from them and set all the hay on fire, trapping them.

This is likely the moment that the birds flew in Birdie's face. There was no way that Birdie could have gotten to the barn in time. She first had to find the fruit farmer who had gathered all the pickers and convince him that something was terribly wrong at home because two birds told her so and that she must rush home. If she had been at Pearl's, though, she would have run into the flaming building. I say this because Birdie was the one who stopped a bulldozer by throwing herself bodily in its path when the New York State Power Authority was attempting to confiscate about one-fourth of the Tuscarora Indian Reservation.

Why didn't the sparrows also fly into Vivian's face? Because Vivian wouldn't have had a clue that they were communicating.

It is true for me that if a bird flew into a windowpane of my house, my cabin, or my car, I knew that someone on the reservation had died. If my children were with me when this happened, they would call my mother as soon as we could get to a phone to find out who had died. I kept thinking that one day a bird flying into a windowpane would just mean that a bird had an accident.

Finally, a time came when we called, and my mother said, "Nobody," to our question "Who died?" This happened in the month of August. We were at our camp in Naples, New York, a remote wooded high place above a valley. A wood thrush hit the front-door window and fell dead. After a month passed, we gave up asking because everyone said, "No, no deaths on the reservation."

A year went by, and I was visiting on the Manawaki Indian Reservation in Quebec. I met a friend, Pete DeConte, who had married a Tuscarora woman, had children there, and lived at Tuscarora for many years. We talked a while and then he asked, "Did you know that my daughter Marlene died in Toronto last year?"

"Was it in August?" I asked.

"Yes."

And that's why the wood thrush knew more than the Tuscaroras.

Each Element communicates in whatever way it can, and I have mentioned just a bit about birds and flowers. We would sorely miss the beauty and the sweet aroma of the flora as well as the heartwarming music, the graceful flight, and the colorful plumage of the birds if one day they were not here.

Another Elemental Communication

There are places in the world where people have gotten lost and never come back alive. The Adirondack Mountain region of New York State is one such place.

Ronnie Mt. Pleasant got to calling himself Beasley, sort of trying to scare people into thinking that he might be part witch or devil. Some people likely did become somewhat apprehensive of him, but others just thought of him as somewhat squirrelly. Squirrelly or not, Ronnie was the first Tuscarora to get a deer with a bow and arrow in "modern times" (after the Tuscaroras migrated from North Carolina). Not only that, he got it in the Adirondacks.

WELL, if Ronnie could get a deer in the Adirondacks, the rest of us ought to be able to get two or three, even with a bow and arrow. I was there the following hunting season with my trusty bow and arrows. I didn't even SEE a deer.

I couldn't believe that I couldn't even find a deer, and each year I went back more determined than ever. "Maybe," I thought to myself, "being too careful of not getting lost has caused me to not go far enough in, into where the deer are."

Actually, hunters from our reservation had been going into this Speculator area (name of nearest town) for so long that names had been given to certain places. Bob Anderson (before I was born) used to have to hire a mule train at Utica and go in by that mode of transportation. There were no paved highways yet. So maybe even Bob had a hand in calling, for example, a certain mountain "the Gray One."

Although I started seeing some deer, I began expecting to maybe even get a bear (more rare), so I ventured farther and farther from camp. On one particular hunt in one particular year (1958?), I came with only one other hunter, a white man named Fran Schwartzmeyer. Fran was afraid of his own shadow, so he stayed within sight of camp (eight-five to ninety yards).

The topographical map showed a trail to the east side of Potash Mountain and not much farther. Here is where I went, crossing the Jessup River and coming to the place where the trail ended, part way up the mountain. I had walked along this side of the Jessup River before, so I expected that if I circled the mountain at this height, I would know I had completed the circle when I saw the river.

All went well, but it was not easy to walk quietly in the bed of dry curled leaves. It takes a while to circle a mountain, and when I began seeing wisps of fog crawling in, I began stepping along rather than pussyfooting. Just the same, I soon found myself engulfed in a fairly thick fog. Vision became restricted to about fifty yards, then forty, then thirty.

I decided to keep going but to drop down to a level that would take me to the trail if I made a full circle. Soon I found myself at base level of the mountain.

Wait a minute! Where was I? Here was a large patch of cattails. I was very sure that I was very close to having circled the mountain. If so, I should have been in an area that I had walked before, but there had never been any cattails anywhere. Maybe this mountain was connected by a gap to another mountain. Maybe I was far off the mark of where I thought I was. If so, to go on was to go "off the map," farther from the trail and camp. Not only that, the heightening inability to see was not just because of a thicker fog. Night was falling.

Without going any farther, I gathered a huge stack of leaves and crawled under it, thinking, "I'M STAYING RIGHT HERE!"

Now it got quiet. I tuned in to the coming night.

"Wait . . . what was that? . . . hmmm . . . men's voices!"

I bet Fran had panicked and gotten someone to walk the trail and look for me. Maybe I'd recognize Fran's voice.

I listened . . . no . . . it's wasn't Fran, but for sure it was two men talking. Well, it didn't seem as though they were on the move, but I thought I'd better go and ask them where we were.

As I moved toward "the talkers," the sound of that talk got louder, but maybe they weren't speaking English.

They weren't. They weren't even "they." It was the gurgling of the Jessup River. I had to follow it but a short way to get to the familiar bridge of the trail.

When I got back to camp, sure enough, Fran was in a panic. He was about to call the National Guard, not so much as to find me, but to be in the company of people and not bears.

War and Peace

My earliest recollections of the nature of people include the "Bill Uh" episode in which I awoke in the middle of the night to hear the sound of army snare drummers marching along the lane that led to an old powder house of the Revolutionary War. Bill Uh was the first person I had ever seen wearing an army uniform, and seeing a man in a uniform "die of a broken heart" left a powerful lasting impression on my little self.

Other than that abstract reference to war, several years went by without my knowing what it was all about. My folks had not the least interest in such things, so for a while I didn't know that such things existed, there being no talk about war.

Maybe we all were in denial, sort of like if you don't think of a dentist and his drill, maybe no toothaches will come.

Maybe I didn't tell you about this incident of mine that reinforces the concept of reincarnation. War, however, was part of it.

As a toddler and preschooler, I would go nuts and scream and yell whenever an airplane flew overhead. I would put my hands over my ears, go running and crying into the house, and crawl under my bed. This experience was especially frightening if the plane was a "double-winger."

Freud may have said that I had been sexually abused by a dragonfly. Anyway, when I got to be forty years old or so, I happened to go to a past-life regression session out of curiosity.

In the first regression (there were three), which was "back to the most recent lifetime," I found myself in Europe someplace, maybe France, and it must have been during World War I because a double-winger airplane flew over and dropped a bomb. All I remember after that was seeing the bomb coming at me and getting bigger and bigger; then I "woke up" from my past-life trance "all shook up." I had been killed in a wartime scenario by an exploding bomb dropped from a biplane, a double-winger. This scenario certainly could account for my preschool reaction to biplanes. It might also account for the fact that, for no real reason, I distrusted people in uniform—policemen, doctors, nurses, and even boy scouts.

I also made two half-hearted attempts to study and speak French. Oui.

The next "indoctrination" I received that spoke of war (after Bill Uh) was a reading by Warren Jack at the Tuscarora Baptist church. Every Memorial Day in May, or the nearest Sunday to it, Warren Jack —whom I now assume was a veteran of some war—would rise from his seat in the congregation and hobble (you know them old vets: somehow, the older they get, the more devastating was the wounding episode . . . the telling of it) to the front of the congregation carrying a ledger book.

He was not a big man, but bigger than Bill Uh. After a couple of "ahems" to clear his throat (or maybe as a three in the Enneagram, he did it to get more attention) he would open the ledger and read names of Tuscarora Indians who had participated in American wars dating back to a surprising long time ago. This book may still be in existence for the benefit of trivia pursuiters. "Hawk" trivia pursuiters maybe.

Interestingly, the older the names, the more biblical many were: Obediah, Zaccariah, and so on. English missionaries must have waylaid the Tuscaroras very early on and dubbed them with English names because, as I mention elsewhere, I could not come up with a Tuscarora surname that wasn't in a phonebook in Oxford, England.

But the whole point here is that the concept of war continued to recur throughout my childhood. Then, of course, the tombstones at the reservation cemetery indicated service rankings of dead soldiers or sailors. Our Memorial Day was called Decoration Day, and we decorated any and all graves, even if the skeleton underneath had never touched a gun. Parades of marching service personnel took place on main streets, even in small towns like Lewiston.

Then came World War II. Grandmother Geese-a-geese would treasure a copy of the *Niagara Falls Gazette* whenever Father bought one, and I could hear her "Ohhh myyying" through the locked doors of her room as the war unfolded. Of course, it was all the more real to her because she had predicted it from seeing the aurora borealis in brilliant "blood" reds. She coined a word for the bombing: *bum-ber-dings.*

Aunt Minnie, a nurse in New York City (and, incidentally, if I have such a poor memory, why do I still remember her address, 575 Riverside Drive?), used to send me books to smarten me up. One was a copy of *U.S. Camera*. In it was a photo of a typewritten letter from Albert Einstein to President Franklin Delano Roosevelt. The part of the letter shown in the photograph contained the words, "I believe that if we bombard the uranium atom we can produce nuclear fission."

I'm sure Albert was thinking of power for peaceful means, but this letter spawned the Manhattan Project and atomic bombs that fell on Hiroshima and Nagasaki. It also produced the naughty place called Love Canal in Niagara Falls, New York.

Love Canal was only a short distance from La Salle High School, where I had "interned." I had played varsity basketball there, and later, when the some-what special fortieth graduation class reunion came about, I decided to attend and see how my past teammates were faring.

Faring? Only two showed up. WHAT? The canal had taken more than we care to think about.

Two Tuscaroras were killed in World War II action, Emmett Printup Sr. and Carl Chew. Sixty-two names are listed on an honoring twelve-kilometer-run T-shirt.

It is amazing what war does to the human psyche. Overnight, all Japanese Americans were the enemy and put in concentration camps. We became little Senator Joseph McCarthys, and to speak against war labeled one a Commie. I was in grade school buying victory stamps, and if I filled up a book, in ten years my $18.75 worth of stamps could be redeemed for $25.00. Uncle Charley could not buy .22 bullets to hunt with, so to keep his mother from starving to death, he acquired the ability to "freeze" rabbits and pheasants by pointing his pointer finger at them, then grabbing them.

Just before the United States declared war on Germany and Japan, and I guess Italy, we boys my age used to prove what good shots we were with a .22 rifle. I think Joe Woodbury started it. He would hold a Pet Milk-size tin can (bottom facing me) at a distance of about that of a bowling alley, and I would put a bullet somewhere near the middle of it. Then I would hold a can up for him to shoot. Of course, this practice also measured our machoism (and our sanity).

Then one day war was declared, and our bullet-buying privilege (which we automatically assumed to be our Christian right and therefore unrevokeable) was gone, and we were able to retain all our fingers. Just the same, I know that by our silliness we were trying to prove to the world that we could accurately shoot a lot of "Krauts," "Japs," and "Guineas" if given the chance. Later, Archie Bunker tried to show us (as grown-ups now) what bigots and prejudiced men we were, but denial just let us laugh and have it go right over our heads.

So next came the threat of the Korean conflict, where we could now shoot "Gooks." Whether or not it was true that we might be drafted into the army, we boys of my age talked ourselves into beating that rap by joining up so as not to become common "straight-leg" soldiers. We would be paratroopers. After high school graduation in 1948 I signed up with a bunch of my peers so that in case of war we would show them how skillfully we great hunters could kill.

Well, I got as far as Fort Bragg, North Carolina. My school records caught somebody's eye, and I became a candidate for riggers school. So right after jump school off I went to Fort Benning, Georgia, to learn to become a parachute maintenance man and be assigned to the Eighty-second Airborne Division at Fort Bragg again; and that's where I spent the Korean War, in Parachute Maintenance Company.

I was issued a second-hand .30-caliber carbine that looked quite small, and, right away, it became suspect as a "killer," what with its short barrel and relatively short bullets. But then, again, when was I ever going to get the chance to shoot it?

The Korean conflict became a lively reality, and "my" company, Parachute Maintenance Company, went twenty-four hours a day packing parachutes. Some huge parachutes, in tandem, had enough "drag" to lower equipment like Jeeps and pieces of artillery. At one of the Christmases we got busy stuffing these small parachutes (packing them for use) so that the "boys over there" could get some goodies. Though we had to be extra careful in packing the 'chutes that men depended on to keep them alive, we packed these little "goodie" parachutes so fast and so any old way that I could picture them falling unopened and hitting the ground like watermelons, burying into some swamp or scattering O-Henry candy bars and cigarettes.

Maybe at one point some bigwig in Washington asked our division commander if we could "fight back" if the enemy snuck up on us because we were ordered out to the rifle range to get some practice. Somehow I got roped into working the pits. That is, somebody (a crew) had to go to the dugout area beneath the targets and with the proverbial ten-foot pole (with a six-inch white circular disc on the end of it) show the shooter where his bullets were hitting. At the end of the day our captain asked if there were any of us who hadn't shot yet. Three of us raised our hands.

"OK, get your weapons and go to the firing line. You have one round to sight in with."

I aimed carefully at the bull's-eye and squeezed off my sight-in shot. The marker told me that my bullet (barely) hit the six-foot by six-foot target in the lower left-hand corner of the whole big frame. This was the weapon I had been issued to help win the war.

That was fifty some years ago, and now it seems best if Warren Jack's list would come to a peaceful closure—maybe trailing off into the aurora borealis, a pure white one with no reddish tinges.

We Indians, recalling our history as it came to us in oral tradition, say that we originated from Sky World, from Sky Woman, who was expelled for "fooling around" and, some said, "with the Fire Lion" and becoming pregnant. However, she was the seed that populated Turtle Island.

Let us allow ourselves to see a "what if."

Let's say that one nice summer morning I'm out behind the house seeing how the flowers are doing in their beds and talking to them when I feel a gentle tap on my shoulder.

I turn around and see a stranger standing there with a nice smile on his face.

"Please don't be alarmed," he says, "I'm a distant relative of yours. I come from the Pleiades, and I've been sent to see how the population of Turtle Island has been faring." Then with a bigger smile, "You look pretty well behaved."

If this is some kind of a joke, then why do I feel only a strong "goodness" emanating from this stranger?

"Obviously," I say, "You know the common language here . . . I take it you can also read?"

"Yes."

"How does this sound to you, then? I'm scheduled to be in Asheville today for most of the day, but why don't you come with me and visit our library there and see in the history books just how things have been going."

"Excellent!"

"I'll bring you back here, we'll have a nice evening meal together, and you can tell me about your observations."

"I would like that very much."

And off we go.

Before I can even come to a full stop to retrieve my "cousin" at the library, I see his long face. It is an hour-long ride back up into the mountains. Cousin is near tears.

"Why the history of mankind is nothing but a series of wars! . . . the rise and fall of great empires . . . and even the word *greatness* is used in association with wars . . . the Great War . . . Alexander the Great. What about Alexander Nevsky? I mean, get this! . . . 'A SAINT AND MILITARY HERO!' . . . the Crusades . . . the Inquisition . . . war on sin . . . the hanging and burning of witches at Salem . . . too much . . . too much.

"I nearly walked out of the library . . . but then I came upon, in the literature section, writings of a counteracting nature. A woman wrote, 'Yes, just let me have an abortion and bingo! . . . now I'm a great sinner, excommunicated. But let that same kid grow up to be twenty and have his head blown off in a war, then, 'Oh sure! Now he's a hero!'

"And this other writer, a man, writing of the aristocracy at the time of World War I, said, 'when war came they welcomed it with a cry of eagerness, as if they had been rescued from the lavender-scented, the nightmare-haunted embrace of a large feather bed.' "

"Well, don't run off just yet and make so wicked a report. I shouldn't have simply sent you to the library. As you must know, the direct descendants of Sky Woman have no alphabet. The people you have been reading about may have originated from a different place. They are said to have come from two people, Adam and Eve. They view the descendants of Sky Woman as uncivilized and unintelligent because of that lack of alphabet and even, at first, calling us savages and heathens. But they do not speak or understand any of the Six Nation languages or any Indian languages and so therefore know nothing about the Great Law of the Great Peace.

"Indeed, from 1100 on, from the inception of the confederacy until 1500, people of the original Five Nations were born, grew up, and died never knowing what war was. I am happy that you will be taking this message back to Sky World.

"And for you, a poem."

ANOTHER FORM OF INSANITY

To those of us whose genes reflect
The insane notion that we possess
A God-stamped permission to kill
To go to war and wear upon the chest
The Congressional Medal of Honor
Whose ribbon dangles so near
The arm-less sleeve of olive drab
That drags against the wheelchair wheel
A symbol that we cannot resist
The grasping of the sword
Ensuring that we will never know
The bliss of Peace.

Love,
Ted

A Sequence of Events

Did you ever experience a sequence of events that by themselves would perhaps be just interesting, but when one leads to another is phenomenal? I have gone through several such sequences, and one was only one day long.

This one-day-long experience might also be called, "Don't pray for too much, you might get it."

What happened was that I have a circle of magical friends, and one of them suffered a disastrous fire that consumed his home. It was no ordinary home. He and his family had worked hard to turn it into an environmental showcase called the Longbranch Environmental Center.

On the evening of the fire I came home about 6:30 P.M., and my wife, Diana, said, "McNaughty called and is inviting you to see a UFO documentary that he is showing." McNaughty is a member of that magical group, and I gave him the name "McNaughty" (in reality, it's Clyde Hollifield) because he is so tricky. Paul Gallimore is the sufferer of the fire. Hobey Ford and Joe Roberts are the other members of the magical group and would also see the documentary. Hobey and McNaughty are puppeteers, and Joe is a drum maker.

Paul lived only two miles from us, but I thought the UFO video was to be shown at McNaughty's. He lives some eighty miles away off Bat Cave Road. Had I left and gone to Paul's immediately at 6:30, I might have seen the first small blaze of the fire because it was some forty-five minutes later that a phone call came informing us that "Paul's place is on fire!"

Everyone was inside viewing the video and had no idea to what extent the fire was raging before it was discovered. They had all they could do to dash out and save themselves. And what could be eerier than to see, through the window of the building engulfed in flames, the UFO video still playing.

◆　◆　◆

301

It was about three weeks later that I had my one-day bonanza. It was a Saturday and the day that a special benefit shindig would be performed at a donated hall to raise money for Paul to rebuild. I had consented to go with Paul to a radio station and plug the benefit.

When I awoke that morning, I was very sad. I couldn't believe it. I just don't wake up that way. I'm a seven in the Enneagram, and all my thoughts are of having fun. So alien and disconcerting was the feeling that I did a prayer/ceremony immediately, the gist of which was, "Get me out of this blue funk!"

After the benefit plug at the radio station, we stopped for a few minutes at Hawk Littlejohn's little Indian flute-making factory. Some flutes were going for around six hundred dollars. I said to myself, "I'd like a flute but not for six hundred dollars." Knowing me, I might toot on it for about twenty minutes, then go looking for some other fun thing.

When I got home, it was near time to get dressed and ready for the benefit. There was a large package on the porch, a UPS delivery with my name on it. As soon as I opened it, I knew it was the answer to my prayer. It was a basket used in disc golf, a game patterned after golf in which a frisbeelike disc is used in place of a golf ball. Whereas in golf the ball is putted into a hole, in disc golf the disc must land in the shallow basket to "hole out." Anyway, there are eighteen-hole disc golf courses around the world, but these baskets can cost three or four hundred dollars each. This one was from my Algonquin friend, Mike Bastin, who lives in South Wales, New York.

The sad feeling I'd had upon awakening had lasted about as long as my prayer, and I was already in good spirits when I opened the package.

Also, present when I got home were two good friends of Diana and me, Ron and Rachael Clearfield. I said to them, "I'm so glad to see you, but I'm so sorry that I can't visit long with you. I have to get ready to go to a benefit for Paul Gallimore."

"Well, you'll wait, though," Ron said, "because we have something for you." He went to his car and came back with something that somewhat resembled a violin case. I smiled because I thought of Al Capone's gang carrying tommy guns in violin cases.

Well, it wasn't a violin case, and it wasn't a violin, and it wasn't a machine gun. When he handed the case to me, I opened it. It was a brand new trumpet.

About thirty years had passed since I had played the trumpet, gigging in dives in Chicago, emulating a style somewhere between Miles Davis and Chet Baker. I'd loaned my trumpet to a granddaughter so she could get into the high school band, and she had promptly dropped it and dented the valve housing. Ron was a concert cellist, and maybe he sensed that every now and then I missed not having a horn. As elated as I was, I knew that I was holding in my hands evidence that I'd prayed for too much.

So off I went to the benefit and walked into the hall, and what do you think happened? Before I could take my coat off, an acquaintance walked up to me and handed me an Indian flute. "I've been wanting to give this to you, but I don't get to see you very often." By now, I'm speechless, and he thinks it's just because of the flute. I wanted to rush out and do another ceremony so that I didn't explode from lack of sadness. Instead, I hugged the man for a long time.

Now, of course, this is too much. Some things shouldn't be told because people will think you're lying. Like when I put a quarter each into three different one-armed bandits at the Sahara in Las Vegas and hit a jackpot on each one. I don't know if there is a law of the Universe that says that one can reach a point of euphoria where no matter what you do, only beds of roses or the equivalent appear. After the three jackpots I probably should have tried for four and then five and so on to see about such a law, but I didn't. I was there for a professional archery tournament, and the Sahara was a cosponsor. I had to get some sleep, and, besides, three jackpots worth of quarters is quite heavy to carry, don't you know?

The reason I advance the theory of the law of euphoria is that perhaps getting a disc golf basket, a trumpet, and a flute all in one day caused a euphoria in me that caused the next thing to happen. Maybe I should have left the benefit hall and gone to Vegas with a bunch of quarters because more did happen.

Let me tell you about something first. Up to the time of the benefit day I had not yet seen any of the Little People whom we call Eh gwess hi yih (a Tuscarora word; see more about the Little People in other parts of this book). After learning that my father wasn't fibbing about his experiences with Eh gwess hi yih and hearing many Elders tell about them, I tried very hard to see them, even at night-time. One night I even offered some of my flesh to them, albeit a very small amount. I could hear them in the leaves at what I'm guessing to be a distance of ten feet, and I couldn't bring myself to shine a flashlight on them, believing Yeats ("when the first light bulb went on in Ireland, the Little People took to the woods and never came back").

One day I told an Elder how much I liked the song the False Faces were singing before they entered the Longhouse on their night. He said, "If you think that song is beautiful, you should hear the songs of the Little People." Not having seen them and therefore not having been invited to join their society, I despaired of ever hearing their songs, songs of the Dark Dance (the name of their secret society).

OK, back to the benefit for Paul Gallimore. Many people came to the benefit, so it was a success. Among them was a Cherokee named Chris. He came up to me and gave me a Medicine staff complete with an eagle feather and all manner of decoration. Then he handed me a book, saying, "And here's something you might like to see. I may want it back."

Most of the lights in the hall had been extinguished except for those on the performers, so I didn't get a good look at the rather small book. Thank goodness the flow of gifts of one day ended with that book. When I got home, though, I looked at it. It was a book of Indian songs with the notes, time, and words where applicable. Well, don't you know, in it were the Dark Dance songs.

I was so excited I wanted to rent a big vault someplace and put the book under extreme safekeeping. I was also scared that Chris would want it back. But in another too strange to believe twist, Chris, handsome and alert at the benefit, died two weeks later.

I had Ron, the concert cellist, record the Dark Dance songs on his instrument for me, and that's all I'm going to tell you about me and the Little People, but I'll tell you why.

Ru chuh'need told me that his little contact said to him, "We're not all good, you know." He also said that another member of that same secret society had told him the same thing about his own contact. So I took that to be a powerful message with various implications. Nevertheless, with a Heyoka-like bent I wrote a poem about it.

EH GWESS HI YIH (THE LITTLE PEOPLE)
I know the Little People
Have been looking at me
They don't trust me yet
And for good reason

I don't always bring marbles
Or red or black squirrel meat
Or leaves of wild Tobacco

But it's sort of a touché affair
Because one of them said
"We're not all good, you know."

Love,
Ted

I sent the poem to Ru chuh'need with no other writings in the envelope. After reading it, he put the poem back into the envelope and handed it to his mother-in-law, Eulale. At that time she was still alive, a fun-loving and superalert person, a Faithkeeper of the Onondoga Longhouse. Not having been told by Ru chuh'need about what his contact said, she read the communication and then she looked up with a very serious look on her face.

"You think Ted's alright?"

An interesting sequence of events in the 1970s started, I suppose, when I found a nice soft leather man's glove on the sidewalk in Rochester, New York. I said to myself, "What a shame. Someone has only one glove now, and who walks around wearing only one glove?"

I took the glove home and cut one finger off and filled it with Sacred Indian Tobacco. This made a nice little Medicine bag, which I tied shut with deerskin thongs and hung around my neck. Why? Who knows?

A weekend later I happened by the Museum of Science on East Avenue and saw a sign, "Folk Festival," so I stopped to look it over. Various groups in the dress of whatever country they represented were set up in separate areas. Some sold

traditional foods, some played music, and some maybe danced to their native traditions. Presently I came to a group wherein the mother of a Seneca Indian family drummed and sang Six Nation social dance songs while her children danced.
The father stood off nearby, so I stopped and spoke with him, introducing myself.
He told me that they came from the Tonawanda Seneca Indian Reservation,
which is about thirty miles from Tuscarora, though I had never met him before.

The following weekend I left Rochester, driving casually toward Tuscarora
with my eye open for a special shrublike Medicine called in the Tuscarora language Ga jeet roo rud gwa ri yit (The-shrub-is-red-in-color). I'd had a teacup
reading by Sally Dubec, who told me that someone, maybe a witch, was seeking
to do me harm in some way. She also mentioned that this person seemed unable
to get to me, that something, or somebody, was protecting me. I did not have my
False Faces yet.

I said to her, "If a witch was after you, what would you do?"

She replied, "Well, there's a powerful protection Medicine that I don't know
the name of, but it looks like a very miniature tree. But it's very rare. It's beautiful.
Its limbs grow in a series of U-shaped crotches." But then she said, "Oh, but I feel
that even if you found it, it would be too powerful for you to use it in the way that
I would. If you did find it, maybe you could just hang it on your wall and tie a
fresh pouch of Tobacco [meaning the Sacred Tobacco] on it each year."

A few years later I realized that I already had this miniature tree. I'd been
bow hunting in Pennsylvania some five years previous and saw this tiny tree. I'd
walked on past it some hundred yards or so, but I couldn't get it out of my mind,
so I went back and got it. I'd painted it white and planted it in powdered Tobacco
in a thin-stemmed milk white vase. Since then, I had been using it simply as a
decoration.

Sally then said, "Oh, I know what you can use, Ga jeet roo rud gwa ri yit. All
you do is make a tea of the bark and wash your hair with it."

Later, a landscape picture came to my mind of the place where this Medicine grew. I couldn't remember if it came in a daydream or nightdream. Anyway,
here I was now cruising in my car toward Tuscarora. As I neared the Tonawanda
Reservation, I began feeling that this "picture" of the Medicine coincided with
the nature of the land of the northern section of the Tonawanda Indian Reservation. So I drove into and through that reservation, south to north.

(Now I just have to tell about this one unrelated thing. Anyone who has ever driven or walked the road on which I passed through has surely been taken by one particular scene. Someone who lived at one of the houses had probably a hundred tricycles lined up in a row like they were doing the Stomp Dance from one end of their lawn to the other. Each tricycle had a fairly large doll on it. This spectacle was always there, rain or shine.)

Pretty soon, what with the twisty roads, I wasn't sure which direction I was going and felt lost. This northern section borders the Alabama Game Refuge, which I wanted to end up passing through in order to see the large numbers of waterfowl that played there, so I stopped at the next house that I came to for directions. When I knocked on the door, who do you think came to it and opened it? The man I had just met at the folk festival in Rochester. Startled, I asked him if he thought the Medicine I was seeking grew nearby.

"There might be some across the road in those bushes," he said. Thanking him after a bit of talk about the weather, I went into those bushes more to be courteous to him than to expect to find what I sought. What I found was another great Medicine of similar description, so I marked that spot in my mind in case I ever needed it.

(What happened later was that when I came looking for this place, for this Medicine, I never could find it. It was as though that house never existed. Opportunity had knocked, and I should have opened the door.)

I drove on with a good feeling. I'd hardly gone a half-mile when off to the right (east) appeared the scene of my dream, with, of course, the very Medicine I wanted. After the proper ceremonial exchange, I took some of it and drove on. Indeed, I passed through the Alabama swamp area and stopped for a short time to watch the waterfowl.

At Tuscarora there grew a Medicine called Nagdees skuh hut de U-twehh. My father sometimes called it Solomon's Timbers, but I have never seen that name in any plant or flower book. The Tuscarora name implies "Good-for-twelve-diseases." With my good luck rolling, I thought maybe I would see some where it grew at Old Saw Mill at Tuscarora. I got into the car and drove to that place.

At Tuscarora I stopped to give a ride to a man who was walking. It was Allen Jack. He was carrying a hatchet and wearing three hats. Some people are afraid of him. He can do strong Medicine (I mean, he could do it—he's dead now). He's the man that two deputy sheriffs put in jail overnight for vagrancy because he wouldn't tell them where he lived. The next day when they released him, he told the two arresting officers and the judge, "You never should have did that," pointing his finger at them. In one month all three were dead of natural causes. For a while after that some of the young people (Indians) would call him "MIS-TER Jack" loudly. He liked that. He'd grin. When he died, he went outside of his house, put a big padlock on the door, then died INside just to show us one more trick. (All his windows were boarded up.)

When I picked him up that day from Tonawanda, I said, "I'm going looking for a great Medicine, want to come along?"

He hopped right in. We tried to drive in to Old Saw Mill from the Million-Dollar Highway, but my Volkswagen bus couldn't make the last steep part of the hill. It stalled and rolled backward, went off the lane, and would have tipped over except it leaned against a tree.

This scared Allen. He said, "What are we going to do!!?"

"Look for Medicine," I said, "and while we're looking we'll think of what to do."

We looked for Medicine, but it hid on us, and Allen said, "I'll walk home from here."

I got Norton Rickard to pull me back up and out with his old tractor. I gave him some of the Medicine that would protect him if he washed his hair with it.

He said, "Let's have a corn roast."

We went to his cornfield of sweet corn, and I noticed that some of the stalks of the first couple of rows were torn down. Before I could ask why, Norton read my mind and said, "Raccoons. They gotta eat, too. Maybe in the fall I'll eat one or two of them."

Norton had an outdoor barbecue cooker, and he threw a big bunch of un-husked ears into a blazing fire. By now it was totally dark except for the fire and stars. Just to see what he'd say, I asked Norton, "Have you ever had anything unusual happen to you?"

"Yes," he said, "One night my phone rang, and it was Beasley. He had never called me before. He asked me if I would go outside and listen. He was hearing a strange noise outside, and would I try to see if I could hear it, too?" (Beasley was the man who might have been half a bubble off; when he died, instead of a bird hitting my windshield, a huge—and I mean huge—black insect splattered on it.)

"So I went outside," Norton continued, "and from behind my barn I could hear something that sounded like someone in the woods below Beasley's place working the handle of an old rusty water pump. I walked without my flashlight on toward the sound. When I got to about twenty paces of it, it stopped making the noise. I turned my light on the spot, and there was nothing there, but now it started again about fifty or sixty yards to my left, so I put the light out and went toward it again. The same thing happened. I got near it, and it stopped. Then it jumped again to another spot.

"I went back home, and I called Beasley back and told him what happened. We both thought it wasn't a good sign. I asked him how his health was, and he said he felt fine. I told him to be careful and hung up the phone. The next day we heard that his mother had died." Norton went into the house and came back with a dish of butter. We sat there enjoying the roasted corn. We must have eaten four or five ears each when Norton said, "Listen!"

In the stillness a periodic sound could be heard that I would have described as a baby Screech-Owl learning to screech. Before I could say so, Norton said, "It's that same sound! The one Beasley and I heard." We sat listening. Presently, Norton said, "It's coming closer, don't you think?"

Before I could answer, his wife, Marlene, came out of the house crying. "Norton! Your friend So-and-So [I can't recall the name] from Kingston is dying! I'm going to call some people and have a prayer meeting." She went back into the house.

Norton said nothing. He got up and walked into the darkness toward the sound. Since the day I had made the little Medicine bag from the soft leather glove and hung it around my neck, I'd forgotten about it. Now, however, as though this occasion was its sole reason for being, I took the bag from my neck and poured the contents of it on the embers of the fire. "That man will be alright," I said.

Then, somewhat as though I came to myself and had scolding thoughts, "What'd you do THAT for? You think you're God?"

After a while Norton came back. "It seems like that sound is getting fainter," he said. We sat and listened. Indeed it was. We sat there until the sound had disappeared into silence. It was a communication of the Elements. But which Element? I had never heard of this particular-sounding Element before or since.

A month passed before I had a chance to ask about the man from Kingston. "He died. Well, he had no pulse, so they thought he was dead. But then, when they were wheeling his body out, he started breathing again, so they rushed him to an oxygen source and put EEG attachments on him overnight. His heart never skipped a beat, so he was released. He's back to work now."

Maybe he was from the Baby Screech-Owl Clan.

Ceremony

Millions of ceremonies have been done for all time—weddings and funerals heading the list of those that we are most familiar with. Many, though, have been forgotten, the priorities of our way of life having been increasingly infringed upon by technology and computerism. How important IS the ceremony?

Here is a lost one. The late Jake Thomas told me of a ceremony that his father performed that had miraculous results. It came about when an Indian lady came to him with what would now be a very unusual request. She wanted to "rescue" her husband's soul.

What happened was the husband was ice fishing on a frozen lake when the ice gave way, and he drowned. Although this great misfortune had just taken place, the wife had the sense not to walk out on that ice or to ask anyone else to "go out there and see what you can find." She knew he was gone. The lake had taken him.

She said, "I fear for his soul. I have a feeling that it has gone down with him and has allowed itself to be trapped down in that water with him. Do you know the ceremony that 'brings back the soul'?"

In the gravity of the situation Jake's father said, "I was only a boy when I saw that ceremony performed. Part of it includes a feast, and one thing in our favor is that I remember, exactly, what foods need to be in that feast. You make up this plate of foods and meet me at the edge of the lake this evening when the sun is half a fist from setting, and I'll do the best I can with the rest of the ceremony." He then told her of the food items to be placed upon that plate.

After the ceremony that evening he told her, "Tomorrow morning you can come back and get your plate."

The next morning, when she got there, YAW-WEEE!!! (a Tuscarora expression that means something like, "This is so scary, I feel goose bumps all the way up my spine").

311

Next to the plate lay the complete body of her husband.

That impressive a ceremony suggests that in order to have a ceremony "do its thing," it needs to be solemnly and precisely done. Well, how about this next one?

One day a few years ago Diana said to me, "Hey, Ted, we have to do a ceremony for the bears!"

"How come?"

"The season on them opens next week."

Well, it was like "the damsel in distress" saying, "Quit watching the football game and come slay this dragon for me."

I knew what Diana was in distress about. Here, bear hunters are allowed to use "bear dogs" to assist them. Maybe at first, before radio collars on the dogs came to be invented and used, a fair number of wily bears led the dogs and hunters on a merry chase, only to escape by being crafty or long-winded. Not so today. The hunters are able to keep track of where the bear is headed by radio contact. Whenever or wherever the "chase" crosses a road, fresh dogs (radio equipped) can relieve the tired ones, and the wild bear doesn't have much of a chance.

But who has the recipe for a bear ceremony?

At the place where we were living at the time there used to be a stuck-together Cedar tree with a three-prong trunk that I considered "Big Medicine." I went out and sat under that tree; maybe it would "clue me in."

So here is what we did. I got my big Medicine drum and some Joss hoo(t) eh weh (the Tuscarora name for the ceremonial Sacred Tobacco). We started in a slow circling of that tree. We tried to walk like a bear walking on its hind legs. Diana was in front of me strewing the Tobacco like Lotus petals for "the Medicine" to get excited about. I drummed that slow "bear walk" beat. Softly. "Dume . . . dume . . . dume . . . dume . . ."

Once we got the circle complete (had "hit" all Four Directions), I began to chant, one tone, probably a tenor's "G":

"URSA MAJOR . . . IS THROWING . . . A TEDDY BEAR'S PICNIIIIIIC!"

Once to each of the Four Directions. Then:

"BEARS IN THE AIR . . . WOOOF . . . WOOOF" (four times).

That was it.

No bears were killed in our area that year. The following year, in the earlier part of summer, Paul Gallimore called us. "Hey! Did you see the article in the paper? Bear population in North Carolina up 3 percent."

Now, just thinking back to singing "Ursa Major is throwing a teddy bear's picnic" makes me laugh. But it also makes me think, "Well, where DID the bears go? Into caves for an early start on hibernation?" But it also makes me think of another thing that might be a different kind of funny (as in, "Funny you should ask").

At one of the Sundances I attended in the West, maybe the GhostHorse one, an old Indian told me about the disappearance of buffalo (American Bison) in the wintertime. He said, "There is, they say, a big hole in the ground somewhere for the buffalo to go into and hibernate in for the winter. This is like a message that has come down through my people from way back. They said in the summer the buffalo were all over the place, but in winter you couldn't find a single one. They all went into a big hole."

Then I got to thinking: "What about the deer on the Tuscarora Indian Reservation?" Can they hibernate, too? Or what if the deer can shape-shift like some people can? Like Isaiah Joseph shape-shifting with one of the Four Winds or Four Directions, they would simply become invisible during the cold winter. Maybe that's what the buffaloes did too then.

Knowing this was all just speculation, I thought maybe some of the old-time hunters at Tuscarora could straighten it all out. The Tuscarora Indian Reservation is only what, about three miles by three and a half miles, areawise? Yet when I asked one good hunter how many deer he had gotten the past fall, he said, "We got twenty-two." Well, even if by "we" he included his son and maybe even another hunting buddy, that's still a LOT of deer. And what was the total number of deer taken by all of the hunters in the winter? Zip. So I asked, "Where do the deer go in winter?"

"Down by the lake [Ontario]. It's warmer down there. Lots of Christmas trees to break the wind."

As it got close to springtime, I went down to the lake area to see if the ice in the streams was gone, to see if the suckers were running (fish that we speared). Yep, here were two middle-aged men near a bridge already in the water in hip boots and carrying spears. I stopped and struck up the usual "any luck?" conversation.

Hey, maybe they were the perfect people to ask about the deer in winter. Maybe I would learn of the whereabouts of this "nice, warm place."

"By the way, I've been wondering where all the deer go in the wintertime. Where DO they go?"

The answer was immediate.

"Oh, they go up on the Indian reservation."

Wait a minute. How did we get so far off the subject of ceremony? Well, that's Medicine for you. Always connected to all other things. Always seemingly wandering off on a different tangent, like the unexpected flashes of streaky lightening fingers. No "Roberts' Rules of Order," no chronology, yet always able to reconnect.

Time, which includes prolonged effort, is sometimes a big factor in ceremony, like the number of "dips" of a tea bag—stronger tea, stronger Medicine, stronger results in ceremony.

For example, the ceremony to become bullet proof became popular among the Indians in the West when the U.S. Cavalry began pushing the Indians into desolate places. When Spotted Tail did that ceremony, he did it for twelve days running. If that was the prescribed minimum amount of ceremony time needed, then it's no wonder so many didn't do it.

In Spotted Tail's case the "plan" called for him not to be shot, especially not right off the bat.

The plan was that the warriors would spread out in a line in thickets near the cavalry encampment. Spotted Tail would ride his horse in the open, outside of that line, yelling and taunting the cavalry to empty their "ramrod" muzzle-loading rifles at the "bullet-proof" rider, at which time the line of warriors would charge!

Unbeknownst to the Indians, the U.S. soldiers were now armed with repeating rifles. So when Spotted Tail finished his run, bullets continued to "zing" all around him like mad little hornets. Back he went then on another run. Still the bullets came. So back again went Spotted Tail a third time, but this time his horse was struck.

Still, the plan worked. If none of the cavalry were able to shoot just one Indian, how could they hit a charging "swarm" of them who were coming now at full tilt? The soldiers fled. Spotted Tail remained unharmed.

Perhaps, then, there are several ways to induce or influence the powers that be to sanction and carry out the request of a ceremony. A large part of it is likely the strength of the feeling of desire or the degree of need in the request. "I don't want to be shot and die for nothing." My people know that this ceremony is a great one.

What about the Sundance? Here, as spoken about in previous chapters, is a week-long ceremony that is far greater than the sum of its parts. It is actually longer than the week of dancing because the preparation includes, for instance, the ceremony of the carrying-in and the "planting" of the Sundance Tree, plus the draping of it with "robes" and streamers and prayer ties. Each dancer does her or his own Vowing-with-the-Creator Ceremony.

Each dance day starts at 5:00 or 5:30 A.M. with a Sweat Lodge Ceremony, and each day's activity ends with another Sweat Ceremony. Each "round" of dancing throughout the day ends with a Pipe Ceremony. At a certain "time" the Sundance "conductor" gets a message from the spirit world, "NOW! Do the Healing Round Ceremony NOW," and that's when that ceremony takes place.

Each song is its own ceremony. The initial Starting-of-the-Fire (to heat the stones) is a ceremony. The Bringing-in-the-lodge of the red-hot glowing stones is a ceremony. The Hoisting-of-the-flags and the Lowering-of-the-flags are separate ceremonies. The Feast at the end is also its own ceremony. In some Sundances, at a certain "time" a Heyoka will come dancing in, backwards, to tease the thirst-parched dancers with water in a Testing-of-faith Ceremony. Sometimes an eagle will appear and convey its own Blessing-on-the-dance Ceremony.

The number of Sundances done around the country each year is growing. You can imagine, then, the countless ESP-type experiences that have happened to Sundancers. Though many "Iroquois" people Sundance, the main intent of this book is to confine the recounting of the ESP-type experiences largely to those that have taken place on the different reservations of Six Nation Indians.

I have, so far, Sundanced only six times, and only at the first one (1991) can I say that I may have had an unusual experience.

Upon my immediate arrival (one day late) to the Ellis Chips Memorial Sundance at Wamblee, South Dakota, I felt that "something not good" was going to happen. I thought maybe I wasn't supposed to be there . . . that maybe I wasn't ready (spiritual-growth-wise) to dance yet.

I went off to a small copse of trees and meditated on this feeling. Then I said aloud (to the Universe at large), "Am I supposed to be here? If so, give me a sign."

Immediately, two Nighthawks flew out of the brightly lit noonday sky and flew a circle around the Sundance Tree. Then, as if that might not be clear enough, a blacktail fawn came up and licked my hand. Well, if those two signs didn't convince me that I was on the right track, an elderly gentleman, whom I met as I neared the arbor, told me something that convinced me that this dance was indeed a sanctified place to be. Noting that I was newly arrived and likely "wide-eyed," he said, "You should have been here when they brought the Tree in. Wild horses never come to people, but when the drummers hit the beat and began to sing to the Tree, a herd of wild horses came thundering in a cloud of dust. They came to the 'keep-out' fence of the dance perimeter and stood like a sacred audience and watched the Tree come in and be planted. We all cried."

Just as I approached the arbor area, the "something not good" happened.

One of the significant Elders who was participating in the dance collapsed in the rest area of the inner dancer's area. This sacred area is not open to the public. (Not having purified in the Sweat Lodge yet, I was still a member of "the public.")

Without thinking, I dashed into the roped-off area and did a healing-with-the-hands on the man's head. In a minute he opened his eyes, laughed, and stood up. Nobody thought anything about my "crash the party" appearance. I snuck back out to where I temporarily "belonged."

Another thing that happened at Sundance was minor and maybe normal. I was so high from a week-long preparatory fast and anticipation that when my back was pierced and the "pins" put in, I scarcely felt any pain—about like the sting of a sweat bee. (A pin is roughly about the size of a three-inch pencil, tapered at both ends. If it is of hardwood, it is likely made from the Chokecherry tree. It might be made from solid bone, tapered only on one end.) The insertion of the pins on one's back (at a place where, if one ever grew wings, the wings would grow out from) is in preparation to "drag the skulls" (seven buffalo skulls tied together to form a line of them). Later, in subsequent dances, it was NO SWEAT BEE putting in them pegs.

The Sundance does more in helping keep the Universe in balance than any one dancer can see (each being so enchanted by the allure of his or her individual dance purpose itself). So many magical incidences have taken place. (This topic might be another huge book all by itself except that, like great Medicine plants, each incident would likely wish to remain anonymous, to hide within the humility that keeps its strength from being diluted.)

Just the same, I am compelled to tell you of an incident that, though it happened at a Sundance, could have happened to you if you have ever served as a Fire Keeper in any capacity.

The term *Fire Keeper* applies to the Tadadaho of the Six Nations, whose job it is to see that the "fire" that kindles the spiritual glow of the strength of Six Nations acting as one never goes out.

Fire Keepers fascinate me. At the Sundance they keep a twenty-four-hour watch on the heating of the stones even when everyone else is sleeping. They can unknowingly become purified by fire, so I think of them as holy men (or women).

On one middle-of-the-night fire watch, the Fire Keeper saw something very big crawling along the ground in the shadows on the other side of the fire. Drawn to the fire as a moth is drawn to a flame, this "thing" continued forward until it came to the large fire's edge. Here, the Fire Keeper could see that it was a snake. A snake? As big around as a stove pipe?

At the fire's edge the snake did not stop. The only thing that broke its path was the mound of glowing stones, covered by fire. On up and over the middle of the searing pyre, with an air of easy unconcern, continued the huge snake. What color was this snake? Zounds! Rainbow colored!

Fascinated, but oddly not terrorized, the Fire Keeper watched the fire-walking snake proceed through the door of and on into the Sweat Lodge.

Time stood still. The Fire Keeper can't recall how long it was before he peeked into the lodge with a flashlight. Nothing.

When he told me of this great sight, all I could think of was seeing some Aborigines of Australia wearing T-shirts with the imprint of a rainbow-colored snake on the back. The snake was shown as creating a large circle, tail in mouth, to signify the birth of creation.

Don't call me and ask for a ceremony. I'm retired. Do your own.

I can't tell you what will work the best for you, what will tickle or charm the benevolent powers that be, or what channel you might choose to help you. I'll just tell you what I do.

First, I don't do ceremony if I feel a bit under the weather. I like to be absolutely all alone. Sometimes, though, as in an emergency, I might go deeper into the woods, yet still hear the neighbor's chainsaw or mower in the distance.

I shower or bathe first, then I assemble the things I use. Medicine drum, drumstick, abalone shell or earthen bowl (smudge pot), sage or cedar, a bowl or plate to hold the Tobacco, and "the problem" or supplication written concisely on a little piece of paper. Maybe it might say, "Burnham Woods to NOT be clear-cut" or "The big meteor headed for earth to change course" or "The cancer in 'So-and-So' to dematerialize" or "Mother-in-law, Jane Doe, to go into Balance, Mind, Body, and Spirit" or, even in a lighter vein, "The headache that kept my sister up all night to GO TO BED!"

You might have more than one of these supplications, each written on its own little piece of paper.

Just remember this: YOU are NOT the "one" causing the miracle of the ceremony to happen. You are only making contact and presenting a problem whose solution and consummation is for consideration. You are contacting the great, great, great Benevolent Force that has a thousand names. I know it's OK for you to speak directly to this power (or it wouldn't be benevolent, would it?), but I use the Four Directions as the message carrier.

Take lots of time wording the request, using as few words as possible, to make sure that you are NOT putting your two cents or even a tiny bit of suggestion into the HOW of the solution.

Do not expect every request to be taken care of as you or the requester wants to have it happen. Maybe a better solution will occur, and maybe you won't know what "better" is. Now you fire up the sage (I like to use that white sage that likes to keep smoldering) and smudge yourself. Then you smudge everything else, like the "problem" paper(s) and the bowl into which you will put the Tobacco. You don't need to smudge the Tobacco; it is already sanctified. Then if you're going to do the ceremony inside a building, you may want to smudge the small floor area where you will be standing.

Many people (many who are a two in the Enneagram) don't need a Medicine drum or rattle (Mother Teresa was a two), but if you do use one, it will become Medicine after the first day you use it. Smudge it.

Now you put the Tobacco (half of a small handful) in the bowl or plate, then the "problem" papers(s) on the Tobacco, and the rest of the Tobacco on top to help keep the paper from blowing away if you're doing this outside. You might even cover everything with another smudged plate if it's windy. Now you are ready.

I'll just tell you how I happen to do it, whether all I do is relevant or not. It's just what works for me.

I used to do this in a benevolent vortex of a spot where a small spring-fed pond lived (see the poem "Sleepy Lagoon" in the poetry chapter) and also where a big White Pine tree leaned toward the East. I would lay back against it, facing the West to start with. In my butterfly-minded head someplace, I decided that the Four Directions, as used by Fool's Crow, would be the best "channel" to the Great Benevolent Powers That Be (of a thousand names), such as Soong gwi oo dee sut eh; and that the West is a woman, my Clan Mother and Principal Direction.

So I aim my drum to "Grandmother" in the West and strike it.

When we do a Tobacco-Burning Ceremony outside, we customarily give a sharp yell into the sky, three times. Each yell is something like, "YOO HOOO! YOU UP THERE THAT CAN DO ANYTHING . . . IT'S US AGAIN THAT NEED SOMETHING AGAIN. Second yell: "YOO HOOO! . . . CAN YOU HEAR US? Third yell: "I KNOW YOU'RE UP THERE . . . SUPPLICATIONS WILL BE COMING SHORTLY!"

When I hit the drum, I know it's saying approximately the same thing, but I don't say anything. Instead, I listen. Each beat has a reverberation wave sound, "Boom . . . 'oom . . . 'oom . . . 'oom. . . ," each echo getting dimmer. After six echoes, I hit the drum again. Three times I do this. Then, listening to the pitch of the sound, I sing in tune first to the West. I sing a slow version of the Four Directions Song as I first heard it at one of Art Horn's sweats. I'm sure I've changed some of the words. I try to sing in the "key" of the drum.

(I'm not a good singer, but one day someone asked me, "Hey, Ted, can you sing?" Just to be funny, I said: "Hey! When I sing, Pavarotti listens.")

What I sing is:

"I see Grandmother sitting in the West
O Sacred Mystery [here I hit the drum once]
. . . She is Sacred
. . . She is looking at us [drum beat]

. . . We pray to Her . . . We pray to Her

. . . She is Sacred

. . . She is looking at us [drum beat]."

Then I put down the drum and drumstick. I pick up the "problem" paper and aim it to the West so Grandmother can read it. (Lately I have seen my dead grandmother, Geese-a-geese, sitting there.)

When I pick up the little paper, I leave a big pinch of Tobacco on it. As I read the "message," I rub the Tobacco on the writing.

By the way, NEVER say HOW you think the problem should be resolved. I have been in the unenviable position of having two opposing factions come to me asking for solutions that counteract one another. So I say to each, "I just do the ceremony. It is up to the Benevolent Higher Power to fix things. The 'fix' is probably guided by 'whatever makes this a better world for the unborn.' "

Now, after reading the "message" and maybe any short clarification that may seem necessary, I say (as much in the Tuscarora language as is possible), "Now you tell North, East, South, and Soong gwi oo dee sut eh what the supplication is so that the fix will take place. Thank you."

Then I take a small pinch from the Tobacco on the paper and throw it at the direction that I am speaking to, and I say, "Gooh! . . . gan nih hess nih, it n'waw joss hoo(t)" (Here, then, we'll smoke on it).

Along with the reading of the little paper, I also usually tell the other Directions, "Three times three times three, big time Thank Yous. Now in our life, energy, Divine Consciousness, we are like one."

The next thing I do—and, remember, after a while, as you find out what works best for you, what brings the quickest and most exciting results (often much trickier than you yourself could have ever thought of), you'll probably end up doing it all your way—is to put the paper back in the Tobacco, pick up the drum, and sing to the North, repeating it all again. After that, you will sing to the East and, lastly, to the South.

Now here is where you have options. You can burn the "ask for" paper or papers and the Tobacco, together, a mini Tobacco-Burning Ceremony. If you do, you should make the fire with wood that came from a tree that was felled not longer than (roughly) twelve months earlier; do not use old building scrap wood.

Another option is to bury the "message(s)" in the ground, in Mother Earth.

I have a Medicine box (I don't know of anybody else who does this) in which I put the little "imploring" papers. This box also contains all the power objects and little things that I went ga-ga over when I saw them or felt them. Or maybe someone just gave me a little prayer tie. I have made this collection over many years, but you can start one any time. Likely you already have some things that you have collected. (Look on your windowsill.)

One of these things came to me when I was at a Crow Dog Sundance.

Each year a certain trusted crew comes in before the dance and gets everything ready. Each person has a specific job and doesn't infringe on anyone else's job. So during the first day's work for the Crow Dog Sundance, somebody started getting hungry and said, "Whoa! Guess what? We ain't got no cook! John died since last year, so nobody is cooking. How we gonna eat?"

Sure enough, it was realized that John, the cook, had not been replaced. He used to bring in the food.

"What are we gonna do?"

"Well (ha ha) we're supposed to be half-ass Holy Men. All we gotta do is pray. Do a ceremony."

This seemed like a better than nothing idea, so all those present at that particular work spot got on their knees and formed a little prayer circle and prayed.

While they were praying, they heard a noise out on the main road, like someone might have lost control of their car, gone off the road, and maybe hit something.

"What was that?"

"Let's go and see!"

Out on the road lay a freshly killed blacktail deer. Someone's vehicle had struck it, and the driver had driven on.

Here was their food!

After the Sundance they gave me the tail of that deer. I put it in the Medicine box.

But something else in there is even more sacred.

One day I happened to overhear a conversation between two little girls. The smallest one was picking her nose.

"DON'T DO THAT!" the little bit older one said.

"WHY NOT?" the little one said back, "GOD IS BOOGERS TOO!"

Well! I had heard of sages saying, "All is One," but I don't know if they would dare go as far as that little girl did.

I went up to her with paper and pencil and got her autograph and put it in that Medicine Box.

And that's all I've got to say about ceremony.

Closing

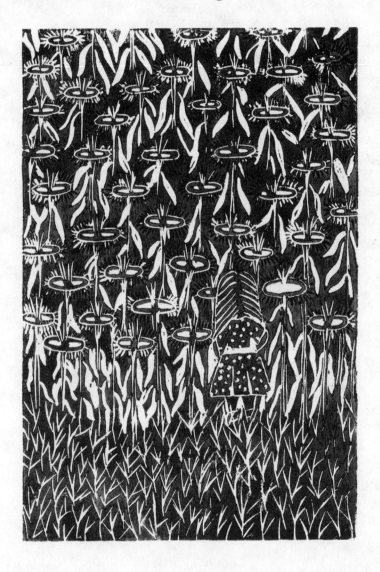

Overleaf: Halo on each ear of corn in elemental communication;
see "Elemental Communication," pp. 286–91, and the poem "Isaiah," p. 328.
Woodcut by Rhiannon Miles Osborne.

Poetry

It has been said that the poet cannot help but lay bare the soul and let the world see the world that the poet sees and is.

One day I was told that Buck GhostHorse was coming from wherever he lived, someplace near Mt. St. Helen's in Washington, to do a Lowanpi Ceremony. I then felt honored to be asked if I wanted to sit in one of the chairs to be healed in this ancient healing ceremony. I said yes, but then I had to say what it was that I wanted to be healed of so that Buck could tell me how many and of what color to make the prayer ties needed.

I said, "Well, I Sundanced to get rid of ego, so now when I speak, let me hear the words of other members of our universal family. Maybe they have the secrets to making this a better world."

As it turned out, I needed four groups of four differently colored prayer ties. More than a hundred in all.

After the ceremony, I waited for some time in anticipation of what would come out of my mouth. In the meantime, at night I started picturing or dreaming of trees. The Four Winds came through the leaves, so I started jotting down on scraps of paper what these whisperings were saying. I'll share them with you now, but I'm not sure in what order they came. I began calling them the "Love, Ted" poems, which, of course, infuriated them. So after this I'll have to make up my own poems.

Love,
Ted

ALL OCTOBERS END
With the turning of the Leaves
And the tree-sap scurrying Earthward
We know that we shall never see
The Dog days of this year again
But Grandmother Moon can scarcely wait
To see this gestation period's ending
When fauna babes will romp the glades
Amid the songs of songbirds.
And we will place within the Sod
Each sacred kernel of White Corn
When the Red Oak's leaves
Resemble a Squirrel's hand

       Love,
       Ted

Sent to friends Debra and Joe Roberts, for the turning of the season (and because they are "tricky").

When the Little Death of Autumn comes
The Little People hold a wake
For the fallen Colors
And the No-see-ums

       Love,
       Ted

Ceremony thrives best in an atmosphere of purification. I found just such a place surrounding a large White Pine in a wooded cove. Next to it was a pond of pure spring water. When winter temperatures came, the pond froze over. That night I heard the big White Pine whisper.

SLEEPY LAGOON
The gelid theft of Summer
Put a hush upon the Bog Pond
Put a curfew on the Frogs
Left the lockjaw Turtle bedridden
'Neath some sunken Oaken Leaves
'Neath a makeshift counterpane
Asleep? . . . well . . . yes
But with one ear cocked
In case the Robin sings.

> Love,
> Ted

COO DEE(T) (OR MAYBE)
I don't know what to do today
I'm retired, you know
Maybe I'll throw a party
Invite only babies
(They haven't learned to fib yet)
Maybe I'll speak to the energy
That dictates the placement of Stars
Maybe I'll go outside
Blow kisses to the Sundance Tree
But then again
I might just lift my sleeve
And blow out the blackfly
Making ready to bite.

> Love,
> Ted

THE FREEMAN WAY
The Day Sun fist high. Westerly
As the Mourning Dove cooed on limbs-end

If his lover came
He would probably go to bed

If the birdhawk came
He would probably go to dinner
Freeman-Sowdening-it all the way.

Love,
Ted

Freeman Sowden was a great Medicine man at the Six Nation Indian Reservation at Osweken, Ontario. One day he was asked why he was late to church.

"Ohhh," he said dreamily, "I walked out to the end of my driveway; if a car came from one direction and gave me a ride, I would go to the lacrosse game. If one came from the other way and gave me a ride, I would go to church."

The passing of Isaiah Joseph—of all mentors, other than my father—left in my life the deepest void.

ISAIAH
Please . . .
May I inherit
The wisdom lurking
In the crowfeet of your eyes
That saw the halo on the corn
At Green Corn Time
As you sang.

Love,
Ted

The Six Nations, and particularly the Onondaga Longhouse, lost a great person when Leon Shenandoah died. He was the Tadadaho, Keeper of the Flame (Fire Keeper) of the Six Nations Confederacy. I miss him dearly, and when I enter the Onondaga Longhouse at Midwinter Ceremonies, I can't help but look at the bench where he usually sat. He might just take a notion to reappear for us.

TO LEON

Grand Council is being called
All the Elements are summoned
And they resonate to the pulse
Of the summoning of the drum

To gather in the vortex
Of the Great White Pine
A place where ego nonexists
Where Grace and Benevolence thrive

And in the hush and glow
Of timelessness prevailing
There hangs a Wampum black
The Tadadaho is dead.

G'wa uhh *
Then from Chief Seattle's Speech
" . . . death did I say?
There is no death
Only a change of worlds."

Love,
Ted

* The cry that the runners utter at each nation when they bring the news.

On January 26, 2004, a dear Elder of the Lakotas left his physical self. His name was Wallace Black Elk.

ODE TO WALLACE
They say he has even made Crazy Horse laugh
And is now working on Spotted Tail
About not knowing they had repeating rifles
Plus he has teased Einstein
For wearing one blue and one green sock
And tho' I could never get a word in edgewise
I love him to the end
Even tho' there is no end

Love,
Ted

OTHER WORLDS
As all days start at night
Grandpa Thunder did some fireworks
In the predawn 4th of July
Ionizing a swath of landscape

Unused road ruts filled with water
Forming long water beds
To incubate a batch
Of 'wogs and water wigglers

So all day long one wiggler
Zig-zagged up and down
Measuring the puddle depth
In quarter inches

But as puddles do, puddles dry
And this was no exception
What then would come to happen
To Miss Mosquito in the making?

Surprise! Surprise!
She metamorphosized!
And whined off singing
Like northern Plains Indians.

But mealtime came
And as luck would have it
The soft nose of a pinto pony
Became her dinner table

But would you know . . .
The pinto pony had a mate
Whose tail came swishing
And sent the diner lifeless to the earth

But in the annals of mosquitodom
It has never been seen
Where a mosquito has ever
Been promised a rose garden

                    Love,
                    Ted

MEDICINE WHEEL

When the Day Sun dazzles the Earth
And the warmth of the sod is so-so
A swarm of Cicadas appear to sing
A song that ripens the Sacred Corn

When an Autumn chill comes wafting in
It watches Milkweed silken seedlings rise
To ride the breath of rale-ing breezes
To fall to Earth . . . to sleep . . . to wake to greenness

When all is white and crystalline
Along the creek bed's murmured reassurings
A prowling Weasel weaves on past
Leaving its paw prints to melt into Spring.

Love,
Ted

The Thanksgiving Address

Let us awaken to our duty to always be thankful . . . and so we greet and introduce into the consciousness and gratitude of our mind and spirit, the Element People . . . for, first of all, if it weren't for our ancestors, we wouldn't be here . . . they have strived to make this a better world for us and all living things . . . and for their having prayed seven generations ahead for our welfare, we must especially be grateful to those who prayed for us, seven generations ago.

And they have passed on to us the Medicine knowledge that cured and healed and kept them alive and healthy so that we were able to be born.

Part of this Medicine came in the form of the great ceremonies in which we were taught the explicit songs and dances . . . including instructions for induction into the various healing societies and other important societies for those of us who received the calling.

We must also be grateful for the instructions regarding the power and the use of all the great variety of food plants . . . and the explicit ones to be used in each of the ceremonies called the Feast . . . also the reverence and use of the great Sacred Tobacco.

And for the many other things we were taught . . . how to communicate with the other family-member Elements . . . to regulate the weather . . . to shape-shift . . . and we must be most grateful to have had expounded to us the Great Law of the Great Peace.

And so we open our hearts to you and tell you, "We love you and wish to thank you for all that you have done for us and for all you have given us."

UH SEH DE UH SEH DE UH SEH DE WA G'YEAH HANNEE'GIH N'YOWWEH HOI(T) . . .

OO'NIH TWEANT IT'NWO(T) DE YOO'REAH DUH'GIHH G'WIN-NEE(T) G'WIHH EHH'JEEH.

(Translation: Three times three times three large, enthusiastic "Thank yous" . . .

Now all of us universal family members, in our Urehdeh—life, energy, Divine Consciousness in all things—are as one.)

And so we greet and introduce into the consciousness and gratitude of our mind and spirit the next Element, our Mother Earth . . . and we can see our Mother as we may have seen her in a vision quest . . . the same as the picture taken by Apollo 17 . . . a blue-and-white opalescent orb . . . gliding gracefully and effortlessly through space . . . as though on a spiritual mission . . . so, so beautiful . . . the blue of the oceans . . . the misty white cloud cover . . . and the white polar caps. So beautiful.

That is our Mother . . . never telling a lie . . . no ulterior motives . . . and she has given us everything we would ever need . . . air, water, food, clothing, shelter, Medicine, love, a Divine Consciousness . . . a wonderful place to live.

So we open our hearts, and we say to her, "Mom . . . we love you very much, and we wish to thank you for all you have given us and for continuing to do so."

UH SEH DE UH SEH DE UH SEH DE WA G'YEAH HANNEE'GIH N'YOWWEH HOI(T) . . .

OO'NIH TWEANT IT'NWO(T) DE YOO'REAH DUH'GIHH G'WIN-NEE(T) G'WIHH EHH'JEEH.

And so we greet and introduce into the consciousness and gratitude of our mind and spirit the next Element, Plant Life.

From the bottom of the deepest ocean to the top of the highest mountain, we have all of these green growing things . . . billions and billions of leaves . . . each producing pure oxygen in photosynthesis with the Day Sun that we may breathe more healthfully . . . billions and billions of leaves . . . each waiting for us to exhale carbon dioxide . . . that they, too, may breathe . . . that this exchange can be perpetual . . . and we know, then, that we are indeed an intricate part of this Divine and Harmonious Universe.

So we honor, first, the Medicine plants . . . knowing that the amount of cure that we can get from them is directly related to the amount of reverence we have for them . . . and knowing that they have always gladly given their lives for ours, and for our ancestral health and ceremonial usage we owe them a great amount of gratitude. Among them the great see-into-the-future Medicine, the great Ga noo du(t) oit . . . the baby-never-die Medicine, the great D'yeh g'yeh guh tu(t) uh . . . the great Sacred Tobacco, the Joss hoo(t) eh weh . . . and many more magical Medicine plants.

And so we open up our hearts and say, "We love you, and we wish to thank you for saving the lives of us people and for all the other magical things that you have done for us."

UH SEH DE UH SEH DE UH SEH DE WA G'YEAH HANNEE'GIH N'YOWWEH HOI(T) . . .

OO'NIH TWEANT IT'NWO(T) DE YOO'REAH DUH'GIHH G'WIN-NEE(T) G'WIHH EHH'JEEH.

And so we greet and introduce into the consciousness and gratitude of our mind and spirit the next Element, the Food plants . . . and they are powerfully represented by the many varieties of the three Sacred Sisters . . . the Corn . . . the Beans . . . and the Squash.

Not only have they been our sustenance and preventative Medicine . . . but they provide the exact ingredients needed to produce the supernatural results of the various Medicine feasts.

And so we say to both the domestic and the wild Food plants, "We love you very much, and we wish to thank you for keeping us alive and well."

UH SEH DE UH SEH DE UH SEH DE WA G'YEAH HANNEE'GIH N'YOWWEH HOI(T) . . .

OO'NIH TWEANT IT'NWO(T) DE YOO'REAH DUH'GIHH G'WIN-NEE(T) G'WIHH EHH'JEEH.

And so we greet and introduce into the consciousness and gratitude of our mind and our spirit the next Element, Water . . . and we can see that water in so many different forms . . . icicles and snowflakes . . . moondogs and sundogs . . . rainbows and clouds . . . glaciers and icebergs . . . oceans and rivers and streams . . . water fountains and waterfalls . . . fog and little droplets of dew on a spiderweb . . . sweat on our brow and steam in a Sweat Lodge . . . and when we become out of balance . . . too materialistic . . . here comes a flood . . . to put us on our knees . . . and balance is restored . . . and when we realize that we ourselves are 85 percent water or more . . . we realize how vital water is to us and to all living things.

So we open our hearts, and we say, "Oh beautiful and precious water, we love you very much, and we wish to thank you for all you mean to us."

UH SEH DE UH SEH DE UH SEH DE WA G'YEAH HANNEE'GIH N'YOWWEH HOI(T) . . .

OO'NIH TWEANT IT'NWO(T) DE YOO'REAH DUH'GIHH G'WIN-NEE(T) G'WIHH EHH'JEEH.

And so we greet and introduce into the consciousness and gratitude of our mind and our spirit the next Element, all Creaturehood, both on land and in the sea . . . from the amoeba to the zebra . . . from the seahorse to the Clydesdale . . . from the lightning bug to the electric eel to the elephant . . . and this enormous family membership is symbolized by the principal member, the deer, whose antlers represent the awareness and alertness of the aggregate of that great family . . . and they have faithfully given themselves that we may have food . . . clothing . . . shelter . . . Medicine . . . companionship . . . oracles . . . a Divine Consciousness, and more.

For all this, we open our hearts to all Creaturehood, and we say, "Oh dear loving family members . . . we love you very much, and we wish to thank you for all you have given us."

UH SEH DE UH SEH DE UH SEH DE WA G'YEAH HANNEE'GIH N'YOWWEH HOI(T) . . .

OO'NIH TWEANT IT'NWO(T) DE YOO'REAH DUH'GIHH G'WIN-NEE(T) G'WIHH EHH'JEEH.

And so we greet and introduce into the consciousness and gratitude of our mind and our spirit the next Element, the Trees . . . and they have given us so much . . . the aesthetic pleasure of the taste of various fruits and nuts . . . the syrup and confections from the sap, or lifeblood of the principal tree, the Sugar Maple . . . the symbolism and Medicine of the Tree of Peace, the great White Pine, which the mere touch of cures depression . . . the Medicine tree, the Basswood, from which the False Faces are made . . . the many other Medicine trees .. and their providing of shade, building material, firewood, love, peaceful companionship, the prevention of landslides, and great beauty, especially in the coloring of autumn.

For this and much more, we open our hearts, and we tell them how much we love them and that we wish to thank them.

UH SEH DE UH SEH DE UH SEH DE WA G'YEAH HANNEE'GIH N'YOWWEH HOI(T) . . .

OO'NIH TWEANT IT'NWO(T) DE YOO'REAH DUH'GIHH G'WIN-NEE(T) G'WIHH EHH'JEEH.

And so we greet and introduce into the consciousness and gratitude of our mind and our spirit the next Element, the Birds . . . and what a drabness would beset our world if it were not for the aesthetic pleasures of the music of their voices . . . the beauty of the colors of their feathers . . . the great grace that they exhibit in flight . . . and they have provided us with food . . . an astounding oracular talent . . . an example of peace and alertness as exemplified in the symbol of the eagle atop the Tree of Peace, guarding the Six Nation Confederacy . . . their contributing portion of the great, great Medicine, the Na go(t) na gaww, the never-die Medicine . . . their example of a Divine Consciousness.

For this and more we open our hearts to all birds and tell them that we love them very much and wish to thank them for all they mean to us.

UH SEH DE UH SEH DE UH SEH DE WA G'YEAH HANNEE'GIH N'YOWWEH HOI(T) . . .

OO'NIH TWEANT IT'NWO(T) DE YOO'REAH DUH'GIHH G'WIN-NEE(T) G'WIHH EHH'JEEH.

And so we greet and introduce into the consciousness and gratitude of our mind and our spirit the next Element, our great family member, the Great Grandfathers, the Thunderers . . . and they have faithfully guarded and protected us against any intruding out-of-balance forces that emerge from time to time to beset us . . . and we have heard them vehemently scolding such existences away so that we would not be influenced . . . and we have even seen the fire with which they do that . . . but we can only imagine the joy and anticipation of the green growing things for the ionized rain that follows to make sure that everything is clean again.

So we open our hearts and say to our Grandfathers, "Oh dear

Grandfathers, we love you very much for your protecting us, and we wish
to thank you."

UH SEH DE UH SEH DE UH SEH DE WA G'YEAH HANNEE'GIH
N'YOWWEH HOI(T) . . .

OO'NIH TWEANT IT'NWO(T) DE YOO'REAH DUH'GIHH G'WIN-
NEE(T) G'WIHH EHH'JEEH.

And so we greet and introduce into the consciousness and gratitude of our mind
and our spirit the next Element, the Four Winds . . . and we know that they
travel about, keeping track of things and aiding the Grandfathers and the rain to
reach their destinations . . . and when we again get out of balance for any of
many reasons, here comes a hurricane or tornado to frighten us back into balance and to remind us that we are not infallible . . . and though we might see
parts of our abode flying up into the sky, we can also wonder how long we would
live without air.

So we open our hearts to the Four Winds, and we tell them how precious
they are to us and that we wish to thank them:

UH SEH DE UH SEH DE UH SEH DE WA G'YEAH HANNEE'GIH
N'YOWWEH HOI(T) . . .

OO'NIH TWEANT IT'NWO(T) DE YOO'REAH DUH'GIHH G'WIN-
NEE(T) G'WIHH EHH'JEEH.

And so we greet and introduce into the consciousness and gratitude of our mind
and our spirit the next Element, the Four Directions . . . a subtle doorway between the physical consciousness and the ethereal world . . . members of our
universal family that transcend molecular structure . . . the means by which nesting birds can fly south in winter and return unerringly to their nesting places . . .
the means by which lost ships can be found at sea . . . a miraculous means by
which we travel . . . always constantly at our disposal . . . the cornerstone of our
equilibrium.

So we must not unconsciously take for granted this great family membership
. . . but instead open our hearts and say, "Oh great Four Directions, we love you
for your everlasting faithfulness, and we wish to thank you."

UH SEH DE UH SEH DE UH SEH DE WA G'YEAH HANNEE'GIH
N'YOWWEH HOI(T) . . .

OO'NIH TWEANT IT'NWO(T) DE YOO'REAH DUH'GIHH G'WIN-
NEE(T) G'WIHH EHH'JEEH.

And so we greet and introduce into the consciousness and gratitude of our mind
and our spirit the next Element, the Night Sun, our Grandmother Moon . . .
and he loves us and, if she could, would like to bounce us on her knee . . . and
when we get too take-it-for-granted of her, she would like to remind us that
she is not just up there whistling Dixie . . . that she is there to remind us that
she will not allow us to be forgotten as a species . . . for she has given females a
time-cycle period called a moon . . . and at a special time in that cycle they
can become fertile and reproduce . . . and for those of us who may not believe
that there is a powerful attraction between our Grandmother and us and
the earth, we can be reassured by watching the rising and the falling of the
tides . . . and we are reminded by the natal ties we have with our beautiful
Grandmother Moon that we are indeed an intricate part of this Divine and
Harmonious Universe.

So we open our hearts and say, "Oh dear Grandmother, we love you very
much and wish to thank you for all you mean to us."

UH SEH DE UH SEH DE UH SEH DE WA G'YEAH HANNEE'GIH
N'YOWWEH HOI(T) . . .

OO'NIH TWEANT IT'NWO(T) DE YOO'REAH DUH'GIHH G'WIN-
NEE(T) G'WIHH EHH'JEEH.

And so we greet and introduce into the consciousness and gratitude of our mind
and our spirit the next Element, our elder brother, the Day Sun . . . and if it were
not for the steadfast love and warmth embracing us each day, we would not exist
. . . we would be cast in the darkness and frozen . . . and we don't know the vast
amount of beneficial vitamins, minerals, and trace Elements that have been radiated to us throughout our existence . . . and so this magical life-giving source is
responsible not only for our existence but for the existence and growth of all of
our family and therefore all of the other necessary benefits that we derive from
our other family members.

So we open our hearts, and we say, "Oh dear elder brother, we love you very
much, and we wish to thank you for all you have given to us and for all you mean
to us."

UH SEH DE UH SEH DE UH SEH DE WA G'YEAH HANNEE'GIH
N'YOWWEH HOI(T) . . .

OO'NIH TWEANT IT'NWO(T) DE YOO'REAH DUH'GIHH G'WIN-
NEE(T) G'WIHH EHH'JEEH.

And so we greet and introduce into the consciousness and gratitude of our mind
and our spirit the next Element, the Stars . . . and their awesome nightly beauty
evokes the astrological influences they have upon us . . . and we can be en-
tranced by them when we lay in the soft summer grass and peer into the sky . . .
a myriad of diamonds, twinkling and winking at us, as though they had some secret to tell us . . . then after a while it comes to us that there just have to be thousands of other solar systems like our own . . . with Day Suns and celestial bodies
orbiting about them . . . then after a while it becomes clear . . . that what we are
looking at . . . is nothing but a replica . . . of the molecular structure of all other
things . . . even the internal workings of an atom . . . of neutrons . . . protons . . .
ions . . . electrons . . . photons . . . each orbiting . . . each smaller particle less
physical than the other . . . until we are speaking of pure energy and Divine
Consciousness . . . the recipe of all that there is, including ourselves . . . and we
can feel a Divine responsibility for the caretaking of this Divine and Harmonious
Universe.

So we open our hearts and say, "Oh beautiful, beautiful stars, we love you
very much, and we wish to thank you for all you mean to us."

UH SEH DE UH SEH DE UH SEH DE WA G'YEAH HANNEE'GIH
N'YOWWEH HOI(T) . . .

OO'NIH TWEANT IT'NWO(T) DE YOO'REAH DUH'GIHH G'WIN-
NEE(T) G'WIHH EHH'JEEH.

And so we greet and introduce into the consciousness and gratitude of our mind
and our spirit the next Element, the Four Protectors, sometimes called the Four
Messengers . . . and now it behooves us to be aware of this great connection with
the ethereal world . . . our own intuitive link with the vast dynamic intelligence
of the Universe . . . a mystical family membership with no molecular structure
. . . and we don't know how many times our lives have been saved by these alert
messengers . . . for instance, at times when we were leaving the safety of our
homes to do an errand, something stopped us at the door, ostensibly to see if we

remember to take everything we might need . . . when we reach the intersection where another vehicle would have struck us . . . THAT vehicle would have already passed through . . . and these great Elements stand ever ready to help transport the supplications of our ceremonies.

So we open our hearts and say, "Oh dear Four Protectors, we love you very much, and we wish to thank you for all you have done for us."

UH SEH DE UH SEH DE UH SEH DE WA G'YEAH HANNEE'GIH N'YOWWEH HOI(T) . . .

OO'NIH TWEANT IT'NWO(T) DE YOO'REAH DUH'GIHH G'WIN-NEE(T) G'WIHH EHH'JEEH.

And so we greet and introduce into the consciousness and gratitude of our mind and our spirit the ultimate Element, Soong gwi oo dee sut eh . . . Creator of this Divine and Harmonious Universe . . . the manifestation of supreme power, goodness, intelligence, and forgiveness . . . and so we owe a great gratitude for there being all that there is . . . and for the constant watching over us . . . and for reminding all things of their duties.

So we open our hearts to this Highest Consciousness, and we say, "We love you very much, and we wish to thank you for all that there is and for all of your benevolence."

UH SEH DE UH SEH DE UH SEH DE WA G'YEAH HANNEE'GIH N'YOWWEH HOI(T) . . .

OO'NIH TWEANT IT'NWO(T) DE YOO'REAH DUH'GIHH G'WIN-NEE(T) G'WIHH EHH'JEEH.

If we have forgotten any Elements and left them out, let them speak for themselves, for all the Elements are more Divine than we are, being as they are unable to tell a lie or have ulterior motives.

Afterword

DEBRA ROBERTS

Many people have asked me about "working on this book" with Ted. It was never work. It emerged from that seamless place of deep friendship that always has more of a sense of the eternal than a "beginning."

Ted and I had been friends for years. I met him just after he had shared the Thanksgiving Address at one of Larry Littlebird's Native American story-telling conferences in New Mexico. I was forever changed by that prayer. On that magical evening we all were.

Ted and I fell into friendship a few evenings later over a dinner for a small group of the Elders. Something about eel sushi, which neither of us chose to order, tickled our funny bones. We laughed our way into friendship (which was cemented, soon after, by the discovery that both of us were sevens in the Enneagram).

About three and a half years ago Ted said he had a story that needed typing. I offered to do it. I type fast. One story led to another (always handwritten on yellow legal paper, never white). And eventually, across the years, the face and form of a second book emerged. This sacred book, *Big Medicine from Six Nations*.

Two things I love to share most with people about "working" with Ted. The first was our typical rhythm in meeting and passing chapters back and forth. Ted would write a while and then call me up to meet for breakfast or lunch. As timely and sometimes as early as I usually was, he'd always be in the restaurant first, drinking coffee. He'd hand me new material, I'd hand him typed chapters, we'd have a little edit session, and then we'd mostly eat and do the big gab.

The end of our ritual often involved another mutual love—dancing. He'd bring a new favorite piece of music, inevitably jazz, along to our meeting. After the meal he'd pop a CD into the player in his car, and we'd boogie. There, on the asphalt, in front of the Home Folks Diner or the Athens Restaurant (and sometimes the Waffle House), we'd hoof it for one tune, happy as clams, and then head our separate ways—he back to his beloved Diana, his world disc golf championships, and his home in the woods, and I back to Weaverville, gratefully carrying another piece of the wealth of the world.

The second thing I love to share is how many times—between typing, editing, retyping, hearing, speaking, and reading—I have experienced Ted's words *the Divine and Harmonious Universe.* Probably thousands of times. It's part of my own language now. Part of my cells. It is a sacred naming that points to sacred living.

Just before Ted went into the hospital, he handed me the last chapter of the book, which was Divine (and Harmonious) timing, of course. None of us knew that his illness would lead to his imminent departure. That he would disappear like a shooting star—joining his beloved Eleazer, Isaiah, Leon, Wallace, and, of course, Empty Cloud.

Diana says that to read Ted's words is to hear him speaking still. It's uncanny how true that is. We both wept as we read this book through one more time before passing it along to the wonderful folks at Syracuse University Press.

And so I say to you, Ted, "Three times three times three big-time thank yous." I miss you. We all miss you. You have left us with your good thoughts, good feelings, good words, and good deeds, all the things you've said are what matter most.

Somehow we know that our love, like your beautiful prayers and words, goes on forever . . .

Love,
Debra